Reformation of the Senses

The Paradox of Religious Belief and Practice in Germany

JACOB M. BAUM

UNIVERSITY OF ILLINOIS PRESS
Urbana, Chicago, and Springfield

1 2 3 4 5 C P 5 4 3 2 1
∞ This book is printed on acid-free paper.

Library of Congress Cataloging-in-Publication Data
Names: Baum, Jacob M., author.
Title: Reformation of the senses : the paradox of religious belief and practice in Germany / Jacob M. Baum.
Description: [Urbana, Illinois] : University of Illinois Press, [2018] | Series: Studies in sensory history | Includes bibliographical references and index.
Identifiers: LCCN 2018020261| ISBN 9780252042195 (hardcover ; alk. paper) | ISBN 9780252083990 (pbk. ; alk. paper)
Subjects: LCSH: Senses and sensation—Religious aspects—Christianity—History. | Senses and sensation—Germany—History. | Reformation—Germany. | Germany—Church history.
Classification: LCC BT741.3 .B38 2018 | DDC 274.3/06—dc23
LC record available at https://lccn.loc.gov/2018020261

E-book ISBN 978-0-252-05093-0

Reformation of the Senses

STUDIES IN SENSORY HISTORY

A list of books in the series appears at the end of this book.

Contents

Acknowledgments

Many people made this book possible. My parents, John and Patty, instilled in me from an early age a discipline that was absolutely necessary to seeing this project through to its completion. My success as an academic has been built on the foundations they laid. As I was growing up in western Michigan, friends and family members shaped me in innumerable ways. There are more to be acknowledged than space permits, but I'd like to single out my siblings, Mark, Laura, and Zach, and my grandmother, Nancy. Also in western Michigan, I owe a special debt to an individual who will remain anonymous here. Growing up Catholic in this part of the United States, I was sometimes reminded of the differences that separated me from the majority (reformed, Calvinist) Protestant culture, never more so than when, in the course of a high school English class discussion on religion, I was confronted with the question: "Don't you people worship statues of the Virgin Mary?" I didn't realize it at the time, but this question sowed the seeds that would eventually grow into this book.

My undergraduate education at Aquinas College was instrumental to my formation as a person and intellectual. Above all, I am deeply grateful to my adviser, Charles Gunnoe, who was a model teacher, channeled and nurtured my interests in German and the history of religion in a variety of courses, and offered sage and sober advice about graduate school. I still look to his example when figuring out how to approach my own classes, and I am glad to call him a friend today. Also at Aquinas, I owe very heartfelt thanks to Katharina Häusler-Gross, the best teacher of German I could have hoped for. I also want to thank Jason Duncan in History, Deborah Wickering in Anthropology, Jennifer Dawson and Rebecca Coogan in English, and Dennis Marshall in Theology. You were exemplary teachers and scholars, and the care you devoted to me as a student influenced not only the writing of this book, but also my development as a person.

As a graduate student at the University of Illinois, I learned much from both faculty and fellow graduate students and became a more mature scholar. Early in my first semester, I probably would have quit my studies if it hadn't been for Antoinette Burton. The course I took with her that semester profoundly expanded my intellectual horizons, and whether she intended to or not, she taught me to take the discipline of history, and myself, more seriously. Similarly, without Carol Symes's early interest and involvement in my work, I'm sure I would not have gotten as far as I have. She's always been more than generous with her time, thoughtful feedback, and enthusiastic support. *Tibi gratia mea infinita*. The friendships I formed with fellow graduate students, especially Ian Hartman, Dave Bates, Nathan Chio, Ashley Howard, Andy Eisen, and Amanda Eisemann, were also essential for survival. I also greatly benefited from opportunities to work with scholars in History, Medieval Studies, German, and Religion, especially Megan McLaughlin, Dana Rabin, Clare Crowston, Bruce Rosenstock, and Mara Wade. Of course, my greatest thanks go to Craig Koslofsky. He first told me about this "new thing" called sensory history. Since then, his steadfast enthusiasm for the project has given me the confidence to keep going with it, and if I hadn't been able to talk through parts of it with him, I wouldn't have been able to sort it all out. His work is always before me as the model of imaginative scholarship that treats difficult and complex subjects in a disarmingly accessible, elegant manner. Here I aspire to that model, and I hope I don't fall too short of the mark.

I conducted much of the research for this book while living in Germany from 2010 to 2012. There I enjoyed the generous support of the Leibniz Institute for European History, which, in addition to financial support, provided housing, a stimulating intellectual climate, and very friendly support from a community of fine scholars: special thanks to Luka Ilic, Henning Jürgens, Irene Dingel, Esther Möller, Lorenz Baibl, and the entire library staff at the Institute. The Center for Library and Information Resources in Washington, D.C., also provided substantial financial support that enabled further research in Germany. Among the many helpful library and archival staff I encountered during my time in Germany, and since then, those at the state and city archives in Nuremberg, the city libraries in Nuremberg and Mainz, the university libraries in Mainz and Frankfurt am Main, and the Herzog August library in Wolfenbüttel, stand out as exceptional.

Since coming to Texas Tech University in 2013, I have had the good fortune of belonging to a welcoming and supportive intellectual community. The Department of History has my deep gratitude. Alan Barenberg, Paul Bjerk, Zachary Brittsan, John Howe, Matt Johnson, Erin-Marie Legacey, Ben Poole, Patrick

Scharfe, and Abigail Swingen all have provided helpful feedback at various stages as this project moved along. Karlos Hill deserves special thanks: not only did he read portions of the work, but I also learned much from our many conversations about the writing process and publishing, and I'm sure I avoided many a rookie mistake as a result. Beyond the History Department, a generous fellowship from the Humanities Center at Texas Tech enabled the timely completion of this book.

At various stages in its development, this book has benefited from the interest and input of many other individuals and institutions as well. Bridget Heal at St. Andrews University has offered many helpful insights over the years. Wietse de Boer read the entire manuscript and offered many helpful suggestions that improved the final product. Joel Harrington, David Whitford, Matthew Milner, Susan Karant-Nunn, and Philip Hahn have all read portions of the work and given tremendously useful feedback. Presenting portions of this work at the Center for Medieval and Early Modern Studies at Stanford University, the Department of History at Vanderbilt University, and the Medieval and Renaissance Research Seminar at Baylor University provided opportunities for challenging and fruitful engagement with other scholars and was instrumental to refining the book's arguments. I am also deeply grateful to Mark Smith, who has enthusiastically supported this project since I asked him to look at a draft of a prospectus. The editorial staff at the University of Illinois Press, especially Marika Christofides, has also been exceptionally responsive, helpful, and a pleasure to work with. Special thanks as well to Lem Skidmore, MA, MPH, who lent his keen eyes and refined rhetorical sensibilities to the project in its final proofreading stage.

Finally, my deepest love and thanks go to my family. My partner, Emily, has been the greatest example of a scholar and good person. I've looked up to her since I met her, and always will. I'm lucky to have had her support all these years, and the opportunity to build a wonderful life together. My daughters, Frankie and Theodosia, were actually not very helpful at all in the process of writing this book. In fact, they were very distracting. For some reason, though, I still love them very much. I dedicate this book to them, and their mother.

Reformation of the Senses

Introduction

Let's begin with an image. In 1532, Erhard Schön (1491–1542) completed a small woodcut titled *God's Lament for the Fate of His Vineyard* (see figure 1). Schön was a prolific artist, and in the context of his whole oeuvre, this was a relatively minor piece. It nonetheless told a powerful story that resonated with many of his peers. Schön was a contemporary of Martin Luther (1483–1546), whose religious disputes with the established Church of Rome (what we would today call the Catholic Church) had captured the imagination of people across the German-speaking world over the previous decade and a half. Schön lived and worked in Nuremberg, where Luther's message took especially strong hold among the city's ruling class and better-educated artisans in the early 1520s. By 1525, the city government had taken the decision to sever ties with Rome and adopt the new Protestant religion. Nuremberg was the first free imperial city to do so, but the Reformation spread quickly, particularly in urban locales, and particularly among the better-educated segments of society.

Schön's woodcut crystallized a core Protestant mythology that was forged in these early years but has proved quite durable over the centuries. This myth, which I call the "reformation of the senses," is the primary subject of this book. It was a simple story, describing the relationship of late medieval and Reformation-era sensory cultures. It held that the late medieval church engaged and manipulated churchgoers in an overwhelmingly ritualized, sensual manner, and that Protestant Christianity represented a fundamental break with that paradigm. In place of late medieval sensuality, reformers put the pure administration of the Word of Scripture. Preaching, Bible reading, and sometimes singing became the keynotes of the new Protestant piety. If sensual at all, this new piety may have emphasized vision and hearing over other sensory modalities. However, the shift was more fundamental, according a central role to linguistic declamation and intellectual

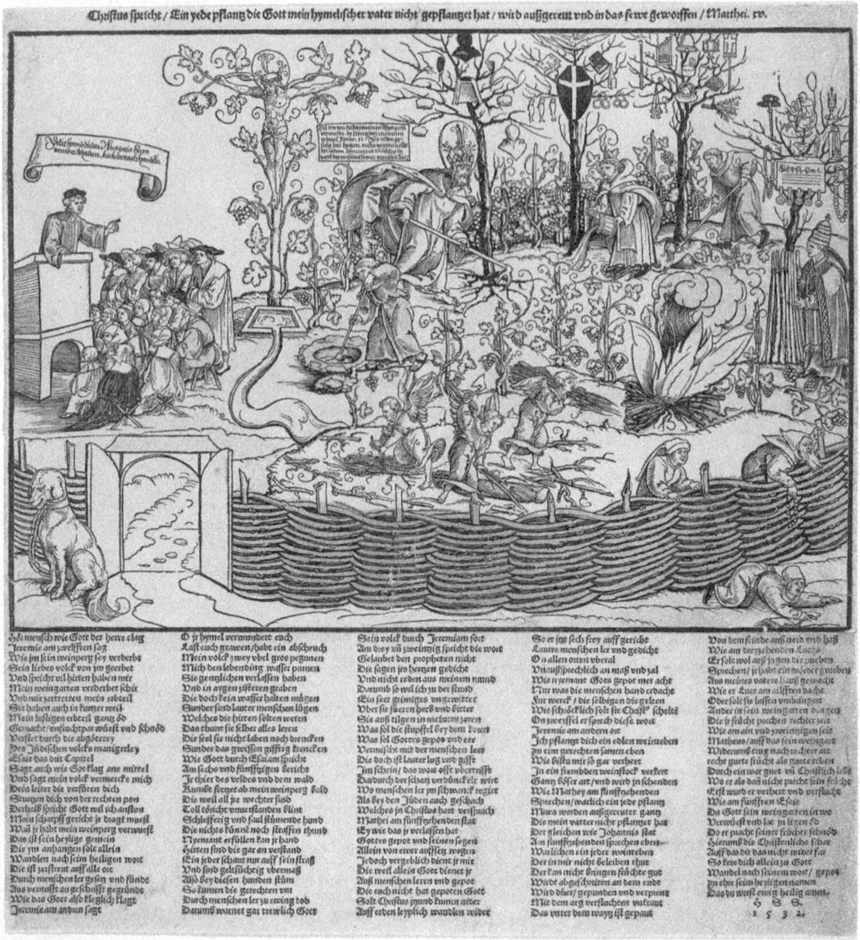
Christus spricht / Ein yede pflantz die Gott mein hymelischer vater nicht gepflantzet hat / wird außgereüt vnd in das fewr geworffen / Matthei. xv.

Figure 1: Erhard Schön, “God’s Lament for the Fate of his Vineyard” (ca. 1532). © Trustees of the British Museum.

comprehension, in contrast to the aesthetic evocation of meaning more characteristic of late medieval Christendom.[1] The intellectual, disembodied, spiritual domains of experience were the only things of real importance in the new religion.

God’s Lament represented this mythology concisely and effectively, depicting two churches divided by an unbridgeable stream. On the left side of the image, Schön presented the epitome of Protestant piety, with a preacher giving a sermon to an audience listening with rapt attention. The words above the preacher declared: “Blessed are those who hear the Word, and keep it, and act accordingly.” On the right side, the material culture of traditional Christian piety was arrayed in all of its overwhelming sensual potency: rosaries, chalices, censers for incense, candelabra, bells, priestly vestments, holy water, vessels for carrying the Eucharist, and images populate the enclosure where monks and popes tend vines. The message was clear: the new Protestant piety had cleared these things out and, in doing so, produced a fundamentally different way of interacting with the bodies of churchgoers than had late medieval piety, or its successor in the Roman Catholic Church. It was somehow less sensual, less emotive, but more intellectual, more interiorized.

This narrative originated in the earliest days of the Reformation in Germany, a product of Protestant propaganda. Despite its very specific geographic and chronological origins, the story of the reformation of the senses has influenced how we think and talk about religious, cultural, and ethnic difference for centuries. In both popular and academic discourse, it's just self-evident that Protestant Christianity is less sensual than its Catholic counterpart. This was true of the Lutheran tradition, the first major Protestant denomination, and it was true of the reformed tradition, or Calvinism. Indeed, late medieval Christianity, Lutheranism, and Calvinism constitute recognizable plot points on a progressive narrative of change over time central to notions of modernity. Late medieval Christendom was highly sensual in its orientation, Lutheranism somewhat less so, and Calvinism, as utterly a-sensual, was the resolution of the plot. As the sociologist Max Weber put it long ago in his famous *Protestant Ethic and the Spirit of Capitalism*, Calvinism typified "an entirely negative attitude . . . to all the sensuous and emotional elements in culture and in religion." In doing so, it laid the foundations for the worldly asceticism and internalized discipline of modern capitalist subjects.[2] Similarly, the theologian and philosopher Ernst Troeltsch considered the ascetic rejection of "the sensual" to be the essence of Protestant Christianity and the cornerstone of modernity.[3] In a related vein, the construction of a mysterious, exotic, and sensual Other, in opposition to the dispassionate Western observer, so apparent in the orientalist discourse from the eighteenth century, and then again in the origins of the modern academic discipline of anthropology, owes a great ideological debt to the sixteenth century. Today, the myth of the reformation of the senses resonates in popular, perhaps more benign, representations of Catholicism as a religion of "smells and bells."[4] As outsiders looking in to these sensory worlds, we are encouraged to take up the sober, intellectual gaze of the Protestant subject. This has become the normative position of western European modernity but has provincial roots in the cities of fifteenth- and sixteenth-century Germany, where the Reformation first took hold.

The story of sensory reformation was and is a powerful one because it draws such sharp, easily comprehensible distinctions that have proved useful for talking about religious difference, and cultural-ethnic difference more broadly. But, to ask a naïve question, was it true? Among some specialists in what might be called the cultural history of the Reformation in Germany, there has been no sustained attempt to answer this question.[5] However, in a variety of projects, historians have touched on the issue from time to time. Recent interpretations of ritual, emotions, and material culture have confirmed the basic thrust of the narrative, if in a somewhat qualified way.[6] On balance, Protestant Christianity eliminated much of the ritual diversity of the late medieval church and thus at least obliquely contributed to the formation of a less sensuous religion. The logic of the argument is intuitively persuasive: less stuff to appeal to the senses obviously means less sensual religion. Paired with that, it's also difficult to deny that, in much of their rhetoric at least, reformers generally seem to have suppressed the positive ways people thought with and about the more affective dimensions of their religious experience, including the senses and emotions.[7]

Others have complicated this view, if not completely abandoned it. Above all, Robert Scribner's later work devoted sustained attention to the problem of visual piety in both the late medieval and early Reformation eras. He found significant continuity, showing that many of the early reformers enthusiastically embraced the visual along lines similar to their late medieval counterparts, although they tended to emphasize the intellectual, rational capacity of the sense of sight more than its pre-linguistic, affective dimensions.[8] More recently, others have challenged the notion of the Reformation as a significant break with the medieval past by shedding light on continuities in the ways leading reformers like Martin Luther and Philip Melanchthon thought about the pious use of the senses of sight and hearing.[9] Additionally, Thomas Kaufmann has pointed to the retention of the sacraments of communion and baptism as evidence that leading reformers continued to value the multisensory appeal of these rites, stressing in particular the fact that these appealed to touch.[10] Still others have challenged us to think about the materiality inherent in Reformation conceptions of the Word of Scripture. The Word, like so many other objects of late medieval devotion, had a "stuffness," or "thingness" unto itself. In the minds of reformers, it was not simply the *message* of Scripture; the Word was also something to be seen, heard, and even touched.[11] The basic idea in these interpretations is that the Word displaced all other traditional objects of devotion. Hence Peter Blickle's oft-quoted rhetorical question: "Why did people in 1515 want to 'see' the [Eucharist] Host, and why in 1525 did they want to 'hear' the plain Word of God?"[12]

These provocative discussions certainly enrich our understanding of Reformation religion's complicated relationship to the late medieval sensory past, but their heavy focus on sight and hearing, historically considered the intellectual senses par excellence, gives the impression that the "lower senses" were either of little consequence or intentionally excluded by reformers from playing a meaningful role in the new religion.[13] Moreover, they often still have a hard time escaping the ideological tinge of progressive narratives about modernity. Blickle, for example, posed his question in the context of a reflection on the Reformation as a process of Christianization.[14] The idea that what came before was not Christianity, but rather a purely superficial, sensuous edifice, was a sixteenth-century idea, yet as we've already seen, social theorists and philosophers like Weber and Troeltsch incorporated it into their understandings of modernity. Leopold von Ranke, too, often regarded as a founder of the historical discipline, adopted a similar mode of thinking, reflecting in his diary on the importance of the Reformation as a shift away from the "objective" to the "subjective" in religion. From here, the entire history of the modern world, culminating in the modern state, could be written.[15]

For the most part, historians of the German Reformation have developed their interpretations of the senses in religion parallel to, but not necessarily in conversation with, the emerging interdisciplinary field of sensory studies. Anthropologists, historians, and literary scholars engaged in the critical study of the senses have all cautioned against uncritical acceptance of binary oppositions of "more" and "less" sensual cultures, societies, or historical epochs.[16] Instead, they have cultivated habits of thinking about time and place that remain vigilant of their full "sensory textures."[17] All human history, so the old Marxian adage goes, is nothing if not a story of the formation of the five senses.[18] Attending to them is the imperative of the sensory historian, and offers a critical means of re-evaluating the breadth, depth, and meaning of human experience in the past, as well as some of the master narratives we tell about that experience. We have only begun to see the first fruits of a cross-pollination between the very old field of Reformation history and the relatively young field of sensory studies. In the German-speaking world, two excellent articles by Philip Hahn have shed light on the complications and ambiguities in sixteenth-century Lutheran practices of bell ringing, and how the senses (mostly vision) constituted an essential aspect of how Protestants conceived of sacred space.[19] For my own part, I have attempted to contribute to the project in a focused study of incense ritual, assessing in socially and culturally contextualized ways the religious meanings its smell evoked in the later Middle Ages, and how early Protestants responded to it.[20] In each case, the sensory history of the Reformation that appears to be emerging is one of partial continuity with the late medieval past.

Still, these are only article-length studies, and the sensory history of the German Reformation remains in its infancy. Why has German Reformation history remained so stubbornly "sense-less," to borrow the expression from George Roeder Jr.?[21] We might chalk it up, at least in part, to what Susan Karant-Nunn has identified as the "deep, often confessional conservatism" that has often characterized scholars' approach to the field.[22] Many Reformation historians have had a vested interest in promoting a particular view of the events of the sixteenth century, usually through a more traditional lens of the history of theological ideas. Another reason seems to stem from the intellectual genealogy of sensory studies itself, with its origins primarily in the Francophone and Anglophone academies.[23] Since Lucien Febvre's famous declaration that sixteenth-century "man" was more attuned to the senses of smell, taste, touch, and hearing than his modern, ocular-obsessed counterpart, French historical writing, particularly that coming from the *Annales* school, has often suggested the importance of the senses in both medieval and modern times, albeit usually in rather cursory or impressionistic ways.[24] Alain Corbin's pioneering work on odors in revolutionary France and bell ringing in the nineteenth-century French countryside developed these early insights into systematic studies and laid the groundwork for subsequent, penetrating analyses of the senses.[25] Beyond the narrow confines of French historical thought, though, it would seem that interest in the senses, particularly the nonvisual senses, has been characteristic of French academic culture more broadly in recent times. As Martin Jay has documented, the denigration of vision among French thinkers of the twentieth century gave rise to some of the most probing criticisms of the senses, particularly shedding light on the ways they mediate various forms of power and authority. The work of Michel Foucault on the disciplining force of the gaze of course exemplifies this trend, but a variety of sense modalities have been of central concern to many others, from Maurice Merleau-Ponty and Paul Lacan to Emmanuel Levinas, Pierre Bourdieu, and Jean-François Lyotard.[26]

Although approaching things from a slightly different perspective, the English-speaking world has gradually come to its senses over the past few generations as well. The ever-expanding collection of studies focused specifically on visual culture is in no small part the result of fruitful engagement with many of the French thinkers mentioned above.[27] Similarly, historians of medicine and historians of the body have taken many cues from the French academy and have uncovered the importance of smell and touch in a variety of contexts.[28] Although not explicitly engaged in the project, historians of music, and musicologists, have often made critical contributions to the history of hearing.[29] Additionally, the work of media theorists Marshall McLuhan and Walter Ong has proved extremely influential in the English-speaking academy. In the 1960s, both McLuhan and Ong theorized about the relationships between the senses, language, and communications technologies, setting the paradigm for subsequent scholarly discussions. Of central import for many historians was the so-called "great divide" thesis: the notion that the advent of moveable type in the mid-fifteenth century, in conjunction with philosophies of the Renaissance and Enlightenment, displaced the traditional oral culture of medieval western Europe with a more ocular-centrist regime. The values we today tend to associate with modernity, including individualism, rationality, and objectivity, were bound up with this large-scale shift toward a culture of the eye.[30] Although sensory historians have since subjected it to heavy criticism on a variety of grounds, the great divide thesis continues to hold sway on thinking about the transition from the medieval world to the modern. Finally, we shouldn't overlook the significance of the fact that when early pioneers like David Howes and Constance Classen defined sensory anthropology and history in response to the developments we've just surveyed above, they did so primarily in the context of the Anglophone academy of North America.[31]

This intellectual genealogy helps account for the fact that, when we want to understand the sensory past of late medieval and early modern Europe, we're usually on much firmer ground in England in the fifteenth, sixteenth, and seventeenth centuries than we are for most other locations in premodern Europe. A critical mass of historical scholarship has built itself up on the firm foundations laid by sensory studies.[32] Most important for our purposes here is the work of Matthew Milner, who has covered much of the same chronological and thematic ground that the present study proposes to do for the German scene.[33] Overall, Milner has told a story of continuity in the sensory cultures of late medieval and Reformation England. He observes that some of the religious practices that appealed to the senses changed, but the underlying culture that conditioned their meaning remained fundamentally the same. "Religious change," to the extent that it took place, "was shaped by persistence of the principles of traditional piety."[34] People thus adapted to their new religious surroundings by means of an older cultural paradigm. The basis of that paradigm was the natural philosophical, or scientific, understanding of the senses and human soul maintained in intellectual discourse. Building on Aristotle, learned discussions fundamentally shaped the meaning of religion in late medieval England, and even motivated the design and performance of worship. The Reformation, far from breaking with this pattern, built on and intensified it. In the practical reforms they introduced to worship, and in their understandings of the meaning of practice, English Protestants embraced Aristotelianism just as wholeheartedly as their late medieval forebears. More recently, Milner has suggested that his findings for England might be indicative of a broader pattern across Europe.[35]

Milner's continuity thesis poses important problems that I intend to grapple with in this study. It is, to be sure, a welcome corrective to the older story of a less sensuous Reformation Christianity. Nonetheless, it also runs the risk of creating a counternarrative that is perhaps more coherent, and more self-contained, than the facts merit. This risk derives in part from the argument's strong orientation toward intellectual history.[36] Ideas about the human senses bind together the fifteenth and sixteenth centuries, and even assume a primary historical agency, moving people to think and act in the peculiar ways they did. This turns our gaze away from other factors external to this system, including how local political economies shaped the forms of worship that communities were able to produce, the power dynamics involved in an intellectual class attempting to impose a hegemonic discourse on the meaning of sensible religion, and the capacities of churchgoers and those situated on the lower rungs of the ecclesiastical hierarchy to respond creatively to the ritual edifice they confronted. It also avoids dealing with the paradoxical matter of religious change: If so much remained the same in the transition from late medieval to Reformation religion, why did so many people like Erhard Schön so consistently perceive the events of the sixteenth century in terms of a profound, world historical rupture?

In this book, I build on the insights of sensory history and anthropology to offer the first systematic study of the senses in the religious landscape of late medieval and early modern Germany. I argue for a more qualified understanding of the coherence of the sensate in late medieval religion, as well as its determining role in the history of the Reformation. Late medieval religion offered up a rich array of multisensory appeals for consumption by churchgoers. The way in which it did, however, was not primarily determined by learned understandings of the senses, important though those may have been. Rather, more pressing, pragmatic concerns confronted those who wanted to put on a good ritual show. People's actions were constrained by local economies in conjunction with liturgical traditions. Intellectuals endeavored to control the meaning of sensuous worship, deploying a largely Aristotelian framework analogous to what prevailed across Europe, but their ability to establish this understanding among more ordinary sorts of people is subject to question. In the vernacular, people played with the language of the senses, and shaped their own understandings of the sensate in religion. When turning to the Reformation, it is clear enough that many, indeed most, leading theologians, pastors, and preachers retained the traditional understanding of the senses from learned culture: immersed in an educational system that retained Aristotelian learning, it was cultivated as a basic assumption from an early age. It forced Lutherans and, perhaps more surprisingly, Calvinists into meaningful engagement with the positive role of the senses in religion until the very eve of the Thirty Years' War (1618–1648). Yet, alongside this continuity were important changes. Aristotelian natural philosophy was not the only lens through which people viewed and acted upon religion. Indeed, at the very core of Protestant identity was the story of de-sensualized Christianity, forged in the rhetoric of the earliest days of the movement. This story motivated liturgical change at least as much as the intellectual discourse, even as reformers encountered obstacles to implementation. Although the weight of the evidence suggests significant continuities in the practice of sensuous worship in late medieval and early Lutheran Christianity, there were also some profound ruptures. Objectively, Reformation religion was not de-sensualized, but it was sensibly different from traditional Christianity.

The focus of this argument is chronologically limited to the period from approximately 1400 to 1600, but many of the developments sketched in these centuries have much deeper origins, extending back to the twelfth and thirteenth centuries, and in the case of the Aristotelian account of sensation, back to antiquity. Developments of the sixteenth century of course resonate well beyond this endpoint, as this period marked a crucial turning point in how western Europeans thought about the social, religious, and indeed, "civilizational" significance of the senses. Geographically, I am primarily concerned with an area that is today roughly contiguous with modern Germany—a political entity at the time known as the Holy Roman Empire. This excludes certain parts of the German-speaking world, including Switzerland, but includes large parts of modern Austria, the Czech Republic, Poland, and the Baltic Sea coast (then parts of Prussia and other North German principalities). Even more specifically, our gaze will rest mostly on the urban communities that dotted this landscape, for, as we will see, the story of the senses in late medieval and early modern Germany is largely a story of the cities.

Within these chronological and geographical limitations, we will deal primarily with late medieval Christianity and its two major Protestant heirs, evangelical and reformed Christianity, usually referred to in popular parlance as Lutheranism and Calvinism, respectively. This necessarily excludes important groups, including Swiss reformed (or Zwinglian, after Huldrych Zwingli) Christianity, which exerted strong influence in many southern and southwestern German towns, and Catholicism (distinct from traditional Christianity as a post-Reformation identity). It also excludes members of the "radical reformation": Anabaptists, and other minorities sometimes referred to as "spiritualists" that splintered from the so-called "magisterial reformation" led by Luther and company. When we reach the sixteenth century, how these people thought about and used the senses is drawn into the narrative for comparative perspective, to set in relief and clarify developments within the Lutheran and Calvinist communities. They are not, however, the subject of this inquiry, important though they might be in their own right as subjects of sensory history.[37]

Thematically, the principal object of concern is the rite of the Mass, alternatively the celebration of the Eucharist, or, as most sixteenth-century Protestants preferred, the Lord's Supper. The reasons for these limitations are both practical and historiographical. Attempting to compass the entire sensory history of religion in this period would require many volumes and would obscure engagement with the major problem at hand. The Mass, however, was undeniably the central locus of the sacred at the end of the Middle Ages, and so its sensory history is entangled with the most important moments in the religious history of this era. It therefore serves as a useful tool for engaging a broader and deeper history of the senses in Reformation Germany. In this respect, I use this ritual as both an object and method of analysis, in order to excavate the religious experience of the past, which, as Wietse de Boer and Christine Göttler have helpfully observed, "is overwhelmingly mediated by sensory discourses and practices."[38]

What follows develops in two parts, intended to grapple systematically with the problem of sensuous religious experience. Taking its methodological cues from the work of Mark Smith, part 1 of this study attends to the key dynamics of sensory production and sensory consumption in late medieval religion, offering a sketch of its complexity.[39] In chapter 1, I situate the sensory production of the Mass, here referring to the objects, practices, and environments that engaged the senses of churchgoers, in political-economic context. By interrogating underutilized ecclesiastical inventories, liturgical books, and the accounts of people who worked in churches, I demonstrate considerable variations in what communities were able to achieve, especially between urban and rural contexts. Chapters 2 and 3 move to the issue of sensory consumption, or the culturally and historically specific ways in which people take in their sensory environments. Here, I show that learned discourse in the fifteenth century consistently asserted a positive role for all five senses in worship, describing the benefits of ritual in terms of the affective, sensuous bond it established with the souls of churchgoers. Talking about ritual in this way reinforced intellectuals' status as ritual experts, but it is important to keep in mind that it was a proposition made to people about the meaning of worship. In chapter 3 we encounter more ordinary sorts of people in cities building on some of the ideas from learned discourse, but also responding to them, and acting upon them in creative ways. Personal prayer book manuscripts, typically overlooked in Reformation studies, form the basis of evidence for this argument. Also here, we see the anxieties this creative use of the senses generated among ecclesiastical authorities, who often responded negatively by disparaging religious sensuality as external to the essence of Christianity.

In part 2 of this study, we assess the relationship between the sensory culture of the later Middle Ages and the Protestant Reformation. The increasingly negative views of sensuality articulated by late medieval churchmen laid much of the groundwork for early Reformation discussions of traditional religion as overwhelmingly hyperaesthetic, and correspondingly dangerous to the human soul. In chapter 4 we turn to this problem, showing how this story formed the basis of a common evangelical identity in the imaginative landscape of the early 1520s. In the printed polemics of this era, rhetoric cast the sensuality of traditional religion as feminine, foreign, and contrary to the new evangelical Christianity taking root in the cities. People imagined true Christianity antithetically as disembodied, masculine, and indigenous to the urban German world they inhabited. This narrative became a keynote of sixteenth-century culture more broadly, grounding assumptions about the history of the church among Protestants and Catholics alike. In chapter 5 we see how this rhetoric motivated early Lutherans to introduce material changes into their worship system, even as a variety of theological, political, and economic considerations intervened to complicate the process. The result was an incomplete and obliquely achieved reformation of the senses, evident in new liturgical ordinances, church inspection reports, and church inventories. Significant continuities with late medieval practice endured, but the full scope of sensuous worship exhibited equally significant ruptures. Finally, in chapter 6, we return to the problem of learned discourse and see how the persistence of Aristotelian natural philosophy formed an important context for how Lutherans and Calvinists alike thought with and about the senses in the religious world of the late sixteenth and early seventeenth centuries. Continued debates about the practice of the Eucharist disclose clearly how these thinkers rejected the notion that external ritual could be a matter of indifference on the grounds that it inexorably affected the souls it touched. Theologians from both confessional camps were especially concerned with the sensory appeal of the rite in general but, perhaps most surprisingly, devoted sustained attention to the importance of the tactile domain of experience.

In making an argument for a more qualified, socially and politically nuanced reformation of the senses, this study proposes to challenge some of the most pervasive narratives about this critical period in the cultural and religious history of Europe and the world. The Reformation was not a force of de-sensualization in the history of Christianity, but neither was it purely a continuation of what came before. Here we set aside unhelpful and overwrought bromides about the sensuality of the Middle Ages and thus see the reality of religious belief and practice through a glass somewhat less obscurely than has previously been the case. On the other side of that glass, too, we see the religion of Reformation Christianity not as an a-sensual inversion of the medieval past, but as series of responses to it, unfolding dynamically in the changing contexts of the sixteenth century.

1 Late Medieval Worship: A Sensory Production

It's a commonplace that the medieval church produced a seemingly endless array of ritual devices to engage the five senses of churchgoers. The seven sacraments of the church, the numerous sacramental processions, seasonal blessings, and other ceremonies punctuating the liturgical calendar, as well as various personal devotions, all self-consciously appealed not only to vision and hearing, but also to touch, smell, and taste. The laying on of hands in the rites of baptism and the ordination of new priests, for example, were manifestly, but by no means exclusively, haptic. Complementing the ritual touch was chrism oil, fragrant with balsam, the vestments of officiating priests and altar cloth framing the event visually, and by the fifteenth century, polyphony and organ music, reverberating throughout often cavernous spaces of Gothic churches. Other rites were similarly intersensorial. Auricular confession was just that—primarily an aural exchange between penitent and confessor, but one can't discount the disciplining gaze of the confessor, as well as the kinesthetic gestures of sorrowful bowing, clasping of hands, and beating of the chest, performed by the penitent. Marriage, too, by the late Middle Ages, had its own ritual formulae that developed according to their own peculiar sensory logics.[1]

Above all, celebration of the Mass formed the beating heart of ritual life in the Middle Ages and mobilized an elaborate multimodal appeal to the senses that sometimes seems to have verged on the chaotic. In Germany on the eve of the Reformation, where devotion to the Eucharist became especially intense, the impression is that no expense was spared. "Even in rural churches and chapels," one historian relates,

> the devout heard the sound of the bell, the intoning of the ritual prayers. . . . They often saw the altar with its cloths and retable, the corpse-laden crucifix, the sheen

> of paten and Chalice, the glint of candlelight, the ceremonial vestments. . . . They smelled the sweat of their neighbors and at the same time the heavenly fragrances of beeswax and incense.[2]

At the center of this environment was the Eucharist, a wafer of unleavened wheat bread and a chalice of wine, each consecrated with the Latin words *hoc est corpus meum*, and *hoc est sanguis meus*, effecting a transubstantiation of the profane elements into the actual body and blood of Christ. The priest elevated these sacred objects above the altar for all to see, and thereafter, occasionally, churchgoers received communion sacramentally—that is, they consumed it orally. More often, however, they were content simply to take in the entire experience and gaze upon the elevated Host, satisfied by their "ocular communion."[3] The image-trope of the *Mass of St. Gregory* (see figure 3), which became diffuse in various media in the second half of the fifteenth century, provides stylized representations of this moment and is often cited as evidence of the overwhelming sensuality of Mass practice.[4] The "theatrical techniques" depicted in such images constituted the production of the Mass as a multisensory event, transporting people from the often disgusting sensory surroundings of their daily lives, focusing their gaze on the Eucharist, and bringing them closer to heavenly things. The Mass, often standing in for the entire medieval liturgy, was eminently sensual and, indeed, *synesthetic*, appealing to multiple sense modalities simultaneously.

There are likely a variety of factors that have given rise to the persistence of this scholarly mise-en-scène among medievalists, Reformation historians, and specialists in sensory history alike. In part, it may reflect a tendency to exoticize the Middle Ages: the primitive medieval world, in contrast to the sober intellectual universe of modernity, was of course highly sensual. As we will see in coming chapters, the determination to see the later Middle Ages in this way is in no small part a legacy of storytelling by the first people who thought of themselves as Protestants. Much as sensory anthropology has rightly criticized this mode of thinking as it applies to non-Western societies, it is imperative to regard its historical counterpart with caution.[5] More charitably, however, there is no denying that ritual practice, regardless of time or place, is always already a sensuous affair. There is also no denying that a lot of evidence suggests medieval ritual practice was intentionally designed to appeal to all five senses. In addition to imagery like the *Mass of St. Gregory*, the proliferation of liturgical texts from the period supports this point. It is also difficult to move beyond the lingering residue of material culture. Collections of sacred vessels and vestments on display in museums, and the remains of medieval churches, radiate sensuality.[6]

The major problem with the current understanding of the sensory production of late medieval worship, however, is that it does not take into account its basis in local political economy. Usually, we implicitly assume that communities had unrestricted access to the multisensory spectacles that so commonly appear in descriptions of late medieval practice. Occasionally, the assumption is made explicit that the sensory actuation supposedly attested in the Mass "was the bare minimum."[7] Was it though? The production of a multisensory environment of such density was an expensive proposition. It was materially dependent on rare commodities such as incense and silk, liturgical furniture fashioned from gold or silver, as well as an entire cast of ritual actors that included priests, deacons, acolytes, choirs, choir directors, and other musicians. This cast also required a "script" for putting raw materials to use: ritual ordinances—above all, those rubrics known as *missals*—provided this script and were costly even after the advent of print technology made them more widely accessible. Beyond this, the full extent of sensory production presupposed an extensive "backstage" support staff to procure, organize, maintain, and provide at the proper time and place the liturgical equipment necessary for performance, as well as a community of artisans with the technical proficiency necessary to aid the support staff in its duties. These demands made producing the Mass as a multisensory experience not simply a liturgical problem. In such contexts, the material world imposed fundamental limits on the sensory production of church ritual, and people largely made do with what they had.

This is not to say that ritual practice in some communities was more or less sensual than it was elsewhere. All religion, and all human behavior for that matter, is always already intersensorial. There was, however, considerable variation in how churches made appeals to the senses, and a major divide is discernible between urban and rural spaces. In the German-speaking world, a handful of large, wealthy, urban communities were best positioned to approximate the ideal extent of sensory production outlined above. Even here, variation prevailed according to the resources available from one church to the next. Neighboring churches in a single city could produce substantially different rituals from a sensory perspective. Practice within a single church, too, varied over the course of the liturgical year, depending on the abbreviations, substitutions, augmentations, or other peculiarities in local observance. In the countryside, church practice smelled, tasted, felt, looked, and sounded rather different. Rural parish churches were, simply put, materially different from their urban counterparts. As a rule, they were physically smaller and financially poorer. Their access to the commodities and furnishings commonly depicted in late medieval church practice was more restricted. As such, the sensory production of late medieval worship was diverse from one context to the next. Communities recognized, and even touted, this fact. As one commentator from the city of Magdeburg noted, the local liturgical calendar was filled with diverse celebrations. Masses, processions, and other practices distinguished themselves from one another within the community, and externally from other communities, "not only by the distinct mode of singing and reading assembled [on feast days], but also by the diversity of bells, vestments, vessels, candles, and the other many things pertaining to divine worship."[8]

This chapter outlines the diversity of sensory production specifically as it pertained to the Mass in late medieval Germany. The Mass is a good place to start because it was unquestionably the most important locus of the divine in the fifteenth century, and because it often serves as a kind of synecdoche for the entire ritual edifice of the late medieval church in scholarly discussions. I argue that, from a sensory perspective, late medieval ritual was highly variable and, if judged against the ideal imagined in recent scholarship, imperfect. From one community to the next, economic circumstances determined the fullest extent, and limitations, of sensory worship. Above all, there were major differences in how wealthy urban communities and their smaller, poorer, rural counterparts produced the sensory appeal of the Mass. Given the resources on hand in most rural parishes, the sensory experience of church ritual was fundamentally different from the urban scene. Since the majority of the population lived in these rural parishes, the fullest extent of sensual ritual in urban communities should not be taken as representative of late medieval Germany as a whole.

I develop this argument by analyzing how local communities constructed the ritual environment from the field of possibilities they had at their disposal. I'm interested in the "raw materials" necessary for the construction process: not simply the speaking of prayers and performance of gestures, but the more immediate problem of the availability of material resources that set such prayer and gestures in context, and were necessary for putting on a good ritual show. The investigation begins in the free imperial city of Nuremberg. As one of the largest and wealthiest cities in the German-speaking world, Nuremberg is a good place to start because it faced relatively few constraints on its acquisition of the material resources necessary for sensory worship. Because of the exceptionally well-organized administrative structure that maintained its two parish churches, St. Sebald and St. Lorenz, Nuremberg also offers an unusual amount of evidence on late medieval piety. The documentary record in Nuremberg provides a baseline for comparison with other locations across late-medieval Germany, from peer cities such as Strasbourg, to medium-sized towns, down to humble parish churches in small villages. Church inventories, ritual agendas, and the notes of pastors and other church officials provide insight into how these communities produced sensory worship. For small rural parishes where evidence from the fifteenth century is rather slim, analysis relies on a "back-streaming" method employed in ethnohistory and historical anthropology: inventories collected during inspections, or visitations, of rural parishes conducted in the sixteenth century by both Catholic and Protestant ecclesiastical authorities supplement the fifteenth-century record.[9] Evidence from this later period, although imperfect, provides insight into the material culture of rural churches in the generations prior to the Reformation. Following a bit of context on Nuremberg and the political economy of fifteenth-century churches, the chapter outlines the extent and limitations of providing for tasting, seeing, smelling, touching, and hearing. To varying degrees, appeals to each of the sensory modalities worked in concert with one another, producing an intersensorial Mass.

The material demands of sensory worship on the eve of the Reformation meant that wealthy urban communities were best positioned to produce the elaborate spectacle commonly depicted in the scholarship. The city of Nuremberg illustrates the upper limits of sensory production in this era. With respect to liturgical furniture, the city's parish churches were well equipped, owning extensive collections of the objects necessary for the production of a multisensory Mass (see table 1). Both churches accumulated most of these objects over the course of the 1400s, particularly in the latter half of the century. They were stored in the sacristies of each church, carefully described in the inventories, accounts, and notes of city officials specifically appointed for these tasks.[10] Additionally, the immobile elements of the structured ritual environment, including church architecture, sculpture, and the large bells in the churches' bell towers, contributed to the sensory production of the Mass. During the fifteenth century, both churches underwent numerous renovations, expansions, and beautification projects to enrich these environments.[11]

Several economic factors contributed to Nuremberg's extensive provisioning for the senses. The city benefited tremendously from its situation at the intersection of several international trade routes running from the Netherlands,

Table 1: Material Provision for the Senses in Nuremberg's Parish Churches: Raw Numbers of Liturgical Furniture in St. Sebald and St. Lorenz.

	St. Sebald	St. Lorenz
Visual Provision		
Chalices	22	34
Patens	29	33
Candelabra	69	9
Images	59	64
Textiles	193	221
Olfactory Provision		
Censers	2	2
Tactile Provision		
Pax Boards	17	27
Aural Provision		
Bells	3	0
Organs	2	2
Gustatory Provision		
Host iron	3	0

Prussia, and Poland in the north and northeast, to Italy, Spain, and Portugal in the south and southwest. Along these routes, spices, silks, textiles, coral, and gemstones flowed into the city.[12] Further, in the fifteenth century, Nuremberg had established control over several mining operations in the *Erzgebirge* in the east-central reaches of the Holy Roman Empire and had interests in others to the south in Tirol, and further north in Saxony.[13] The metals stripped from these mountains eventually found their way into the local Nuremberg market, where they were usually finished by the city's master craftsmen, renowned for their metal work, particularly ornamental and liturgical items.[14] This system often benefited the churches of St. Sebald and St. Lorenz via the patronage of wealthy patrician families who dominated the city council.[15] In exchange for donations of vestments, liturgical furniture, and other religious art, the churches added numerous new services and feast days to commemorate and pray for patrons and patrons' families. Thus, as the material complexity of Nuremberg's liturgical furnishings grew, so too did the complexity of the ritual calendar.

At the same time, Nuremberg's city council had managed to wrest effective control of most ecclesiastical matters from the bishop of Bamberg, who technically held authority over the city's parish churches. The council developed a centralized administrative structure to manage the growing complexity of ritual life in St. Sebald and St. Lorenz. The offices most immediately relevant to sensory production were the church master (*Kirchenmeister*) and sacristan (*Mesner*). The church master managed finances, a large proportion of which was dedicated to the maintenance, repair, or beautification of church property. This required cultivating a network of artisans, including goldsmiths, tinsmiths, stonemasons, carpenters, glassmakers, sculptors, and painters. It also required accounting for all donations received, whether in the form of money, liturgical furniture, or other kinds of wealth.[16] Below the office of church master were the sacristans. The sacristans were primarily responsible for overseeing the cleaning of church interiors and managing the property held in the sacristies of each church. In cooperation with the church masters, they kept inventories of all liturgical furniture, books, and vestments. Twice a year, these officials would inspect the sacristies to ensure the fidelity of these inventories. Additionally, it was the sacristans who supplied priests and other ritual actors with the vestments and liturgical furniture appropriate for the particular feast day being celebrated. The "sacristan's books" produced in the last two decades of the fifteenth century document the extraordinary complexity of this task and provide invaluable insight into the extent and limits of the sensual in late medieval practice.[17]

While considerably wealthier than most of its urban counterparts, the basis of Nuremberg's extensive provisioning for the senses nonetheless exemplified political economic trends in late medieval German cities more broadly. Beginning especially in the late thirteenth and early fourteenth centuries, many other large cities consolidated power and authority over church property and appointed secular officials to manage it.[18] At the same time, the growing popularity of patronizing churches with donations significantly contributed to the complexity of ritual life and its sensual appeal. In Strasbourg, for example, 7,803 donations were made to the cathedral from the middle of the fourteenth century to the early sixteenth century. While liturgical furniture and other devotional objects constituted only approximately 3 percent of donations, this represented an outsized impact on ritual life, as these objects were regularly used throughout the liturgical year.[19]

Closer scrutiny of this material substratum reveals how communities produced the sensory appeal of the Mass in highly differentiated ways. Even the wealthiest urban parishes had to confront very real limitations imposed by the material world. Sensory production in these places was, properly speaking, the art of making do with things ready to hand, rather than any rigid, mechanical adherence to the ideal of an overwhelming spectacle. Variations, especially between town and country, were apparent with respect to each of the five senses.

In the fifteenth century, perhaps more than any other time in European history, eating and drinking dominated religious belief and practice. In Germany, there is no denying that the Eucharist was the central object of devotion. Despite this, scholarly interpretation has generally struggled with the role of taste in late medieval religious practice. With the exception of fasting, Robert Scribner observed, "it is often difficult to see where taste had its place."[20] Much of this has to do with the challenge of finding the sense in the primary source record: ritual ordinances such as missals, for example, seldom offer details on the material composition of the Eucharist bread and wine, and therefore nothing on their gustatory properties. More descriptive accounts are virtually nonexistent, at least in the form of what we would today classify as reliable "ego-documents"—letters, diaries, and other private writings.[21] Despite these difficulties, it is possible to establish some facts on the provisioning for taste, if only on a preliminary basis.

To some extent, the church attempted to legislate the gustatory experience of communion. The first comprehensive vernacular explication of the Mass, which appeared around 1480, dictated that the Eucharist Host be "clean," "pure," thin, and made without the addition of salt. It should be made exclusively from unleavened wheat, which "in its nature is sweet."[22] The somewhat surprising description of unleavened wheat reflects theoretical expectations of the gustatory experience of the Eucharist, addressed more extensively in the following chapters. Of more immediate concern, the potential of communities to produce a Eucharistic experience to these standards was highly varied and dependent on local economic circumstances. Wheat cultivation was fairly widespread in late medieval Germany, but quality and quantity could fluctuate widely from region to region.[23] Access was therefore by no means equal; consequently, the adulteration of hosts with other grains happened with some regularity. The famous humanist bishop Nicolas Cusanus (1401–1464) complained about this during a series of inspections of the parish churches under his care in the late 1450s, where he observed many neighboring dioceses selling hosts "made not from pure wheat, but a mixture of spelt and other kinds of grain." Cusanus condemned the practice as "dangerous" and attempted to maintain some degree of consistency in his territory by requiring that the cathedral directly oversee all host production in the diocese.[24] Realistically, however, the material composition of the Eucharist Host remained heavily subject to local grain production, and its taste varied accordingly.

The production process introduced other potential variations. The paper-thin Eucharist wafers required a specialized oven, or "host iron." Such host irons tended to wear out rather quickly, which also affected the quality of the hosts they produced.[25] Hosts were very easy to burn, and burning food produced a bitter taste—the unhealthy and polar opposite of the sweetness so essential to the Eucharist, according to the predominant understanding of how flavors worked.[26] A host iron that burned wafers was therefore a serious problem, and church masters devoted significant time and energy to ensuring their tools were in good working order. Sebald Schreyer, the master of the church of St. Sebald in Nuremberg from 1482 to 1503, was constantly paying for repairs to the three host irons owned by the church.[27] As a result of these economic challenges, even communities of considerable means often had to purchase finished hosts from larger neighboring cities. The Rheinland town of Koblenz, for example, acquired hosts from Cologne, while in Franconia, Windsheim got its hosts from Nuremberg.[28] Even Nuremberg occasionally had to purchase finished hosts. In 1490 and 1491, Schreyer twice recorded payments for hosts "because of the dearth of wheat."[29]

Because wine cultivation was restricted to relatively few regions in the German-speaking world, provisioning for it was even more problematic than the production of hosts. Wine used during the Mass was supposed be "pure and clear," produced strictly from wine grapes. It was not to be sour, but nor could it be overly sweet or fortified with sugar.[30] However, even communities of considerable means made do with what was on hand. Some churches, such as those in Rothenburg and Freiburg, owned vineyards that provided a reliable, local supply of wine.[31] In most places, wine had to be imported. In Nuremberg, this responsibility fell to the church masters. In the church of Our Beloved Lady in Ingolstadt, the major institutions in the city, such as the university and trade guilds, enthusiastically saw to it.[32] In Göttingen, the city council provided wine directly to the churches, free of charge.[33] Under such circumstances, the quality of the wine varied drastically. Even the wealthy churches in Nuremberg occasionally struggled to provide acceptable wine. Upon taking the office of master of St. Sebald in 1482, the city council charged Sebald Schreyer with the task of keeping a consistent supply of red wine in the sacristy. As the mandate the explained, the need arose from the "great failure" that had "previously allowed considerable, frequent, great, and serious negligence and harm, when on several occasions Mass had been celebrated with water alone, and without wine."[34] Schreyer appears to have taken his charge seriously, spending a substantial amount on wine, Eucharist Hosts, and a new host oven, in the following year.[35]

Provisioning for taste in this manner was a significant concern in urban communities like Nuremberg, where large numbers of people received sacramental communion with unusual frequency. As the humanist Johann Cochläus (1479–1552) observed, Nuremberg's "common" men and women communed sacramentally as often as six times per year.[36] The sacristans' books for St. Sebald and St. Lorenz document the provisioning of wine for major feast days, and roughly agree with Cochläus's impression: six days were singled out in the St. Lorenz liturgical calendar, while the sacristan in St. Sebald noted seven.[37] Specific numbers of communicants are not available for Nuremberg, but the sacristans' books provide some sense of the extent of sacramental communion. The most extensive communion occurred during Holy Week. From Palm Sunday to Easter Monday, the total of wine provided in St. Lorenz amounted to 187.54 liters; in St. Sebald it was somewhat less, at 165.85 liters. Both churches received their largest numbers of communicants on Good Friday: in St. Lorenz, sacristans were to provide 62.87 liters of wine, while in St. Sebald it was 59.62 liters. In addition to Holy Week, other important days for sacramental communion included Christmas (presumably in both churches, although only the St. Sebald sacristan's book indicates provisioning for wine), All Saints' Day in St. Lorenz, and in St. Sebald, the Annunciation of the Virgin, and Pentecost.[38] It is also likely that Corpus Christi and the feast days of the churches' patron saints, Sebald and Lorenz, were important days for communing as well.[39] Similar patterns prevailed in other urban communities of scale: the most extensive communion occurred during Holy Week, followed by Christmas, other locally important feast days, and occasionally the Sundays during Lent. In major cathedral seats like Trier and Mainz, as well as parish churches in Ulm, Göttingen, and Ingolstadt, the numbers of communicants on these days was quite impressive, sometimes reaching the thousands.[40]

Such extensive communion, however, was exceptional, and if taking into account the whole of late medieval Germany, one must conclude that the taste of the Eucharist was a rare thing indeed. The Eucharist was administered throughout the year, but those who communed at times other than the major feast days were among an elite class of the devout, usually in some way connected with a religious order. In southern Bavaria, Cistercian brothers received the sacrament "as is custom each first Sunday of the month; in Advent and in Lent, every Sunday."[41] Dominican sisters in some parts of Germany communed every week, while in others, fifteen times per year.[42] The Carthusian Dionys Ryckel (d. 1417) paints a general picture of female communion in the fifteenth century, writing that "in many convents and congregations . . . the sisters receive communion very often, namely in Advent and Lent on every Sunday. Otherwise they receive communion every two weeks."[43] Some lay members of religious orders communed sacramentally even more frequently—in some cases on a weekly or daily basis. Moreover, such cases of frequent communion were largely restricted to the urban milieu or, if in the countryside, monastic communities.[44] For the vast majority of the population, who lived in rural parish churches, sacramental communion was sporadic and inconsistent, compelling authorities like Nicolas Cusanus repeatedly to command rural parishioners to receive sacramental communion at least once per year.[45]

Unlike taste, the importance of vision in late medieval piety has been discussed rather extensively in the scholarship. As Scribner explains, "There was no celebration of the Mass, indeed almost no prayer, which did not involve a relevant image, while the major feasts of the liturgical year were celebrated by a 'dramatized liturgy' in which images played a major role."[46] The focal point of people's gazes was the ritual elevation of the Eucharist during the Mass. Held aloft by the priest following the words of consecration, the Host and (to a lesser extent) the chalice were the laity's primary point of contact with the sacred—as Scribner called it, the "densest" and "most pregnant" expression of late medieval visual piety.[47] The evidence supporting the popularity of this practice is substantial, and its centrality will not be disputed here. However, scholarly interpretations run the risk of painting a picture that is overly coherent and consistent. Practical variations in the visual production of the Mass abound.

The elevation of the Eucharist took place during the Canon of the Mass but involved a number of staging gestures in the precedent and antecedent portions of Mass, beginning with the Offertory and ending with Communion. Collectively, these portions of the Mass composed the "liturgy of the Eucharist" (see table 2). Somewhat surprisingly, the deep significance of this moment in late medieval piety did not translate into consistent liturgical usage. Of a sample of fifty-one printed missals for German dioceses between 1470 and 1520, only twenty-four (47 percent) include explicit instructions for the ritual elevations during the Canon.[48] This does not mean that the elevation was not performed or that it was unimportant; rather, it likely reflects the fact that the elevation was well-enough established by the late fifteenth century that printers, and the episcopal officials who approved the prints, did not find it necessary to

Table 2: Outline of the Mass in Late Medieval Germany (based on *Missale Bambergense*) (Bamberg: Sensenschmidt, 1490).

PREPARATIONS
1. Celebrant Preparations
2. Introitus

LITURGY OF THE WORD
3. Kyrie eleison
4. Gloria
5. Collect
6. Epistle
7. Alleluia/Tract
8. Sequence (Prosa)
9. Gospel
10. Credo

LITURGY OF THE EUCHARIST
11. Offertory
12. Preface
13. Sanctus et Benedictus (Canon and Elevations)
14. Pater Noster
15. Pax Domini
16. Agnus Dei
17. Fraction/Distribution
18. Communion

DISMISSAL
19. Postcommunion (prayers/chants)
20. Ite missae est
21. Placeat tibi
22. Benediction

include instructions, and that a certain degree of latitude was necessary for the peculiarities and practical variations that emerged in local observance. More than anything else, these ordinances were, to borrow the phrase from Matthew Milner, "proposals for liturgical praxis."[49] Communities had various resources at their disposal and therefore could accept and implement these proposals with varying degrees of consistency.

The parish churches of Nuremberg provide a case in point. Officially subject to the authority of the bishop of Bamberg, there is some evidence that the churches combined the official usage proposed by the diocesan missal with elements from other usages, or at the very least had the resources to do so. The sacristies of both churches acquired multiple copies of the Bamberg usage over the last two decades of the fifteenth century; St. Sebald alone held twelve.[50] In addition to the Bamberg usage, however, the Nuremberg churches had a number of other missals at their disposal. As a center of early print culture, the city produced missals for many other dioceses, including Naumburg, Magdeburg, Hildesheim, Brandenburg, Passau, and Salzburg, as well as editions of the Roman missal (*Missale romanum*).[51] The Roman missal presented itself as the norm of practice throughout the late medieval church and provided one of the most elaborate usages of the late fifteenth century. St. Sebald owned at least one copy: an edition appears attached to the altar of St. Peter in the church in 1517.[52]

A comparison of the Bamberg and Roman missals suggests the range of Eucharistic gestures in Nuremberg on the eve of the Reformation. Both required a paten (essentially a large plate) for holding the Host, and a chalice for the wine. In the Bamberg usage, consecration of the elements during the Offertory involved raising the Host on the paten, making the sign of the cross over the chalice, raising the chalice, and the returning the chalice to the altar before bowing. During the Canon, the elevation instructions delineated six procedures: bowing to the altar, signing the cross over both elements, elevating the Host in the hands, executing a cruciform extension of the arms, placing a hand over the chalice, and completing the rite by folding hands in prayer. The fraction began after the Canon, with the priest accepting the Host on the paten, breaking it into three pieces, and mixing a small piece into the chalice of wine while singing the *Agnus Dei*.[53]

The Roman missal paralleled certain elements of this usage, while considerably elaborating others. The Offertory was virtually the same but added a ritual hand washing near the end. The usage for the Canon was much more elaborate, involving the priest's signing the cross three times over the Host and chalice together, followed by separate individual signs of the cross first over the Host, then over the chalice; receiving the Host "reverently" (*reverenter*) and elevating it with two hands; returning the Host to the altar and receiving the chalice; returning the chalice to the altar and holding it in the left hand while blessing it with the right; lifting the chalice again and returning it to the altar; making three signs of the cross over both elements, followed by one over the Host and one over the chalice; bowing, kissing the altar, signing the cross once over each element again, and completing the rite by crossing himself. The communion portion of the Mass was also considerably more involved. The priest received the paten, crossed himself with it, and then placed the Host on it. Thereafter, the chalice was uncovered; the priest reverently broke the Host and returned it to the paten with his right hand. He then took up the chalice with his left hand while his right hand took a piece of the Host, used it to make a sign of the cross over the chalice, and then place the Host fragment into the wine. After several more bows and ritual kisses, the priest raised the chalice and then paten "a little bit" (*aliquantulum*), and he took up the Host in his right hand and held it reverently over the paten for another prayer. Thereafter, the priest signed the cross over the Host and received it in his mouth, then drank from the chalice.[54]

In practice, variation and improvisation were the rule, and the Nuremberg churches likely produced something between the usages delineated in the Roman and Bamberg missals. An approximation sufficiently familiar to actors and spectators gathered in the church was all that was required to make the ritual efficacious. As Gerd Althoff has observed, this attitude produced wide ritual variability throughout the Middle Ages.[55] The variability of elevation usages in other dioceses reinforces this point. In Cologne and Würzburg, usage was virtually the same as in the *Missale romanum*, but Würzburg added the use of cloth on which to place the chalice and paten and to wipe hands while handling the Eucharist.[56] In Mainz and Worms, usage also closely followed the Roman missal, while innovating a "double-elevation" of the Host during the Canon.[57] Other dioceses such as Brandenburg, Magdeburg, and Halberstadt provided more detailed instructions on covering and uncovering the elements with additional textiles.[58]

The material resources required for this moment added to the seemingly endless variations and, from a sensory standpoint, produced visibly different rituals. With sixty-two patens and fifty-six chalices between them, the churches of St. Lorenz and St. Sebald could produce a variety of Eucharistic spectacles throughout the liturgical year. Parish churches and cathedrals in other urban communities of scale approached or in some cases exceeded the variety found in Nuremberg. The church of St. James in Rothenburg ob der Tauber owned seventeen chalices in 1410 and likely accumulated more later in the century. The minster of Ulm possessed seventy-one chalices, and the collective inventories of all churches in Lübeck accounted for 339 chalices on the eve of the Reformation.[59] In Strasbourg, the cathedral, three collegiate churches, as well as the chapel of the great hospital could boast a combined sixty-five chalices and fifty patens.[60] No doubt the large numbers were in part necessary to meet the needs of those administering sacramental communion in urban centers: the distribution of the Eucharist following the elevations was executed by the priest with the assistance of deacons, acolytes, and the laity on days when the numbers of communicants were especially large.[61] However, it is also clear that they contributed to the visible diversity of elevation practice throughout the liturgical calendar. The most valuable chalices and patens were usually matching pairs designated for use on specific feast days, such as the large gilded silver set with fine etchings, owned by St. Sebald.[62] This particular set was used on Good Friday, when the church received its highest numbers of communicants.[63]

By comparison, smaller towns and rural parishes produced far less variety. The churches of St. Willibrord and St. Nikolaus in Wesel, a medium-sized but regionally important city on the lower Rhine, acquired five chalices, and probably at least as many patens, over the course of the fifteenth century.[64] By comparison, in the Duchy of Braunschweig, of the 392 parish churches inspected in the early 1540s, only 234 (59.7 percent) documented one or more chalices in their inventories. In the adjacent duchy of Kalenberg-Göttingen, a larger percentage of communities owned at least one chalice (72.6 percent).[65] In most cases, parishes typically owned one chalice, which was only very rarely paired with a paten.[66] Similar numbers appear elsewhere. In the 320 parishes visited in Brandenburg over the course of the sixteenth century, 92.2 percent documented at least one chalice, while only 3.7 percent of communities documented one or more patens. The maximum numbers of chalices and patens owned by a single parish church in Brandenburg were six and two, respectively.[67] In Saxony, 95 percent of parish churches owned at least one chalice, while 45 percent owned at least one paten. The maximum numbers of chalices and paten in a single community were twelve and one, respectively.[68] In general, the chalices used in these rural parish churches were not the fine silver and gilded implements found in wealthier towns: many were fashioned from tin, brass, and, in some cases, wood.

Similar patterns of variability are apparent with respect to other items that elaborated the visual setting of the elevation, including candelabra, textiles, and images of various types. Candelabra, or candlesticks, supplemented the natural light that shone through church windows. In Nuremberg, while inventories documented relatively small numbers of exceptionally valuable silver or gilded candelabra, evidence from the sacristans' books suggests that the churches owned substantially larger collections. St. Sebald, for example, owned at least twelve additional gilded candelabra made to resemble angels.[69] Beyond these, the churches likely owned a number of wooden candelabra. The illumination of the church interiors varied significantly, depending on the particular celebration and the materials on hand. On ordinary Sundays in St. Sebald, both the high altar and the altar of the Blessed Virgin were illuminated with two angelic candelabra apiece. These were lit before the first Mass of the day and allowed to burn through vespers in the evening.[70] In St. Lorenz the picture is somewhat less clear, but it appears that perhaps two to four candelabra, fashioned from brass or tin, illuminated the high altar.[71]

Additional layers supplemented this baseline illumination according to the liturgical calendar. In St. Sebald the sacristans equipped other altars with candelabra and candles for 81.8 percent of the feast days celebrated throughout the liturgical year.[72] In practice, this usually meant lighting the high altar as well as the altar consecrated to the saint whose feast day was being celebrated. In both churches, for example, festivals honoring Mary involved illuminating the altar of the Blessed Virgin. Occasionally, all the altars in the church were lighted, as was the case for New Year's Day, All Saints' Day, the Lord's Ascension, and the Presentation of Mary in St. Lorenz.[73] In the late fifteenth century, subsidizing special "transubstantiation candles" became a popular means of ritual participation among wealthy laypeople and fraternal organizations. The masters of both churches received numerous bequests to endow altars with candles for "illumination when the holy sacrament is transformed during the holy mass."[74] Holy

Week required illumination on a different scale. Transubstantiation candles were essential for Masses on Maundy Thursday, Good Friday, and Easter Sunday: in St. Lorenz the high altar was bedecked with two, while seven were placed on the high altar in St. Sebald.[75] In addition to these transubstantiation candles, both churches provided a single, massive, Easter candle. St. Sebald added yet another layer to this picture, commissioning a wooden frame on which to mount its twelve angelic candelabra for a special display at Masses on Good Friday.[76]

An array of textiles, including priestly vestments, altar cloths, tapestries, and banners, further elaborated the visual topography of the Mass. Given the sheer volume of such items held by each church, the number of permutations was considerable. With respect to vestments, the sacristan of St. Lorenz identified the use of thirty-five different chasubles, mantels, or full sets of regalia; in St. Sebald the number was seventeen.[77] These were fashioned from silk, velvet, satin, damask, or taffeta, and embroidered with gold or pearl tracery, as well as images of saints or the arms of patrician donors. The color palettes were rather similar in both churches: the most common colors were red and white.[78] Black vestments were also fairly common, as were green, and blue, although St. Lorenz appears to have favored these latter two colors considerably more than St. Sebald.[79] Officiants in St. Lorenz also occasionally wore brown or gray.[80] Certain colors were consistently worn at certain times of year—for example, white for Marian feast days, black for All Souls' Day—but most major feast days involved multiple Masses with changes of wardrobe in between.[81] At Easter in the church of Lorenz, for example, the priest wore vestments of red silk with pearl images for the first Mass, green silk with golden floral patterns and a crucifix for the second, black silk with gold for the third, and a set of white silk regalia with extraordinarily ornate golden tracery for the High Mass.[82]

In addition to priestly vestments, both churches deployed extensive collections of cloths, tapestries, and banners to festoon the high altars and choirs. A Mass in St. Sebald involved at a minimum four red banners, along with a huge woven tapestry detailing the life of St. Sebald, at the high altar. Two other large tapestries serving as a backdrop were placed in the choir.[83] As with candelabra, the use of these items was typically denser on important feast days, such as Easter and Christmas, during which sacristans furnished the "best" altar cloths and "all banners" on hand for the choir, while on other occasions, such as the Marian feast days, during which the choirs of the churches were adorned similarly with all banners, but "common" (*schlecht* or *gemein*) altar cloths were used instead.[84] Special tapestries, too, adorned the altars on certain days, such as the linen cloths with images of the Passion draped on the high altar at Easter. The color profiles of these textiles differed significantly between churches: in St. Sebald the predominant colors were blue and green, while in St. Lorenz such textiles were mainly white and gold.[85]

One final category of objects that augmented the visual appeal of the Mass included devotional images, monstrances, and crucifixes. Each of these objects was used in distinctive ways outside the context of the Mass, particularly in the myriad processions that prefaced, ended, or sometimes interrupted celebrations of the Mass throughout the liturgical year.[86] Within the Mass, however, they had more or less the same visual utility, ornamenting the high altar as it framed the elevated Eucharist.[87] In Nuremberg most of these items were fashioned from silver, or gilded silver, and most contained and displayed a relic of some kind.[88] The variety of visual settings these items helped cultivate was substantial. For most Masses in St. Sebald, the minimum number of such objects placed on the altar would include the gilded silver head of the church's patron saint, along with two other unspecified images.[89] Occasionally, crucifixes or monstrances supplemented these items.[90] The church also had a set of large gilded silver images of Saints Peter, Paul, and John the Baptist, favored on feast days of these saints, as well as days dedicated to other apostles, and the church's patron, Sebald.[91] The church of St. Lorenz often decorated the images with small articles of clothing. This was generally restricted to images of female saints.[92] On St. Margaret's day, for example, an image of the saint was dressed in "virginal cloths," crowned, and draped in a garland before being set at the altar for Mass.[93]

The collections of candelabra, textiles, devotional images, monstrances, and crucifixes in the Nuremberg churches were rather exceptional. Notwithstanding peer cities like Strasbourg, most communities in late medieval Germany had comparably few resources for producing the Mass as a visual spectacle of such scope, intensity, and variability throughout the liturgical year. Whereas chalices and patens were immediately necessary for the performance of the Eucharist, candelabra, textiles, and other altar ornamentation were, technically speaking, of secondary importance; that is, they were not formally prescribed as part of the liturgy of the Eucharist in diocesan missals. The contrast between Nuremberg and communities of lesser economic means was therefore even more marked with respect to these items than it was with respect to chalices and patens. In medium-sized towns such as Wesel, inventories for the church of St. Willibrord from the second half of the fifteenth century document the acquisition of twelve wooden candelabra: three at the high altar, three at the altar of the Holy Cross (the second most prestigious altar in the church), and six larger standing candelabra for the choir. In neighboring St. Nikolaus a total of eight candelabra were added during the same period—all of these items were fashioned from various metals, including one iron candelabrum with a special glass container, purchased in 1494.[94] The parish church of St. Martin in the free imperial city of Biberach owned gilded angelic candelabra similar to those found in Nuremberg, but only two. They were designated to hold the transubstantiation candles during Mass. As the superintendent of the church, Joachim von

Pflummern (1480–1554) noted, "One lit them when one had elevated our Lord God."[95]

In smaller rural parishes the contrast was even more pronounced. In Braunschweig, for example, only 33.9 percent of parish church inventories documented monstrances, and only three communities reported candelabra. In nearby Kalenberg-Göttingen, inventories document similar numbers: 28.4 percent of communities owned at least one monstrance, and 12.6 percent owned at least one candelabrum. No single parish church in Kalenberg-Göttingen owned more than two monstrances, and the maximum number of candelabra owned was twelve. In Brandenburg 53.4 percent of communities documented monstrances, 1.5 percent candelabra, and 25 percent at least one textile, whether it was a priestly vestment, altar cloth, or banner. The maximum number of textiles in a single parish in Brandenburg was four. Inventories occasionally indicated that textiles were made of silk, or that they were a specific color (most commonly green), but provide no details beyond these. In Saxony, numbers were slightly higher: 34 percent documented at least one candelabra, 5 percent at least one monstrance, and 68 percent at least one liturgical textile. The maximum numbers of objects owned by single communities were four candelabra, two monstrances, and twelve textiles. The significant differences in material culture available in larger, wealthy cities, and their poorer, rural counterparts, translated into different ritual practice, at least from a purely visual standpoint.

These highly variable manipulations of material culture also unfolded in visually diverse spatial environments. In the Gothic churches that dominated the landscape of late medieval Europe, massive windows flooded church interiors with light, directing sightlines primarily toward the choir and high altar, where the elevation of the Eucharist usually took place. Unlike in England, rood screens separating the nave of the church from the choir and high altar were uncommon in Germany.[96] Church masters devoted special care to the installation and repair of windows, particularly those in the choir, occasionally known as "sacrament windows," often considerably more expensive than other glass in the church.[97] The size of these churches also had an appreciable visual impact. The minster of Ulm, physically the largest parish church in fifteenth-century Germany, boasted some of the largest windows, and the exceptionally vibrant light that filled the space left a deep impression on visitors.[98]

Altars, sculpture, and other permanent art fixtures also populated these spaces. The church at Ulm contained a staggering fifty-two altars.[99] The churches of Sebald and Lorenz in Nuremberg contained a more modest eighteen and fifteen altars, respectively.[100] Elaborate altarpieces typically adorned these locations. The most impressive were placed at the high altar, constituting yet another element in the visual appeal of the Mass. For example, the exceptionally well-preserved *Twelve Apostles' Altar* (see figure 2), installed in 1466 at the high

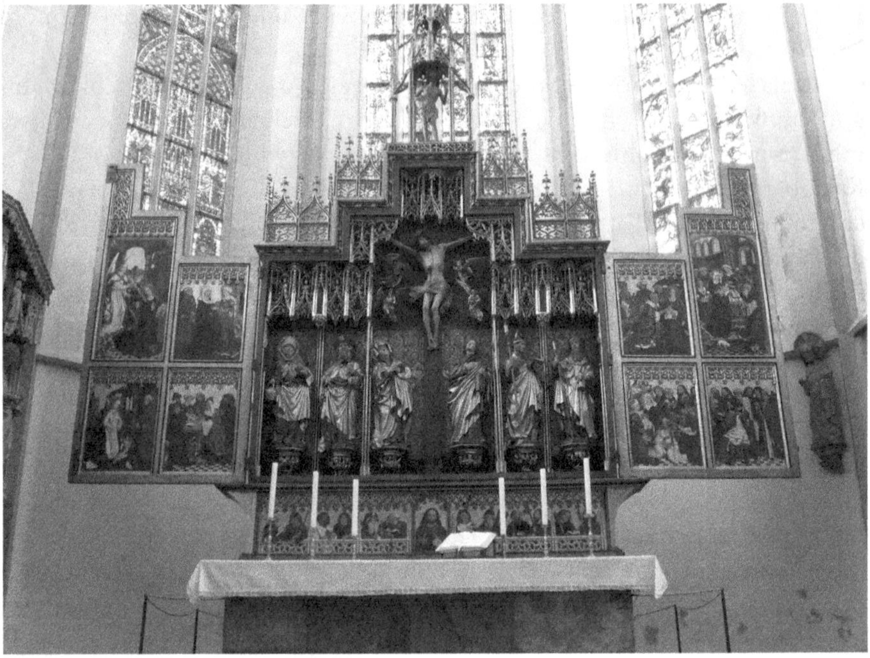

Figure 2: Friedrich Herlin, "Twelve Apostles Altar" (1466). Church of St. James, Rothenburg ob der Tauber. Photo courtesy of the author.

altar in St. James church in Rothenburg, framed the elevated Eucharist and enshrined the miracle of transubstantiation with a visual narrative that quite literally directed the eyes toward the heavens: the base of the altarpiece depicted the Last Supper, its central focal point was the Crucifixion, and at its highest point Christ ascended into the heavens. It should go almost without saying that the material and organizational resources needed for the construction, expansion, and beautification of altars and church interiors skewed heavily toward urban parishes. In the second half of the fifteenth century, in particular, such locations saw considerable increases in these activities, managed by the careful guidance of secular officials and heavily financed by endowments from wealthy individuals and families, as well as religious confraternities and trade guilds.[101]

Since the Reformation, the sense of smell has evoked Catholicism, and arguably medieval Europe more broadly.[102] Traditional Christianity marshaled a variety of fragrances for ritual purposes, but the most important of these was unquestionably incense. Its actual use in church ritual, however, is poorly understood. Most commonly, incense has been treated as one among a litany of theatrical "tricks" subordinated to the "visual theophany" of the elevated Host during the Mass.[103] Some evidence from this period seems to support a connection between the elevation and incense: images of the Mass of St. Gregory, for example, such as that found in the early sixteenth-century prayer book of the Frankfurt patrician Claus Humbracht (see figure 4 in chapter 3), occasionally represent acolytes holding censers near the altar during the elevation. While it may suggest something of the primacy assigned to vision in normative perceptions of ritual, such evidence is far from descriptive of actual sensory production in any straightforward manner. Closer critical scrutiny of how communities across late medieval Germany produced the olfactory dimensions of the Mass—incense in particular—discloses a much more problematic relationship between smell and sight in church ritual on the eve of the Reformation. Producing incense ritual required liturgical books, the fragrant substance itself, and the proper liturgical implement in which to burn it—a censer. Communities across late medieval Germany had highly unequal access to these material resources, and as a result, this particular olfactory dimension of the Mass was diverse and variable at best, nonexistent at worst.

Incense use was, normatively speaking, a significant part of the structured ritual environment of the Mass from at least the eleventh century. However, usage was never primarily in the service of the elevation, at least according to ritual ordinances. Rather, the principal deployment of incense occurred just before and during the Offertory. Occasionally, it was also prescribed for the Introit and just prior to the reading of the Gospel, during which the presiding priest censed the text itself.[104] By the fifteenth century, this general pattern of usage appears to have been rather loosely observed in many communities, if contemporaneous missals are any indicator. Of the sample surveyed here, only 37 percent provided any kind of instruction on censing, or "thurification." The absence of such prescription is not definitive proof that no censing took place. However, it may be a stronger indicator of actual practice than, for example, the absence of prescriptions on elevation practice in this same body of evidence, as detailed above. While Eucharist elevation was essential to liturgical practice across Europe by the fifteenth century, incense was never, technically speaking, anything more than *adiaphoron*—a liturgical-theological term meaning a matter of indifference. Ritual practitioners could, and probably did, exercise considerably more discretion in its use during the Mass.

For the parish churches of Nuremberg, the official rubric of usage, the missal of Bamberg, provided no instructions on censing during the Mass. As we have already seen, however, church officials had a wide range of other usages at their disposal, including the *Missale romanum*, which outlined a basic paradigm for liturgical censing. Thurification in the Roman rite conformed to the historical tradition mentioned above: incense accompanied the opening procession during the Introit, was used to cense the Gospel text, and reached its densest application during the Offertory at the beginning of the liturgy of the Eucharist (see table 2). During the Offertory, thurification began after the priest had prepared the elements of bread and wine by performing a series of blessings, prayers, and signs of the cross over them. At this point incense was placed in the censer (or thurible), the priest spoke a prayer, censed the elements, spoke another prayer, censed the altar, and spoke a final prayer before passing the censer to the deacon. Several intervening phases separated the end of thurification during the Offertory from the ritual elevations of the Canon, including a sequence of ritual hand washings, bowing before the altar, and prayers, leading into the Preface: a call-and-response exchange between priest and congregation, followed by a sung prayer that could vary in length, depending on the particular feast day being celebrated.[105] These intervening phases therefore attenuated somewhat the connection between incense and elevation.

Observation of this paradigm varied in other rubrics. Some religious orders, such as the Augustinian Hermits, followed the Roman usage exactly, while in Augsburg and Konstanz, usage closely paralleled it but omitted censing of the altar.[106] In Brixen and Naumburg, censing occurred after preparation of the elements—like the Roman rite—but was further separated from this procedure by more ritual prayers and bows before the altar.[107] In Basel, Strasbourg, and Meissen, thurification occurred during, rather than after, the preparation of the elements.[108] Other dioceses made clear that censing along the lines of the Roman model was optional. In Hildesheim, for example, priests were provided with instructions for Masses in which "you wish to thurify" alongside "un-thurified" Masses.[109] Still others added their own innovations. In Mainz, thurification began "immediately after the Gospel" and continued through the next several portions of the Mass leading up to the Preface.[110] A fairly constant flow of fragrance therefore characterized the middle portions of the Mass. Some rubrics failed to provide for any incense whatsoever during the Offertory but instituted it elsewhere in the Mass. The diocese of Havelberg, for example, provided for censing only during the Introit.[111] In Freising, censing was stipulated immediately after the Introit during the Gloria, and at the beginning of the Credo, which preceded the Offertory.[112]

The variations suggest that communities paid close attention to incense and may even have taken a degree of local pride in liturgical distinctiveness. Local pride notwithstanding, incense use specifically during the Mass actually appears to have been relatively infrequent throughout the entire liturgical year. To be sure, incense was a significant presence in religious life, generally speaking. As the Nuremberg church superintendent Anton Tucher noted in 1509, the Holy Ghost chapel owned two censers, the smaller of which "is used daily."[113] However, in light of more extensive evidence in the neighboring churches of St. Sebald and St. Lorenz, it seems unlikely that Tucher here referred to the Mass. Incense usage was noted for 42 percent of all feast days throughout the year in St. Sebald, while in St. Lorenz that number was 36 percent; moreover, the sacristans of both churches only explicitly referenced incense-use Masses five times throughout the liturgical year.[114] More regular incense use therefore seems to have taken place during evening services of vespers and matins, which accounted for 24.6 percent of incense usage in St. Sebald and 70.4 percent in St. Lorenz.[115] The use of incense in these services was primarily sacramental—that is, directed toward a particular altar, object, or (occasionally) person, as a kind of blessing or benediction.[116] Other contexts included processions (5.5 percent in St. Sebald, 18 percent in St. Lorenz), and the daily canonical hours (4.1 percent in St. Sebald, 6.8 percent in St. Lorenz).[117] Both churches displayed the tendency to increase provisioning for incense use in these contexts during the season of Advent, as well as Holy Week.[118]

A broader survey of the evidence elsewhere reinforces the significance of sacramental uses of incense outside the Mass. Other ritual ordinances, known variously as *Ordinarius*, *Obsequiale*, *Rituale*, or *Agenda*, frequently prescribed incense for annual blessings of salt and water, in addition to a variety of other seasonal blessings. In Magdeburg, for example, it was a constant presence in vespers services, processions, and canonical hours, and particularly acute during the seasons of Advent and Holy Week.[119] In Augsburg it was used in blessings of candles on the feast of the Purification of the Virgin, palms on Palm Sunday, fire during the Easter vigil, wine on the feast of John the Evangelist, herbs on the day of the Assumption of the Virgin, and foods such as cheese, bread, eggs, and cakes during Pentecost.[120] Additionally, many dioceses observed the blessing of homes with incense during so-called *Rauchnächte*—the twelve evenings between Christmas and the feast of the Epiphany.[121] In Mainz the practice appears to have been especially important, with clergy proceeding through the town and fumigating the homes of prominent citizens. The culmination of this period occurred with the annual blessing of incense on the feast of the Epiphany.[122] While these benediction rituals shared a good deal in common from one location to the next, they too exhibited important variations.[123]

Unequal access to material resources further inflected variations in incense ritual across late medieval Germany. The substance itself—incense—was a rather elusive item. The limited number of previous studies on religious incense use in medieval and early modern Europe assume the presence of what we today identify as incense: the resin collected from trees of the *Boswellia* genus. Cultivated in the southern Arabian Peninsula, the precious substance was transported by merchants to Europe, where it then found application in church ritual.[124] Unfortunately for fifteenth-century Germany, there is little actual documentation of incense trade. In contrast to spices like pepper, cinnamon, nutmeg, saffron, or sugar, which regularly appeared in merchants' accounts from the period, "incense" as a commodity was almost invisible. It is possible that spice merchants failed to indicate incense specifically and instead classified it under the general category of *Spezerei*, which could refer to consumable spices but also could include other dry, nonperishable goods, most often fragrant animal and plant products.[125] This documentary absence notwithstanding, the accounts of masters of churches in larger cities occasionally indicate expenditures for incense as frequently recurring. This was the case in Nuremberg, where Sebald Schreyer documented regular payments for incense throughout his tenure as master of St. Sebald church. In order to have incense ready to hand for the complex liturgical calendar in Nuremberg, it had to be purchased often, sometimes more than once per year.[126] Important feast days often required additional purchases of incense. In the Göttingen parish church of St. James, for example, incense for the feasts of Easter and Corpus Christi alone accounted for 37 percent of all church expenditures for incense in the years 1523 and 1524.[127] Similar patterns prevailed in other communities such as Bamberg, Wunsiedel, Wertheim, Dresden, and Siegen, where church masters documented special purchases of incense for Christmas, Easter, and other locally important feast days.[128]

Even in cases where church officials documented expenditures for incense, the term "incense" did not strictly refer to the resin of *Boswellia* trees, further complicating the notion that there was much consistency in the olfactory appeal of church ritual. The medical and culinary literature of the period identified multiple things as incense, including "white incense," "black incense," "Venetian incense," and "Jewish incense."[129] Accounts from the church of St. Martin in Bamberg indicate the purchase of both black and white incense, the latter intended for use at Christmas.[130] Moreover, there is considerable evidence of communities making do with substitutions with more local fragrant substances. Saffron, for example, cultivated in parts of southern France and Spain, was easier to acquire than true incense and appears to have been used as a substitute on occasion.[131] Many churches utilized a substance known as *thymian*, an oil derived from the herb thyme. Churches in Münster, Bielefeld, Dresden, Wertheim, and Windsheim used this oil in combination with other kinds of incense. Parish churches in the town of Koblenz used the oil exclusively as a substitute for the more commonly recognized forms of incense.[132]

Beyond the fragrant substance itself, communities had varying access to censers, also necessary for the olfactory production of the Mass. Censers, or "thuribles," handled by priests, deacons, or acolytes, had been documented since late antiquity, although they appear with greater frequency in the late Middle Ages, when churches across Europe began to take more detailed inventories of their liturgical furniture.[133] These objects were typically made of copper, brass, or silver, composing a half-sphere basin where incense was placed, as well as a more ornate cover, often made to resemble a church or ornamented with gilded leaves or floral patterns. A chain affixed to the basin-cover assemblage allowed for officiants to carry and swing the object according to proper usage. Church inventories carefully document the presence of censers and therefore provide good evidence of the extent and limits of olfactory provisioning on the eve of the Reformation.

The evidence from church inventories suggests a sharp division between urban and rural practice. In Nuremberg, the churches of St. Sebald and St. Lorenz each owned two ornate silver censers, which appear consistently in inventories from the middle of the fifteenth century through the early sixteenth century.[134] Other major institutions in Nuremberg acquired their own censers at this time as well. The church of Our Lady documented one silver censer starting in 1435.[135] The chapel in the Holy Ghost Hospital had acquired two by the early sixteenth century.[136] Records of the church attached to the Franciscan convent in the city indicated that it owned one silver censer in 1448.[137] In other large urban centers such as Strasbourg, provisioning for incense ritual was similarly consistent. The inventories there document three silver censers in the sacristy of the cathedral, one silver censer in the collegiate church of St. Thomas, one silver censer and one gilded silver censer in Young St. Peter, one silver censer in Old St. Peter, and three brass censers in the great hospital.[138] In smaller cathedral seats, such as Bamberg, the holdings were less ornate: both of the town's parish churches owned a brass censer apiece. The records of parish churches in medium-sized towns like Wesel and Koblenz document the acquisition of brass censers in the fifteenth century.[139] The rural scene drew a marked contrast to the consistent provisioning of censers in urban communities. No censers were documented in the small parish churches in the duchies of Braunschweig or Kalenberg-Göttingen, and only two were identified in the parish churches of Saxony. In Brandenburg, fewer than 2 percent of parish churches owned censers.[140] In the south, one censer was identified in the rural parish churches of the dioceses of Salzburg, Chiemsee, and Freising.[141] Without these liturgical tools, it would seem that incense was simply not a part of ritual life in many rural locations.

Passing references to people receiving the Eucharist, as well as handling relics or other holy objects, suggest in a somewhat impressionistic way that the sense of touch was significant in the Mass. While little serious consideration has been devoted to the sense, touching and being touched nonetheless constituted ritual practice in two immediate, albeit paradoxically interrelated, respects. First, some communities utilized specialized liturgical devices to mediate and minimize human contact with the sacred in the Eucharist. Second, such measures were surrounded by highly intimate, visceral practices of touching, including the ostentatious tearing of the consecrated Eucharist Host, as well as several different kinds of ritual kissing. Because many of these practices were dependent on material resources that were unevenly distributed, producing tactility in the Mass, like other modes of sensory production, was a highly variegated phenomenon in late medieval Germany.

The use of liturgical vessels such as chalices and patens was not simply a matter of visual appeal but also one of producing the Mass as a tactile experience. Once the transubstantiation of the bread and wine had been effected, these containers formed a barrier between the flesh and blood of Christ and that of humanity. In some rare cases, this imperative to maintain strict separation of the sacred and profane produced unusual liturgical devices, such as the sacrament "hooks" found in inventories of churches in Wesel and Koblenz. Also in Wesel, clergy used a special kind of straw when taking the wine. This straw minimized the danger of spilling, and further mediated contact between God and human.[142] The use of cloths known as corporals to wipe the hands of those who handled the sacrament underscored this division still further.[143] The textile collections in sacristies of wealthy churches such as those in Nuremberg were filled with such items. The church of St. Lorenz, for example, held sixteen, fourteen of which were made from velvet. Most were also embroidered with pearl images or interwoven with golden thread.[144]

The paradox in these provisions to mediate human contact with the divine was that they always failed: prior to communion, all liturgies of the Eucharist incorporated the act of *fraction*, in which the priest ostentatiously tore the Host into small pieces. Beyond that, the Host was of course received on the tongue of communicants. Pushing this paradox still further, several kinds of ritual kissing punctuated the liturgy from the Offertory to Communion, playing on the intimacy of touching and being touched. As noted above in the discussion of visual production, the priest kissed the altar multiple times during these portions of the Mass. In the Roman missal, the first of these occurred during the Offertory, following consecration of the elements and a ritual washing of the hands: the priest was to "stand erect for the kissing of the altar, and then turn to face the congregation."[145] Another kiss of the altar was inserted between the elevation of the chalice and the final signs of the cross over the elements near the end of the Canon.[146] Thereafter, the priest was also expected to kiss the altar during the *Pax domini* and *Agnus Dei* portions of the Mass.[147] One final kiss of the altar concluded the liturgy of the Eucharist, immediately after the priest had communed.[148]

The timing, quantity, and objects of these kisses varied considerably from one community to the next. Many dioceses, for example, incorporated an additional kiss of the paten on which the Host rested during the *Agnus Dei*, usually just prior to the fraction rite.[149] In other dioceses, missals provided an image that substituted as the object of the kiss. Typically depicting Christ's face, Christ as the Lamb of God, or simply a crucifix, these images were widespread in both manuscript and print missals in the fifteenth century. Similar parallel images even appeared in private devotionals and prayer books, used in church by ritual spectators. The considerable wear and degradation of such images in otherwise well-maintained texts attests to the fact that people actually kissed them, and that they did so often and enthusiastically.[150] In Würzburg a similar practice endured. The *Pax* began with a kiss of the altar and was followed by the priest kissing an image of the arms of Christ, printed in the missal. Similarly, in Brandenburg the object of the second kiss was the chalice instead of a printed image.[151]

The *Pax* ritual itself merits somewhat more detailed consideration, because, unlike the other kisses during the liturgy of the Eucharist, it involved the whole congregation. As a gesture of goodwill and charity toward one's neighbors and fellow parishioners, churchgoers kissed one another following recitation of the *Pater Noster* prayer. By the fifteenth century, specialized liturgical equipment known as "pax boards" became widespread, transforming the kiss of peace from an interpersonal moment of touching and being touched into a conjunction of human flesh and a cold, metal thing. The missals provide some sense of how this practice unfolded in dioceses that owned pax boards. After kissing the altar, Eucharistic vessels, or special images provided in missals, the priest distributed the pax board to his deacon or acolytes, who kissed the object, and in turn passed it to the congregation.[152] The first vernacular explication of the Mass described the practice in detail, noting that after the priest had kissed the pax, the deacon or altar server followed suit, and then

> carries this same kissed tablet to the other priests in the choir to kiss. And each kisses it with devotion, one after the other. It is also in many places the custom that the altar servant carries about this kissed tablet to all those who during the service or mass stand or kneel, for each to kiss. And this is called the *osculum pacis*—the kiss of peace.[153]

Communities had uneven access to the material resources needed to produce the tactile dimensions of the Mass. Of course, no church lacked an altar, and so priests in urban and rural communities at least had this in common as an object of the kiss. However, other objects were much less consistently on hand. With the exception of corporals, the use of specialized devices to mediate contact with the Eucharist was extremely rare, although they do appear occasionally in rather unexpected places. In Brandenburg, for instance, Eucharist straws were documented in four rural parish church inventories.[154] The distribution of missals containing *Agnus Dei* or *pax* images, too, was highly uneven. Of the sample surveyed here, only 25 percent contained such images. Pax boards were still more problematic. In large, wealthy communities like Nuremberg, inventories attest to diverse collections of such objects. The object of the kiss, therefore, constantly fluctuated throughout the liturgical year. Moreover, in such communities the use of multiple pax boards on days of high Mass attendance produced a fundamentally different ritual, at least from a tactile perspective. The sacristan of St. Sebald, for example, documented the use of three cruciform paxes on the feast of the Lord's Ascension.[155] Instead a single object coming into contact first with the lips of the priest, then his ministers, and finally each member of the congregation, the use of multiple pax boards in wealthy communities seems to have produced a ritual that was more suited to symbolizing these communities as assemblages of individual parts, rather than cogent, unified wholes.[156] Smaller communities, by contrast, usually worked with one pax board or none at all. In the duchies of Braunschweig and Göttingen-Kalenberg, 5.7 percent of churches documented a pax board, and only one held multiple pax boards.[157] In Brandenburg the frequency was rather high, with approximately 41 percent of communities documenting pax boards. In Saxony, small towns occasionally owned substantial collections: Schmiedeberg, for example, claimed seven pax boards.[158] However, this was rather exceptional, as no other parish church in Schmiedeberg's administrative district or its two neighboring districts owned even a single pax board.

The gustatory, visual, olfactory, and tactile dimensions of the Mass nested within and constantly interacted with the soundscape of church space.[159] The soundscape comprised the ecology of speech, music, and ambient noise within church space. Singing, organs, and bells worked in concert with one another, interacted with church architecture and with other sensory dimensions of the structured ritual environment. As with all material resources affecting the sensory experience of the Mass, provisioning for the soundscape could be rather costly, and costs fluctuated considerably according to local political economic circumstances. These practical challenges notwithstanding, the aural engineering of the Mass on the eve of the Reformation favored what Emma Dillon has recently identified as "supermusicality."[160] In churches with the necessary resources, parishioners were immersed in a soundscape designed to obscure the verbal clarity of the spoken or sung portions of the rite and to direct their aural attention to the various layered sounds working in concert or in tension with one another.

Church architecture shaped the soundscape of the Mass just as profoundly as it inflected its visual topography. In design and material construction, the Gothic church was effectively a massive musical instrument.[161] The concave shape of choirs functioned as a resonating chamber, where the words of the liturgy, often sung by the priest and accompanied by an assembly of vicars or schoolboys, were amplified and projected down the elongated nave of the church. The high ceilings and hard stone construction of large churches like those found in Nuremberg reflected these sounds, producing a "cascade of echoes" that added fullness and power to the sound of the liturgy. As Richard Cullen Rath's thought-provoking reconstruction suggests, "sounds bounced around echo upon echo rather than reaching the listener's ears all at once. This created a powerfully moving effect, one that amplified the voice and enriched the tone, but at the cost of clarity."[162] In English churches, rood screens acted as something of an acoustic baffle, disciplining and channeling the noise somewhat. In Germany, however, this element of the built environment was often absent, and so the cascade of echoes was likely even more chaotic. The humbler parish churches dotting the countryside differed considerably: not only were they a good deal smaller, but they also diverged in material construction and design. Stone suitable for building a church was not universally available across Germany and was, as a result, expensive. Large cities like Strasbourg, Freiburg, Ulm, Lübeck, and even smaller towns like Wesel had the financial and organizational capacity to import large quantities of stone from long distances and to commission teams of stonemasons to plan and construct these spaces.[163] Rural parishes, however, often relied much more on locally accessible materials, supplementing stone with wood and plaster, which absorbed more sound. The floor plans of many of these churches were also significantly rounder than Gothic structures: shallower choirs produced less resonation and did not project sound down an elongated nave. Lower ceilings also limited the reverberation characteristic of larger structures. The rural parish church was therefore a very different acoustic environment than its urban counterpart.[164]

Choral singing further distinguished urban and rural ecclesiastical soundscapes. As Milner points out, English churches in the fifteenth century experienced something of an "aural revolution" with the introduction of polyphonic choirs.[165] The same revolution also transformed liturgies in the German-speaking world, and churches that could afford to train and support a polyphonic choir did so enthusiastically. The resources necessary to undertake such a project were considerable and simply did not exist in rural parishes. First, polyphony entailed a heavy commitment of personnel. Vicars, or deputies to the chief parish priest, could and did serve in polyphonic choirs. The number of vicars in St. Sebald in the late fifteenth century fluctuated between twelve and nineteen, while St. Lorenz had between sixteen and twenty.[166] These were actually rather modest numbers for churches of such prestige. The minster of Ulm, by comparison, provided eighty-nine seats for clergy in its richly carved choir stalls.[167] Choral singing constituted a regular obligation for at least some vicars, although it is unclear whether all participated. The polyphonic choir also required a school: unlike vicars, all students were compelled to join. Both parish churches in Nuremberg had Latin schools, and in 1500 the city council passed a new ordinance recognizing the provision of chant and polyphony as one of the essential functions of the school choir.[168]

Someone also had to train and direct the choir—a complicated task that required extensive musical training as well as organizational acumen. The responsibility typically fell to the parish schoolmaster. In especially large cities like Nuremberg, the schoolmaster's responsibilities went well beyond directing the choir, and so assistant cantors had to be paid to help with music instruction. Schoolmasters received a base salary, as well as additional compensation for singing multiple Masses and additional services on major feast days.[169] The sacristans of Nuremberg noted fifty-nine total days in the city's liturgical calendar that met this criterion.[170] The office of schoolmaster was also a rather prestigious one: in the large urban centers of late medieval Germany, the growing influence of humanist culture elevated the importance of music. Alongside public visual art, the high quality of a city's musical soundscape became a mark of local identity and pride. Those officials charged with the task of directing choirs were therefore among the best-educated individuals in the German-speaking world and were very often internationally recognized cultural luminaries in their own right.[171]

Beyond personnel for performance, polyphony required additional liturgical texts.[172] At the beginning of Advent the sacristan of St. Lorenz reported delivering lectionaries and antiphonaries for the winter season to the schoolmaster and the vicars who sang in the choir.[173] In St. Sebald the sacristan was to deposit two special songbooks on the altar specifically for the performance of the Passion play on Good Friday.[174] Wealthy patrons in the community usually subsidized these performances, either by purchasing and donating the texts with musical settings or simply by paying the church master for the performance of a polyphonic Mass on the desired date. In Nuremberg both modes of endowing polyphony exploded in the second half of the fifteenth century.[175] As with other forms of patronage that contributed to ritual sensory production, this practice was widespread in wealthier urban communities in the late fifteenth century.[176] Usually in Nuremberg, polyphonic practice involved four-part harmony—soprano, contralto, tenor, and contrabass melodic lines complementing one another.[177]

Although the enthusiasm for liturgical polyphony was apparently very high, this did not mean that it completely supplanted traditional, monophonic chant (what we usually recognized today as "Gregorian" chant). Rather, it is apparent from the surviving musical settings that the two musical modes existed side by side and very often complemented one another in the performance of a single Mass. This further contributed to the diversity of Mass liturgies from one location to the next, as well as the internal complexity of a single community's liturgical calendar. Each portion of the Mass detailed in table 2 could potentially be sung, either monophonically or polyphonically. A wealth of evidence from fifteenth-century provincial synods, church councils, and surviving musical settings attests that the two modes were frequently intermingled, that portions of the Mass were truncated or omitted, and that in some cases vernacular songs were substituted for Latin hymns.[178]

Given the institutional and material demands, polyphony in Masses was very strictly an urban phenomenon. How then did singing constitute a keynote in rural soundscapes? The fifteenth century offers very few sources to answer this question, but studies relying on more detailed evidence from the sixteenth century suggest that rural parish churches largely practiced monophonic congregational singing, albeit on a very limited basis.[179] Parish churches relied on ritual spectators or auditors—the small gatherings of rural parishioners—rather than professionally trained musicians, to produce this element of the soundscape. However, as Herl argues in his study of sixteenth-century congregational singing, the results were often inconsistent. Many of the same truncations or omissions apparent in urban practice likely prevailed here too, and there was almost certainly a good deal more vernacular singing. People attended church rather sporadically, and when they did participate in song, it was often unenthusiastically and rather poorly.[180]

Like polyphonic choral singing, the presence of organ music in the ecclesiastical soundscape was a strictly urban phenomenon. Also like polyphony, organs represented an "aural revolution" in their own right, composed of some of the most advanced technology available in the late medieval world. Around the mid-fifteenth century, major advances allowing for louder, clearer, and richer resonation produced a new, larger class of instrument. Churches that could afford to acquire them rapidly did so. As a result, wealthier urban parish churches, as well as cathedrals, commonly documented older, "small" organs alongside new "great" organs.

The expense of acquiring and then maintaining this new technology was prohibitive for most communities. Assembly and installation were extraordinarily difficult and time-consuming, involving hundreds of moving parts and requiring structural accommodations within the church (such as canals, air chambers, pipe fittings). The task typically took between two and five years to complete under the guidance of an expert technician, known as an organ master, with assistants. Once installation was complete, bellows constantly needed to be cleaned, repaired, and replaced.[181] In Nuremberg the church of St. Sebald retained an organ master to check the instruments four times a year.[182] In 1490 this "Master Nikolaus" spent thirty-nine weeks repairing the church's large organ, for which he was paid 85 gulden.[183] To put this in perspective, the church's total expenditures in the same year were approximately 979 gulden—in other words, Master Nikolaus's thirty-nine weeks of work accounted for almost 9 percent of all documented expenditures. In the same year, Nikolaus also traveled several times to Leipzig, where he had been contracted to build one of the city's new organs.[184] The demand for Master Nikolaus's services and the premium price they commanded were representative of a broader pattern in the fifteenth century. Finding an organ master proficient with the new technology was exceptionally difficult, and sometimes impossible. In 1497 the city of Dresden failed to find someone who could repair one of its organs, and it sat unused in the church. Retaining an organ master on a permanent basis was even more challenging. The city of Wesel practically had to beg the organ master who had constructed its new great organs to remain in town. His work was so valued that, in 1488, the city council granted him a lifelong pension.[185]

An organ in proper working order required a team of people to operate it. Most important, an organist was needed. The technological advances required organists to have advanced musical training was well as specialized technical competence with the machinery. Occasionally officials with some musical training or inclination—usually schoolmasters, but occasionally sacristans—could operate the older, smaller instruments, improvising and "faking" a melodic line for liturgical performance. The new, larger instruments of the fifteenth century, however, were simply too complicated for anyone who was not a specialist. As a result, the prestige and cost of a good organist increased exponentially on the eve of the Reformation; in many parishes, the organist was therefore often recognized as a peer of the foremost nonreligious officials, including the schoolmaster, sacristan, and church master. The organist could not perform his task alone, however. Due to the large size of the bellows of the new organs, "bellows-treaders" had to be hired to operate the instruments. In some places, a single assistant could manage the task; in other churches, such as St. Sebald in Nuremberg, instruments required a team of four assistants. Occasionally, students, bell-ringers, or other members of the "backstage crew" responsible for producing sensory ritual stepped in to handle this task. In some locations, the organists were expected to hire and direct a team of bellows-treaders.[186]

In the few communities that could afford them, the use of these instruments varied throughout the liturgical year, although some general patterns are observable. Larger organs did not supersede the older, smaller instruments; rather, both served distinct liturgical purposes. In 1483–1484, the church master of St. Sebald paid bellows-treaders sixty-five times for assisting with the small organ and forty-two times for assisting with the great organ.[187] This is because communities regarded the sonic differences between small and large instruments as serving a meaningful liturgical purpose. Nuremberg's acquisition of its organs reinforces this point. In both churches, it was rather the opposite of many other communities in the fifteenth century: the great organs were installed first in 1444, followed by smaller organs in both churches in the 1470s. In the decades following the installation, great and small organs had liturgically distinct usages in the Mass. The sacristan of St. Sebald mentioned the use of organs on thirty separate occasions. The great organ accounted for 33 percent of these occasions, the small organ for 63 percent (one entry fails to specify which organ was played). These references usually only mention the fact that one or the other organ was played during a particular liturgical service—most commonly the Mass, vespers, and matins. The differentiated use of both organs for separate services on a single feast day appears five times; each entry indicates the use of the large organ for Mass and vespers, and the smaller organ for matins.[188] Generally, organs paralleled choral polyphony during the various parts of the Mass, alternating phrase by phrase with the choir.[189] In the Nuremberg churches, this appears to have been the case most of the time.[190] However, neither sacristan identifies organ playing in Masses during Holy Week or Christmas, when appeals to most other sensory modalities were generally elevated. It seems in this case that the absence of organ playing was intended to create more space for choral polyphony, as both sacristans described much more extensively the details for this mode of aurality at this point in the liturgical calendar.[191]

Church bells were fundamentally important in premodern daily life, as a growing body of excellent scholarship demonstrates.[192] In contrast to choral singing and organs, bells were quite widely distributed between town and country. Within the confines of the Mass, there were two basic categories of bells: small, handheld bells, and the more familiar large bells mounted in belfries. Handheld bells, rung at the altar during the elevation, were a distinctive element of late medieval ritual life across Europe, appearing only in the thirteenth century.[193] By the late fifteenth century, they were widespread in Germany. The inventories for St. Lorenz in Nuremberg fail to indicate these devices, but St. Sebald's church claimed three in the early sixteenth century (see table 1). Churches in larger and medium-sized towns, such as Coburg, Wesel, Biberach, Dresden, Koblenz, Mainz, Rothenburg ob der Tauber, and Ingolstadt, also documented these bells, occasionally identifying them as "transubstantiation bells."[194] The complement of large bells in wealthy urban communities was rather extensive. Both parish churches in Nuremberg appear to have been equipped with four large bells, explicitly identifying a "mass bell," "sermon bell," and "storm bell."[195] These names probably refer to the different tones, pitches, or timbres of each bell, as they do not seem to indicate a particular, restricted usage: all were deployed liberally and variously throughout the liturgical year for benedictions, processions, canonical hours, and, of course, Masses. Throughout the German-speaking world, most communities with the means possessed several large bells.[196]

In the Mass, usage varied considerably according to the liturgical calendar. Generally speaking, a single bell rang at the beginning of High Mass on fast days in St. Lorenz. The second Mass included one ring of the sermon bell if the epistle was read, and three bells rung simultaneously if it was sung. On feast days, an additional, single stroke of a bell would be added at the moment of elevation.[197] Similar patterns can be found in St. Sebald, although they are only indicated on special feast days.[198] Throughout the liturgical calendar, however, usage diverged significantly from these basic patterns. Most commonly in both churches, all four bells were rung simultaneously.[199] Bell-ringers also manipulated volume on certain feast days: 9.6 percent of celebrations in St. Lorenz and 19.5 percent in St. Sebald required that bells be rung "loudly" (*schreck*).[200] As with other modes of sensory production, the most elaborate and differentiated usages of bells occurred at times of extensive sacramental communion, particularly Holy Week and Christmas. High Mass on Maundy Thursday in St. Lorenz involved, in addition to the typical bell ringing described above, a special blessing of the "holy grave" in which a consecrated Eucharist was stored until Easter. Following the consecration and elevation of elements during the Canon, three iterations of the *Agnus Dei* prayer were sung at the high altar. After the third *Agnus* was sung, all the bells rang simultaneously. The grave (also at the high altar) was blessed, and again all the bells rang together. Thereafter, the sacristan indicated, "no one rings a bell, whether large or small, until our Lord rises." Bell ringing only resumed at Mass on Easter Sunday, when the sacrament was removed from the grave and placed on the high altar.[201] The silence of the bell towers in St. Lorenz during this period contrasted starkly with St. Sebald, where ringing continued during and between Masses.[202] At Christmas in St. Lorenz, an exceptionally complex pattern of ringing prevailed. For the first Mass of the day, only one bell was used. Throughout the High Mass, the storm and Mass bells rang, becoming especially dense during the singing of the preface, just prior to the Canon. During the Canon, bell ringing ceased, and then at the moment of the elevation, a single toll underscored the visual gesture. This usage was repeated in Masses on feast days for the next two weeks, until the feast of the Epiphany.[203]

Bells were quite widespread in late medieval Germany, and the differences between urban and rural communities appear less dramatic. In part, this is likely due to the dual sacred and quotidian utility of church bells. They not only served a liturgical purpose; they were also a vital communication technology, rapidly relaying information about time or potential threats (natural, human, or supernatural) to the community. As with the altar itself, large bells were essential to the basic fabric of rural church life, and there is little reason to doubt their presence in smaller communities.[204] The handheld transubstantiation bells, too, appear with considerable frequency in some parts of Germany. In Saxony, for example, an impressive 86.1 percent of communities owned at least one such bell, and several owned as many as four. There were, however, some important material, economic, and institutional factors that limited the scope and variety of bell ringing in rural locations. First, it is unlikely that many communities matched the full complement of large bells found in cities like Nuremberg, and so patterns of ringing were less complex and diverse throughout the liturgical year. Further, the more elaborate interplay of multiple bells required personnel, who had to be paid and instructed. In Nuremberg and other large cities, churches hired teams of bell ringers.[205] In St. Sebald, bell ringers each received a quarter portion of wine, six loaves of bread, twelve eggs, and a piece of cheese for their services.[206] Added to this, the expense of maintaining multiple large bells was considerable: because they were used so frequently, the bells and the wooden structures on which they were mounted deteriorated rapidly and cracked constantly. In Nuremberg the church masters kept smiths and the city carpenter on retainer for this purpose; similar patterns prevailed in other cities with large numbers of bells.[207] The financial demands bell ringing placed on communities were thus substantial and would have curbed the diversity of liturgical practice.

Producing the Mass as a multisensory ritual was a highly variegated phenomenon across late medieval Germany. Even in a community like Nuremberg, which faced few constraints on its access to the resources necessary for such a project, appeals to each sense modality in the five-sense sensorium fluctuated rather widely throughout the liturgical year. The wealth of Nuremberg and the handful of German cities that could call themselves its peers, however, were exceptional. Most people in the fifteenth century experienced religion in small, rural parish churches, which made do with far less. With this in mind, then, it is necessary to revise one of the most basic premises of the popular narrative of desensualization that often accompanies the Reformation in the popular and scholarly imagination. The ritual edifice of Christianity looked, sounded, smelled, felt, and tasted rather different from one location to the next. If the material cultural record is any indicator, rural practice articulated a different sensorium than its urban counterpart. This does not mean it was any less sensuous. A humble wooden chalice elevated alongside a plain Eucharist wafer by a priest in drab vestments, speaking the Latin words of consecration in a quavering and uncertain voice appealed to multiple sense modalities and could be a profound aesthetic experience for churchgoers. This of course does not account for the many other environmental factors that certainly impinged on people's senses: the body odors of congregants, the smells of the rural world filtering into the church, the half-hearted attempts at congregational singing, and even the bodily pain of bowing or standing during the service were all part of people's sensuous experience of worship. These were not, however, the intentional sensory design, or production, of the ritual. In this domain, communities confronted real material constraints on the kind of ritual show they could put on—constraints that we typically overlook when we talk about the "sensual" Middle Ages. The reality of late medieval practice was far more diverse, as should be apparent from even a focused consideration of a single rite like the Mass.

Two criticisms to the argument developed here are worth considering briefly. The first is a methodological consideration: one might observe that much of the evidence for rural communities is drawn from sixteenth-century inventories, many of which were taken down by evangelical Protestant authorities. The use of this "regressive" method might be seen as inappropriate because it fails to appreciate historical change from one epoch to another. Protestants, after all, got rid of much of the "sensuous residue" of late medieval practice, often aggressively in the form of iconoclastic riots; maybe the paucity of liturgical furniture in these locations reflects this paradigm. There are, however, good reasons for disregarding this as a possibility in this particular instance. First, those territories studied here that eventually broke for the Reformation in the sixteenth century were evangelical—or Lutheran—and not particularly zealous iconoclasts like their reformed counterparts, and so the amount of material change introduced to liturgical practice is quite debatable, as we will see in chapter 5. The numbers of communities studied here further militate against this presenting a serious criticism: the duchy of Braunschweig alone represented almost four hundred parish churches, and while it may have been the case that some relieved themselves of significant portions of the liturgical furniture so essential to late medieval sensory ritual, it is highly unlikely that all did. It is also unlikely that these items were simply overlooked: the authorities who took down these inventories did so carefully because they had a vested interest in knowing precisely how much wealth these parish churches had, and wanted to get a feel for local liturgical life. Finally, contemporaneous inventories of rural Catholic parishes document similarly modest liturgical furnishings. Given that these parishes actively sought to maintain the material culture they had built upon in preceding centuries, their similarities with their rural Lutheran counterparts are highly significant. We must therefore conclude that the fullest extent of sensory worship, often depicted as broadly representative of the medieval church in general, was primarily a wealthy urban phenomenon, a fairly exclusive segment of late medieval German society.

The second criticism is more substantial and will be addressed systematically in the following chapters. As Mark Smith, Constance Classen, and David Howes have argued, merely documenting sensory production is methodologically and conceptually insufficient to the project of sensory history. Here we have attempted a reconstruction of the range of sensory objects available to those who participated in the late medieval Mass, but a larger set of questions remains: What meanings did people assign to these objects? How did cultural context shape people's senses, or "tune their neurons," to borrow Howes's evocative turn of phrase? Or, to build on Smith's language, what was the historically specific mode of sensory consumption in Germany on the eve of the Reformation? In chapters 2 and 3 we turn to this issue. In chapter 2 we consider the ways in which intellectual discourse formed a key context to sensory consumption. Thereafter, chapter 3 concludes part 1 of this study by examining the significance of sensuality in vernacular understandings of late medieval religious practice. In both cases, the story unfolds in the wealthier, better-educated urban scene of the Holy Roman Empire. Here, sensory practice and discourse about its meaning constituted each other dialectically. To borrow the well-worn phenomenological expression from Edmund Husserl, consciousness was always already consciousness of some*thing*.

2 The Senses and Sacramentality in Late Medieval Intellectual Discourse

"Objects," claimed the popular preacher Johann Geiler von Kaysersberg (1445–1510), "go into a man through the windows of his five senses so that he becomes moved towards them and the desirous force strikes, such that he would have otherwise never pondered them."[1] Kaysersberg made this statement while delivering a sermon from the pulpit of the Strasbourg cathedral at the turn of the sixteenth century. His immediate aim was to admonish members of his flock against sin, but this particular utterance drew from a much deeper reservoir of discourse that extended geographically across Europe and chronologically back to the late twelfth century and into the thirteenth. In the intervening generations, intellectuals produced an understanding of sensory perception that was fundamentally different from modern scientific accounts. Fusing theological concerns with what would today be considered matters of physiology, psychology, and physics, sensation was a problem in a much more encompassing discourse—a true "science of the soul," to borrow the evocative phrase from Sander de Boer.[2] In this science, sensation was corporeal, mobilizing the body and its sense organs, but also immaterial, involving operations of the soul and its internal powers. From the perspective of the perceiving subject, the whole process was a passive experience. Objects projected their sensible qualities into the environment; these qualities struck and moved the appropriate sense organs and affected the internal processes of cognition, emotion, and the formation of moral dispositions and habits. Sensation therefore constituted a powerful affective bond between object of perception and perceiving subject—a bond with implications for the narrative of salvation and how the church intervened in this narrative.[3]

This narrative was deeply paradoxical.[4] Desires, emotions, and internal dispositions produced by objects of sense perception could be virtuous or vicious. The connection between sin and sensuality in Christian thought is well known, with origins in the very beginnings of the church. By the late Middle Ages, it found particularly forceful rhetorical expression in such influential works as Peter of Limoges's *Moral Treatise of the Eye*.[5] In fifteenth-century Germany, intellectuals commonly classified sins according to the senses they affected.[6] Visual art, too, presented similar patterns: the senses inclined toward bodily sin and, by the end of the fifteenth century, were increasingly associated with the female sex.[7] Sensuality was a fact of life and, as such, an all-encompassing threat. Kaysersberg thus paraphrased the prophet Jeremiah, lamenting that "death got in through the windows of my five senses."[8] True apprehension of God was purely spiritual and therefore required sensory transcendence. For those engaged in actual pastoral work, however, this position was of little use. Indeed, pragmatism required it be set aside: humans were by nature sensual beings, and as a result, any kind of universal, intellectual truth—spiritual or otherwise—was accessible in this world only in an imperfect, particular, and sensually mediated way. The issue was not to withdraw from the senses but to understand and instrumentalize them properly in order to cultivate virtue and save souls. Even Kaysersberg recognized this in his jeremiads: the senses were perilous, but they could be tamed and put to good use, particularly when church liturgy became their object.[9]

The same mode of thinking about the senses that heightened concern over human proclivities to sin therefore constituted an essential context when intellectuals confronted the ritual edifice of the late medieval church. This became especially important in the fifteenth century, when questions about the relationship between theology and piety—or, in modern anthropological terminology, religious theory and religious practice—came to the fore.[10] What were sacraments, and how were they efficacious? How could the eminently corporeal and material nature of these things mediate divine grace, itself disembodied, immaterial, and spiritual? How did the practices of the church interact with and affect the bodies, minds, and souls of churchgoers? Could the sacred truly be present in and experienced through the profane, material world? These questions were put to the myriad sacramental and paraliturgical rites that punctuated church practice as often as they were to the seven institutionally recognized sacraments. Taken together, the answers to these questions represented a comprehensive theory of sacramentality, defining ritual practice and describing its function.

The fifteenth-century theory of sacramentality relied on contemporaneous understandings of sensation for its coherence. All five senses were implicated in this discussion. Gabriel Biel (1418–1495), perhaps the most prominent professor of theology in the German-speaking world at the end of the fifteenth century, articulated a multisensory sacramentality in his sermons, defining sacraments as "sensible signs effectively signifying by divine institution the grace of God, or the gratuitous effect of God."[11] The sacraments were one side of the "sensual coin" of humanity: of course, sensuality tempted people with sin in daily life, but its presence in church ritual was a pragmatic necessity. Humans were inherently carnal beings, and so sensuality served as the basis of "cognition of, desire for, and attainment of invisible grace." Sacraments were "vessels of grace and efficacious medicines" that mediated virtues by "imprinting" themselves on the souls of churchgoers.[12]

Biel represented a "harvest of late medieval theology," synthesizing many of its diverse strands and exposing many of its tensions. His statements on the affective bond of sacramentality were part of a discourse widely distributed in contemporaneous intellectual circles, so much so that it appears as a commonplace in variety of texts from apparently disparate genres, from natural philosophical treatises and mystical theology to vernacular sermons and devotional writings.[13] Like Biel, these intellectuals commonly deployed the language of "imprinting" virtues onto the soul to describe sacramental efficacy. The language was not accidental, nor was it an evocation of some mystery of faith: it was a technical statement, referring to the affective bond between perceived object and perceiving human subject in the structured ritual environment produced by the church. The same account was applicable in any context, sacred or profane.[14] However, in the fifteenth century, it became especially compelling for learned elites to talk about church ritual in this way for several interrelated reasons. Most obviously, many of those who commented on the matter were also engaged in the actual work of designing and performing within the ritual environment detailed in chapter 1. From their perspective, it was self-evident that religious practice was multisensory in its appeal to churchgoers. This appeal varied significantly from one location to the next but always constituted some intersensorial combination of visual, aural, olfactory, tactile, or gustatory stimuli.

The common denominator was that the church could reach out and positively shape churchgoers internally by engaging their external senses. This spoke to a fundamental pastoral concern in an age when the church prepared priests to administer sacraments but often neglected to mold them into effective preachers. By the same token, fifteenth-century learned discourse on the sensuous element in religious worship also played an essential role in consolidating the institutional authority of the church. It was a strategy for asserting the clergy's status as a class of what Catherine Bell identifies as "ritual experts": a group whose authority extended not only over the actual production of ritual practice, but also one with special access to the intellectual resources that defined reality and formed the cultural context in which ritual was consumed.[15] The "science of the soul" offered a privileged domain in which religious authorities could work to define the meaning of sensuous practice for the population more broadly.

This chapter excavates the discursive formation of late medieval sacramentality, tracing its genealogy in the late Middle Ages before turning to more focused analysis of each sense in the five-sense sensorium. The discourse most prominently drew upon Aristotelian natural philosophy, although extraneous elements of Neoplatonism and late medieval mysticism had their places as well. It emerged in the thirteenth century, at the same time that urban churches began to accumulate extensive collections of liturgical furniture. By the late fifteenth century, the discourse was widespread, promoting a positive role for the senses in religious practice, although each sense fit into the machinery of church ritual in distinct ways. In Latin and in the vernacular, the discourse wound its way into wider social circles, at least in urban communities, and formed a crucial context for how people understood their relationship with the church in the world and with the divine. As we saw in chapter 1, producing sensory worship in practice was a highly variegated enterprise. By contrast, the accumulation of intellectual discourse established a relatively consistent, and even elegant, mode of thinking and talking about the significance of ritual practice on the eve of the Reformation. Most centrally, this thinking revolved around the affective bond established between subjects and objects of perception. The sensuality of church ritual was good because it actually changed people's souls, inculcating virtue and opening the door to salvation. Intellectual discourse promoted and reinforced this position as a means of consolidating the institutional authority of the church.

How and when did the dominant form of sacramental discourse emerge? Certainly, isolated elements were present well before the thirteenth century, and there is no shortage of interpretations suggesting that Augustine anticipated virtually all developments in medieval and modern theories of sacramentality. Others posit that that a major shift occurred in the thirteenth century, with the ascendancy of Aristotelian faculty psychology especially in the thought of Thomas Aquinas (d. 1274), which provided a fundamentally different account of sensation than what had prevailed in previous centuries.[16] The truth is somewhere in the middle. Although the thirteenth century produced some profoundly important developments in late medieval sacramental discourse, the foundations for its dominant form appeared already in the twelfth century. The tension between Augustinian doctrine, influenced by Neoplatonism, and Thomistic doctrine, influenced primarily by Aristotelianism, was also much less acute than we are often given to think.

In fifteenth-century Germany, the work of Hugh of St. Victor (1096–1141) formed the cornerstone of intellectual discourse on sacramentality. With few exceptions, preachers, theologians, and university professors cited his theory as the most complete account of what church ritual was, and how it worked.[17] Hugh's theory, most fully developed in his magnum opus *On the Sacraments of the Christian Church*, was self-consciously multisensory in its foundational premises. Although a committed Augustinian, Hugh considered Augustine's theory of sacraments as visible signs of invisible grace to be too narrow. "If anyone wishes to define more fully and more perfectly what a sacrament is," he wrote, "a sacrament is a *corporeal* and *material* element set before the *senses* without, representing by similitude and signifying by institution and containing by sanctification some invisible and spiritual grace."[18]

When thinking through how church ritual actually worked, Hugh, like his intellectual successors, took a pragmatic, anthropological view of the matter. The materiality of sacramental practice was a necessity arising from the cognitive limits imposed by human nature, partly due to the corrupting power of original sin.[19] More important, however, was that knowledge of any kind of object always implied a causal chain that linked the abstract ideas or forms in which physical objects participated, the appropriate sense organ, the data conveyed by the sense organ, and the soul of the perceiving subject.[20] A sketch of this theory was already present in Hugh's earlier work, the *Didascalicon*, which construed all theatrical performances, and their affective power, in terms of how they appealed to the senses. By the senses, he explained, the human soul "lays hold upon all things subject to sense . . . through sense impressions it rushes out toward the visible forms of bodies and, having made contact with them, draws them into itself."[21]

Here, Hugh related what sensory historians have called an "extramissionist" theory of sensation, most characteristic of Augustine and other Neoplatonic thinkers throughout the Middle Ages. On this theory, the sense organs projected aspects of themselves into the environment, which in turn laid hold of the object of perception and drew it back to the perceiving subject. Hugh remained an extramissionist, in contrast to post-thirteenth-century thinkers, who overwhelmingly adopted Aristotle's "intromissionist" perspective, detailed at the beginning of this chapter, which basically inverted the Augustinian paradigm and made sensation a passive phenomenon.[22] To be sure, there were significant debates between intromissionists and extramissionists in the later Middle Ages. However, when applied to understandings of church ritual, such differences were largely set aside. Instead, late medieval thinkers came to agree with Hugh that a profoundly powerful affective bond was established with each act of sensation; this had important implications for thinking about and talking about church ritual.

Hugh's theory was not strictly limited to the official sacraments of the church but rather represented a more global view of ritual. It made room for other kinds of "sacramentals"—a plurality of "corporeal species" necessary for exercising body and mind and thereby cultivating virtue. In these latter categories, Hugh provided such examples as aspersion water, ashes distributed on Ash Wednesday, palms, candles, and other signs "by whose sounds the faithful are called together," among other things.[23] Hugh's sacramentality was also transhistorical: recognizing humanity's sinful, corrupt nature, God had "from the very beginning of the world . . . proposed to man the sacraments of his salvation." Some accepted the proposal, others rejected it in favor of sacraments offered up by the devil, "wherefore it is clear that from the beginning there were Christians, if not in name yet in fact." Hugh viewed sacramental practice as responding dynamically to historical circumstances. The ancient Israelites were actually "Christians" in the sense that they practiced a coherent set of rites divinely instituted for a particular historical epoch; the early Christian church represented a different set of rites, again divinely instituted, but for a different historical context.[24]

Hugh's persistent emphasis on the sensibility of sacramental practice differentiated it from anything like a symbol in the modern, typically linguistic sense of the term. Sacramentality was not representational in any straightforward way: the relation between sign and signified was much more fraught because it involved and interacted with the human body. It actualized a more immediate communion with the divine because God had created the sensuous materiality that constituted the structured ritual environment.[25] The divine "institution" of sacraments—that is, their performative demonstration in Scripture—pointed to divine grace inhering as potential in this material. "Sanctification," effected by priests' words and gestures of benediction, transformed potential divine grace into actual divine grace. Finally, sacraments were not merely representational because they accomplished ends "with" and "in" things: they effected actual changes in the human soul. Here again, the theological and anthropological overlapped. As Hugh explained, "since the whole man had been corrupted . . . sacraments had to be sanctified in things that the matter of man might be sanctified, as works in deeds, as words in speech; in that way the whole indeed may be holy, both what is man and what is of man."[26]

Hugh's theory was transmitted to fifteenth-century German intellectuals via major liturgical thinkers of the thirteenth century—namely, Albert the Great (d. 1280) and William Durandus (d. 1286), and to a somewhat lesser extent Thomas Aquinas (d. 1274). Each of these thinkers built on Hugh's work, rejecting the older theory of sacramentality associated with Augustine and advocating a definition that embraced the whole domain of the sensible. This was merited because, as Albert explained, "a sacrament is [both] a corporeal and visible element, signifying by similitude and conferring grace by sanctification."[27] Durandus agreed that Augustine's formulation was insufficient because the signifying power of sacraments rested in their "stuffness" or "thingness," which impressed itself upon all the senses (*ingerit sensibus*).[28] This was a pragmatic observation. In his commentary on the Mass, Durandus provided a fairly comprehensive overview of the various "persons, works, words, and things" that constituted sacramentality. Persons included "celebrants, ministers or aids, and assistants"; works were "gestures, acts and movements"; words encompassed "prayers, modulations of the voice, and lessons or readings"; and finally, things were "ornaments, instruments, and elements."[29] This was the salvific side of Biel's "sensual coin" of humanity. Durandus thus allegorized the windows of the church to the "senses of the body . . . which ought to be shut to the vanities of the world, and open to receive with all freedom spiritual gifts."[30] Against the vanities of the world, church ritual, and the Mass in particular, intervened: "The five bodily senses are exercised altogether, that is: sight, sound, taste, smell, and touch, through the figure, odor, flavor, breaking, and reception [of the Eucharist]." The exercise of the bodily senses affected and transformed the soul, inculcating spiritual understanding, obedience, discretion, love, and a disposition to do good works.[31]

The discourse was widely distributed in fifteenth-century Germany. The work of Albert the Great and Aquinas was of course well represented in various print editions in German-speaking cities from 1455 to 1520.[32] Additionally, manuscript sources were mainstays in monastic libraries across Germany and objects of intense scrutiny in the leading universities of Cologne, Leipzig, and Erfurt.[33] Hugh of St. Victor's treatise on the sacraments also appeared during this period in two print editions.[34] Durandus's *Rationale divinorum officiorum* was especially significant, published at least twenty-five times in German-speaking cities alone.[35] Across Europe, the work went through forty-five editions before 1501 and another fifty-three in the sixteenth century.[36] It was also one of the most copied liturgical treatises of the late Middle Ages, proliferating in both Latin and vernacular versions across Europe. A German translation appeared in the mid-fifteenth century and circulated throughout southern portions of the Holy Roman Empire.[37]

More important than the numbers of print and manuscript copies in circulation was the actual use of this multisensory sacramental theory by German intellectuals on the eve of the Reformation. The theologian Johannes von Auerbach (d. 1469) cited Augustine's classical definition in his own treatise on the sacraments but agreed with Hugh of St. Victor that a broader understanding of the sacraments was more complete and preferable. Sacramental efficacy meant the performance of spiritual truths through the combination of "material elements, the forms of words, and the intentions of sacramental ministers." It was therefore appropriate to conceptualize sacraments as more broadly sensible. Like many of his late-medieval contemporaries, Auerbach described the reception of sacraments as a process of "imprinting" their gifts on the bodies, souls, and intellects of ritual participants.[38]

Contemporaneous sermons reflect the same multisensory view. The popular Franscican preacher Konrad Grütsch (d. 1475), active in southwest Germany and Switzerland, taught that sacraments were composed of "sensible signs" (*signantia sensibilia*) of invisible, internal grace. Put another way, a sacrament was anything that "under the cover of sensible things, the power of God secretly effects the salvation of souls."[39] Likewise, the sermons of Heinrich Herpff (d. 1478) argued that it was not only the visible form that concealed (*latebat*) the invisible power of Christ and the angelic Word of God, but also sweet tastes, smells of nature, and all aspects of sensuality. Sacramental practice made use of this sensuality to affect people's internal dispositions and prepare them to receive grace.[40] Nicholas Cusanus explicitly enumerated the each of the five senses when describing church ritual as "books of the senses": "If you proceed by way of touch, taste, smell, sight, and hearing, and if you consider carefully how each sense has a power of knowing, then you will find that all objects in the perceptible word are ordained to the service of cognition . . . [and] in these different ways the manifestation of the divine intellect is so very wonderful."[41] Preaching "on the governance of the exterior senses" at Passau, Paul Wann described sacramental practice as critically important to protecting the soul from corruption and infusing it with grace.[42]

While the origins of the discourse lay in the twelfth century with Hugh of St. Victor, the intervening centuries added several layers of significance to what it was fifteenth-century intellectuals thought ritual practices did to the human body and soul. In particular, the development of an extensive commentary tradition on Aristotle's *De anima* (*On the Soul*) made for a more articulated discussion of ritual's appeal to the five senses.[43] The natural philosophical tradition developed in dialogue with extraneous elements as well, most prominently Neoplatonic philosophy and mystical theology, two traditions that paradoxically asserted a sensorially transcendent union with God as the ultimate end of Christianity yet at the same time talking about that union in language especially evocative of the "lower" senses of smell, taste, and touch.[44]

In Germany, the promiscuous tendency to blend traditions was in no small part due to the enduring influence of Albert the Great as a mediator of Aristotle. Albert had been the first to work through and comment on most of Aristotle's natural philosophical work. Trained primarily in the older, Neoplatonic tradition, Albert brought the philosopher's insights into conversation with this school of thought, as well as closely related strains of mysticism, to a far greater extent than his successors had, including his student Thomas Aquinas.[45] By the first decades of the fifteenth century, a decidedly Albertine science of the soul had established itself in the formal educational system. In many of the town schools, students were introduced to thinking about sensation through a compilation of Albert's natural philosophical work known as the *Philosophia pauperum*. A new generation of intellectuals, trained in Paris, took up positions in the rapidly expanding German universities and reinforced the primacy of Albertist teachings, beginning in Cologne but exporting them to Heidelberg, Leipzig, and even as far east as Krakow.[46] Even at the university of Erfurt, individuals nominally in opposition to any teaching associated with "scholasticism" were heavily reliant on the wide-ranging work of Albert the Great when developing their theories of human sensation.[47]

The influence of Albert and the syncretistic tendencies in discourse on the human soul and senses in the German-speaking world was somewhat unusual. As Milner has suggested, Aquinas's teachings on these problems were normative for England and much of continental Europe.[48] The Albertine approach also laid the groundwork for the reception of new strains of fifteenth-century Italian humanist and Neoplatonic philosophy into the discourse by the end of the century. Most notably, the Leipzig polymath Magnus Hundt and the prior of the Carthusian order in Germany, Gregor Reisch, put the teachings of Marsilio Ficino (d. 1499) into conversation with traditional religious and natural philosophical sources in the commentary tradition. Their major works—Hundt's *Anthropology of the Nature and Dignity of Man* (1501) and Reisch's *Margarita Philosophica* (1496)—aimed to describe the totality of human experience in a single, religiously centered, system.[49]

Although drawing on perhaps a wider range of traditions than other regions of Europe, German intellectuals were very consistent about the primarily religious purposes of understanding the senses correctly. Gabriel Biel, who trained and worked at the universities of Heidelberg, Cologne, Mainz, Erfurt, and Tübingen, composed a commentary on *De anima* in the middle of his career, around 1470.[50] Biel's treatise brought natural philosophical content into conversation with interlocutors from a range of intellectual traditions, naming Hugh of St. Victor, Boethius, Anselm, Averroes, Porphyrius, Henry of Gent, Augustine, Avicenna, Aquinas, Duns Scotus, William of Ockham, and early-fifteenth-century intellectuals like Jean Gerson and Pierre d'Ailly.[51] Biel began the treatise by explaining the devotional rationale for such a study: in this life, one could only honor God and comprehend Holy Scripture and the miracles of saints with the powers of the soul, and so proper understanding of these powers was essential.[52] The same rationale underlay other focused commentaries, as well as more expansive works like Hundt's *Anthropology* and Reisch's *Margarita philosophica.* Hundt thus justified the study of sensation with the simple observation that "I experience God through the effects of my senses, which reason approves."[53] Reisch remarked, as had his contemporary Johann Geiler von Kaysersberg, that sin and death enter the windows of the soul, "and the windows are nothing other than the eyes, ears, nose, mouth, and hands."[54] Nonetheless, sensory pleasure could also be a good thing: good tastes, for example, indicated the nourishing power of food.[55] Religious worship inserted itself into this dynamic. Reisch described it as "care for the soul," which "happens in the heart through devotion and mental prayer, in the mouth through prayer and voice, in the body through worship, genuflection, prostration, inclination, and in work through offerings of first fruits, tithes, sacrifices, and the sacraments." Understanding the body and sensation was therefore a pragmatic matter, facilitating both "cognition of God, and delight in God," as Reisch put it.[56]

"Cognition" and "delight" in the divine: Reisch's final utterance drew attention to the two basic dynamics at play when fifteenth-century intellectuals conceptualized ritual's affective power. Through the sensible objects it presented to the bodies of churchgoers, ritual impacted the intellect, performing a cognitive function by signifying spiritual truths and knowledge about God. Commenting on the natural philosophical writings of Aquinas and Albert the Great, Cologne theologian Heymerich van den Velde (d. 1460) thus argued that the sensibility of sacramental practice mediated the divine to the human intellect, noting that "nothing in its operation can naturally rise above the grade of its creation, and so the faculty of rational understanding cannot naturally be released from blending with the senses."[57] Rather than philosophizing about transcendent union with the divine, the diligent pastor ought to embrace the fact that the cognitive process was inseparable from the body and could never fully escape its grounding in the sensible world.[58] Other Cologne intellectuals, including Gerhard von Herrenberg, Johannes Hulstadt von Mechlin, and Gerhard von Harderwijck, articulated similar positions in their own natural philosophical commentaries.[59] Cologne reflected intellectual culture across fifteenth-century Germany more broadly. After the middle of the century, the discourse decisively affirmed thinking about cognition in strongly materialist terms: the intellect was inescapably dependent on the sensitive powers of the soul for its existence, requiring bodily organs of perception as its objects.[60] By the end of the century, this was normative. Even in places like Erfurt, where the principle of economy maintained by the so-called "nominalist" school of thought (commonly referred to by the shorthand "Ockham's razor") held considerable sway, cognition was unavoidably dependent on sensation.[61]

More immediately relevant to and pervasive in discussions of church ritual was Reisch's second point about the relation between the senses and delight. This was largely because it provided a compelling account of what ritual did to bodies at a prelinguistic, affective level. To a certain extent, this was already built into the language of passive sensation: affection, affliction, passion, and suffering were all terms used to describe the relation that objects of perception established with their percipients. Scholars often interpret this to mean that the power of sacraments to sanctify people could stand for an actual transfer of supernatural grace from ritual object to perceiving churchgoer along the natural avenues of the senses.[62] At a somewhat more mundane level, however, sensory physiology and psychology simply explained how ritual moved the power of the soul known as the will and shaped people's everyday moral dispositions. In contrast to the intellect, the will governed desires, appetites, and passions. The will naturally inclined toward what theologians considered "the good" but nonetheless also functioned in dynamic relation with daily life.[63] As Magnus Hundt explained, "It is proper to humans before other animals to have a sense of good and evil, as well as justice and injustice, and other similar of these things," yet these moral inclinations could be manipulated and cultivated by sensual appeal to the will.[64] Humans were unique among organisms with sensitive souls in their ability to attach ethical sentiments to these experiences. Only in the human subject "are body and soul mutually transformed" by the "delightful forms" of objects.[65] This provided an opportunity for the church to deploy ritual as a tool of moral or ethical formation: through "worship" and "examination" of God, the will could be transformed and effectively "christianized."

The kind of moral formation under discussion here was prerational, or prelinguistic, in nature. It was what contemporary theologians referred to as habitual conscience, or as Gabriel Biel put it, "the actually or habitually adhering awareness of dictated conclusions, that is, signifying in particular that something good and praiseworthy is to be done or (its opposite) avoided."[66] Here, Biel and his contemporaries wholeheartedly embraced the traditional Aristotelian understanding of how one became virtuous. Cultivated in the soul through repetitive engagement with the objects of concern in daily life, habitual conscience stood for the acquired and internalized set of rules—a kind of software—for responding to specific situations. It was a dynamic of the faculty of the will, and as such it was more intuitive than cognitive processes of the intellect. Thus, with respect to moral philosophy, the science of the soul was considered "among the natural sciences of philosophy more principal and worthy."[67] By explaining the underlying sensory psychology and physiology, the science effectively mapped how people became moral agents. The dynamics of sensitive appetites, desires, and emotions worked on the body and soul in conjunction with the materiality of the surrounding environment. Internal moral dispositions could be affected and improved significantly by controlling and manipulating these factors.[68] This was a powerful tool in late-fifteenth-century Germany, when learned culture became increasingly preoccupied with the idea that the human relationship with the divine was ineffable, affective, and ultimately resistant to capture in language.[69]

Why was this particular account of church ritual so compelling at the time in the German-speaking world? Ultimately, from the perspective of learned elites, it served to reinforce the authority of the church as the caretaker of people's souls, which was an increasingly pressing issue in the fifteenth century for two closely related reasons. First, as a matter of practice, what we might think of as the two major pastoral duties of the clergy—preaching and administration of the sacraments—were more or less distinct offices, performed by two different classes of people. Unlike in modern Catholicism, where one expects to encounter some form of preaching in the course of attending a Mass, the sacrament and the sermon were usually separate ritual events (even when homilies were inserted into Masses, they were typically performed in Latin). The majority of the clergy were not engaged in preaching, nor were they trained for this purpose. Rather, they busied themselves primarily as ministers of the sacraments.[70] With rare exceptions, such as the Strasbourg preacher Geiler von Kaysersberg, the clerical hierarchy was clear: sacramental ministers were in charge, whereas preachers were more or less hired servants—aids to the main pastoral efforts of the institutional church.[71] Johannes Schoup, Geiler's predecessor, frequently observed as much in his sermons and did not hesitate to turn a critical eye to this state of affairs.[72] Over the course of the century, however, enthusiasm for preaching mounted in the cities, motivated in particular by the observant reform movements in the monasteries and the new practice of wealthy lay patrons' endowing permanent preaching positions, like Geiler von Kaysersberg's in Strasbourg. With this development, preaching, especially in the second half of the century, tended to focus more on meeting the pastoral needs of the laity. Doubtless also related to surging humanist interest in rhetorical eloquence, the craft of moving people with words took on new prominence and became a means for preachers to assert their own pastoral value. The surest path to salvation, some argued, was not attending the Mass but was, instead, sitting quietly and listening to the preacher during the so-called "pulpit service."[73] This demanded a response from sacramental ministers, which the discourse on sensuous sacramentality provided. The ritual cult was efficacious in itself: through its multimodal appeal to the senses, it could affect the soul just as profoundly as any sermon, if not in a more primary, visceral fashion. The entire educational system favored this point of view, and even preachers like Geiler von Kaysersberg had to concede that sacramental ministers could play just as important a pastoral role as preachers.

Beyond this, the theory of sacramentality endorsed by learned elites also formed something of a response to claims of religious authority grounded in the private experiences of more ordinary sorts of people. As we will see in chapter 3, significant portions of the laity, especially in literate, urban enclaves, embraced religious sensuality in a variety of ways, in no small part due to the very campaign church authorities had executed over the course of the late Middle Ages. With increasing certainty and consistency, the church had asserted the positive affective dimension of the senses in religious practice at the same time that urban churches developed increasingly elaborate, sensuously variegated liturgies. Both religious women and laypeople made use of this new culture in their own ways, which continuously raised questions about the meaning of religious sensuality and personal experience in the minds of many church authorities. What was going on in the souls of these people? Did the Holy Spirit, or Satan, move them? These questions were put to pilgrims traveling to popular shrines like Mont-Saint-Michel in northern France, Wilsnack and Regensburg in Germany, as well as to visionary religious women like Bridget of Sweden, who claimed a more direct connection with the divine and criticized the priesthood's role in mediating salvation.[74] To be sure, church officials often saw a subsersive, perhaps even diabolical, challenge to the church.[75] Others, like Heymerich van den Velde, remained sanguine about the potential of the sensible church in the world. In response to condemnations of Bridget of Sweden at the Council of Basel in the mid-1430s, Heymerich argued that it was impossible to know with certainty what was going on in the souls of these people, yet he nonetheless expressed confidence in the power of sensible sacramental practice to affect positive internal transformations of the soul. In this respect, the clergy played an essential role in shaping morality and opening the door to the higher spiritual truths of salvation[76] Similarly, the repeated assertions of church intellectuals throughout the fifteenth century suggest the need to control the meaning of church practice and its relation to the mind, body, and soul, as well as to consolidate their own status as ritual experts.

Whatever the underlying reasons for its prominence, the affective theory of sensation determined the basic understanding of sacramental efficacy in the late fifteenth century. The discourse spilled beyond the boundaries of natural philosophy, finding its way into the pulpits, convents, and streets of fifteenth-century cities. Ritual objects of the church were never neutral, nor did they simply point to or symbolize spiritual truths, at least not in any straightforward manner from a modern, linguistic perspective. The underlying assumptions about the natural world, the human body, and its soul prohibited this as a possibility. Burdened by an unavoidable sensuousness, late medieval worship by definition affected changes in the minds and bodies of churchgoers. This diverse array of things appealed to each of the modalities recognizable in the traditional western European five-sense sensorium in a variety of ways, but the interior effects of such appeals remained remarkably consistent.

Many, of course, gave pride of place to the sense of sight. In his later work, Robert Scribner suggested that images like the *Mass of St. Gregory* woodcut by Nuremberg artisan Wolf Traut (see figure 3) disclosed the "intensely visual nature" of late medieval Eucharist ritual. The practices represented in the woodcut, with the elevation of the Eucharist occupying the center of late medieval piety, cohered around a few common epistemological principles, or "ways of seeing." Late medieval ways of seeing assumed that the visible world signified the invisible, and that one attained knowledge of the divine through sensual engagement with the natural world. Further, images contained a form of sacred power or virtue and were not merely passively beheld by ritual spectators; rather, they formed an affective and affecting relationship with their viewer. In popular culture the

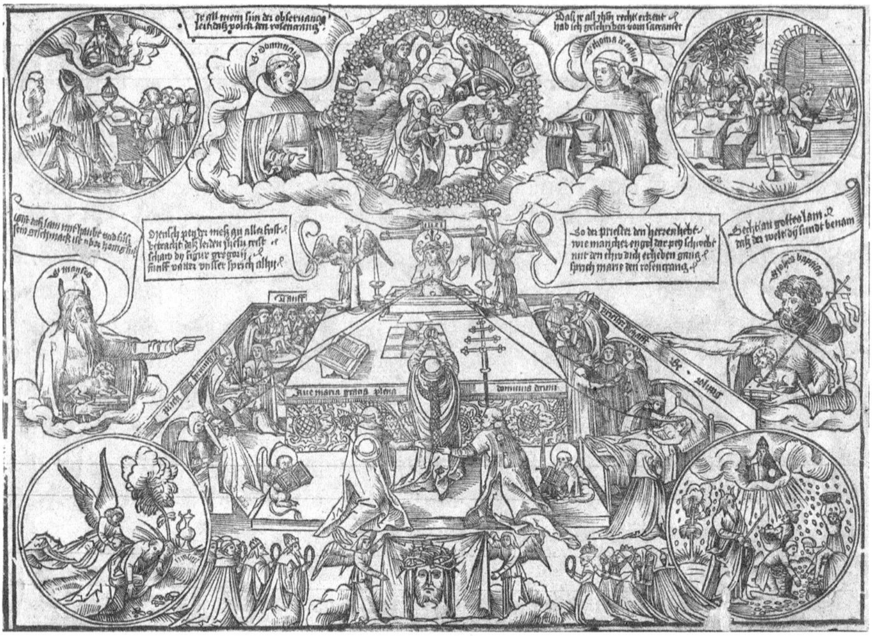

Figure 3: Wolf Traut, "Mass of St. Gregory" (1512). Karlsruhe, Badische Landesbibliothek, Cod. Kb 21. Abb. 3.

clearest expression of this was the popularity of the "sacramental gaze." At the moment of elevation during the Mass, the real presence of Christ was "made real" by the affective bond the Eucharist as an object of vision established with its spectators. The experience impressed itself into the souls of common folk.[77] By the fifteenth century, ocular Communion was widely considered an acceptable substitute for sacramental (oral) Communion.

This same affective sensory dynamic defined the power of various visual media that helped stage the elevated Eucharist during the Mass—candles, textiles, icons, reliquaries, chalices and patens, among others. Images of all kinds, which became increasingly popular objects of devotion after the thirteenth century, were held to affect the bodies and minds of devotees in profound ways.[78] The devotional emphasis on vision in the thirteenth century was reinforced by the natural philosophical discourse that emerged contemporaneously, and the dynamic, affective theory of vision promoted by the new Aristotelian learning became a structuring principle of late medieval theories of religious practice, especially those relating to the Eucharist.[79]

Much of the evidence for the popularity of visual piety in the late Middle Ages comes to us in the form of complaints by clergy. William Durandus, for example, complained that many people ran to Mass only after hearing the ringing of the bell that signaled the elevation.[80] Similarly, the Augustinian Hermit Gottschalk Hollen (d. 1481), active in northwestern Germany, lamented those who "come when they hear the bells, then enter the church, see the elevation, and when it is over, they go, running and flying, as if they had seen the devil."[81] He also complained of laypersons, especially females, pressing close to the altar to catch a glimpse of the Host because of the extraordinary power ascribed to it. Such compalints were widespread in the fifteenth century.[82] Ecclesiastical legislation provides further evidence of the popularity of sacramental gazing. The 1451 synod at Mainz ordered "lest the people's devotion cool down due to frequent viewing of it, henceforth, the sacrament shall not be carried visibly in monstrances except on the octave of Corpus Christi, and even then only during the divine office." Similar proscriptions appear in the decrees of synods at Cologne (1452), Salzburg (1456 and 1490), and Schwerin (1492).[83]

Somewhat paradoxically, the same authorities who complained about sacramental gazing simultaneously promoted its efficacy. According to the popular Franciscan preacher Stefan Fridolin (d. 1498), one of the most important dimensions of Eucharistic experience "consists in the clear viewing of [its] divine beauty."[84] Another Franciscan, Pelbart of Temesvar (d. 1504), preached that ocular Communion was a fully valid substitute for the *viaticum* one received during last rites. The Eucharist also had the power to turn one away from sins, increase faith, grace, hope, and love. Pelbart even claimed that it protected one from physical harm with the appropriate accompanying prayer (*prosit mihi ad tutamentum mentis et corporis*).[85] Many of the most important preachers in Germany made similar claims: Jakob von Jüterbog (d. 1465), Johannes von Werden (d. 1437), Johannes Paltz (d. 1511), Johannes Herolt (d. 1468), and even Gottschalk Hollen expounded corporeal and spiritual the benefits of gazing at the Eucharist.[86] The clergy paid close attention to the visual appearance of the Eucharist Host, carefully and precisely dictating its size, color, and shape in important pastoral manuals such as the *Manipulus curatorum*.[87] The Hosts were to be thin, small, round, and white: as the first vernacular exposition of the Mass explained, these characteristics signaled the "beauty," "purity," and "cleanliness" of the Host.[88]

Beyond sermons and ordinances, mystical literature promoted the visual potency of the Eucharist. In his *Little Book of Eternal Wisdom*, a handbook intended as a devotional guide for a popular audience, the Dominican Henry Suso (d. 1366) provided instructions and prayers for "how one should lovingly receive" the sacrament, which dwelt on the Eucharist Host as a "red rose," "gem," "clarity," and "light," all of which were "most beautiful to my soul" and "to the eye the most beautiful."[89] Suso and other mystical authors like him flourished in the fourteenth century but were most widely copied and read in the fifteenth.[90] A visual campaign accompanied the mystical literature and preaching efforts of clergy. The *Mass of St. Gregory* trope, along with other popular imagery, played a central role in this campaign.[91] Christ's presence in the Eucharist was a visible reality, accessible to any with eyes to see.

The evidence for the importance of vision in late medieval theories of religion is extensive, although it would be misleading to argue it provides a comprehensive view of the problem. As we have already seen, intellectual discourse self-consciously and systematically rejected a narrowly visualist interpretation of sacramental efficacy. A complete explication therefore must consider each of the remaining sensory modalities in the traditional five-sense sensorium.

In the western Europen sensorium, hearing was often considered nearly as important as vision. The Nuremberg artisan Albrecht Dürer wrote in 1510 that vision was "the noblest of all senses" but could not be separated from hearing, for people "grasp something even better when it is both heard and seen."[92] Here, "grasping something even better" had to do with both the intellect and will, as they were defined in the discourse on the human soul. The intellective, or cognitive, role of hearing had been well established since the time of Albert the Great.[93] By the late fifteenth century, the humanist celebration of the word, written and spoken, resonated with and heightened the cognitive importance of the sense in learned discourse. The study of ancient texts, alongside the disciplines of rhetoric, grammar, history, poetry, and morals, were all part of a project primarily concerned with promoting written and spoken eloquence. The most famous humanist of the era, Desiderius Erasmus (d. 1536), thus explained particular word choices in his translation of the Gospel of St. John (1519) as a matter of aural aesthetics. Discarding St. Jerome's use of *verbum* in favor of *sermo*, for example, was justified because the more mellifluous sounds of *sermo* and its declensions would better "persuade the ear to the Christian faith."[94] This was critical because, as Erasmus explained elsewhere, "things are not learned by any other means than through signs of sounds (*per uocum notas*)."[95]

The matter was not purely restricted to reason and intellect, however: as Erasmus himself pointed out, aurality was profoundly affective, appealing to bodies and minds in a more primary way. Again, the discourse had dwelt on this basic fact for centuries. Serious consideration of the problem had begun in the musical thought of Hildegard of Bingen (d. 1179) and was elaborated in the following centuries by theologians and natural philosophers.[96] Sounds were vibrations that affected bodies and souls in material and immaterial ways: by definition, they were qualities capable of being suffered (*passio*). While commentators had made various attempts to parse sound's effects on the soul into intellectual, immaterial, bodily, and sensual categories, such distinctions tended to collapse or, at best, become very confused in the discourse on church ritual. This was true of all the senses, but in the late fifteenth century it became especially problematic with respect to hearing, due largely to the influence of Marsilio

Ficino's view on the matter.[97] Ficino drew upon traditional understandings of the sense of hearing primarily to explain the affective experience of music. In particular, he emphasized the concept of spirit as an air-like power of the soul capable of receiving sounds conveyed by air. The material similitude between the spirit (as power of the soul) and song or sound (as "animated air") is what allowed for hearing to establish an especially powerful affective bond. Thus, he wrote, "if the vapours exhaled by merely vegetable life are greatly beneficial to your life, how beneficial do you think will be aerial songs to the spirit which is indeed entirely aerial, harmonic songs to the harmonic spirit, warm and thus living to the living, endowed with sense to the sensitive?"[98]

Hearing's affective potency framed discussions of the aural dimensions of church ritual. This is apparent in the commonplace that late medieval people generally considered their experience of the Mass to be primarily aural: one did not go to Mass as a spectator; rather, "heard" Masses. This wasn't simply a colloquial expression: theologians actively promoted the benefits, or "fruits," of hearing a Mass. Like sacramental gazing, the passive aural experience of the soundscape constructed by church officials had the potential to shape the soul and transform churchgoers' internal dispositions. As both Wessel Gansfort (d. 1489) and Johannes von Werden explained, the proper devotional mode of the laity during the Mass was silent listening, which opened the soul to the spiritual gifts of Christ's suffering and foreclosed the possibility of noises disrupting the souls gathered in the church, or the priests performing the rite.[99]

The various elements that constituted the soundscape of the Mass—church architecture, bell ringing, and liturgical music—resonated with affective significance. The fifteenth-century German translation of Durandus's *Rationale* described interior church spaces quite simply as the place where "people hear and pray." Hearing the liturgy cultivated communal sentiments of charity and devotion.[100] The text explained the reason for bell ringing along similar, affective lines: through the bells' tone, "the faithful are summoned together to their reward, and the devotion of faith grows in them . . . [and] the souls and bodies of the faithful are protected . . . and thus those who hear the bells flee into the lap of holy mother of Christendom, before the banner of the crucifix."[101] The text underscored the bodily and spiritual benefits of listening to bells by drawing attention to their power to repulse violent enemies, hail, thunder, lightning, and the evil spirits that stirred up storms.

Of all the components of the ritual soundscape, the affective potency of music elicited the most detailed attention in intellectual discourse. In the *Margarita philosophica*, Gregor Reisch drew upon the late antique theory of music developed by Boethius. Reisch began by describing music's effects on the human soul as "tormenting" and "enflaming with desire."[102] He went on to quote Boethius at length, who foregrounded the affective dimensions of hearing. The sense, Boethius explained, "can apprehend sounds in such a way that it not only judges them and recognizes their differences, but it very often takes pleasure in them if they are in the form of sweet and well-ordered modes, whereas it finds displeasure if the sounds heard are unordered and incoherent."[103] From this, it followed that "music is related not only to speculation but to morality as well."[104] This was not a theological argument, Reisch pointed out, nor was it necessarily specific to western Christendom. It was, rather, an anthropological observation: the "affective quality" of music was in evidence in all historical epochs, across social estates, and divisions of gender and age. It was in human nature to find "sweet modes" (*dulcibus modis*) soothing, and dissonant chords aggravating. The feelings inspired by these aural experiences affected the internal morality of the hearing subject. Reisch moved to explain this phenomenon by reference to Ficino's discussion of the physics and physiology of hearing: all forms of music were efficacious when

> . . . natural air placed in motion moves the body; [then] through purified air, aerial spirit is agitated in the soul at the corporeal nodes; through affect it simultaneously impresses sense and soul, [and] through signification moves to the mind; [it] vigorously penetrates through actual motion of subtle air; at the same time it fondly caresses, [and] through qualitative similarity . . . imbues a certain natural delight [that] simultaneously seizes and claims for itself the whole man, both spiritually and materially.[105]

Under this theory, the primary significance of the liturgical soundscape was its power to delight the body and inform the soul. On the eve of the Reformation it became especially clear that, prior to any communicative function, which would have appealed directly to the intellect, the affective, prelinguistic dimensions of sound had a profound power in and of themselves. This explanation proved especially compelling in the context of a ritual environment characterized by its supermusicality, as discussed in chapter 1. The aural engineering of the Mass simply exploited a fact of nature.

The understanding of smell closely paralleled that of hearing in late medieval intellectual discourse. Like hearing, smell was considered a mediated sense; likewise, discussions about smell at the end of the fifteenth century were profoundly influenced by the thought of Ficino. Thus, smell became particularly important in how people conceptualized the affective bond cultivated by the olfactory dimensions of late medieval religious ritual.

In certain respects, modern science and anthropology have vindicated fifteenth-century discourse by demonstrating that the intimate connections between smell, emotion, and memory have roots in both nature and culture. Although they approached the problem very differently, intellectuals on the eve of the Reformation observed the profound affective power of smell and recommended its application in ritual practice. As I have argued elsewhere, the late medieval German theory of ritual smells revolved around the notion of olfaction as an essential means of evoking feelings of boundary demarcation and transition.[106] Olfactory ritual helped define spatial and temporal transitions from profane to sacred contexts. The pleasant smell of incense in the Mass was necessary, as Aquinas explained, "in order that any disagreeable smell, arising from the number of persons gathered together in the building, that could cause annoyance, might be dispelled by its fragrance."[107] The German translation of Durandus's *Rationale* elaborated the role of incense during Vespers services as demarcating the transition between day and night, arguing that the practice had a Biblical mandate detailed in Exodus 30:7–8, which instructed Aaron to burn incense both in the morning and evening.[108] In these instances, ritual elaborated upon everyday experience and established a privileged distinction with it.

Underlying the power of ritual smells as boundary markers was a more complex understanding of olfaction as an aesthetic sense. Fragrant scent stimulated desire and attracted the perceiving subject to its source. This aesthetic potential led Hundt, Peilicke, and other late-fifteenth-century commentators to conceptualize smell as a sense "necessary for living well."[109] Under this view, ritual incense had a positive power to affect and delight both body and soul in more profound ways. Complemented by incense, sacraments possessed a greater affective power to leave lasting imprints of the love of Christ on the heart and mind. For this reason, Heinrich of Herpf interpreted the imperative of Ecclesiastes 38 to "give sweetness" as a specific reference the use of incense in Eucharistic practice.[110] Hundt agreed: the affective power of odors "is the very same reason why priests use aromatics for invocations of the divine, for they extend upwards, and those that are delightful comfort souls."[111] The so-called *Book of Art*, a vernacular text popular in print and manuscript in the late fifteenth and early sixteenth centuries, explained that the good smell of incense signified that through devotion "the soul may be purified and anointed." While its fumes "hovered before the heart," prayer "is ignited in love."[112] The practice of devotion more generally involved savors that produced "bodily and joyous devotions" in the soul, which "bring much grace of virtue."[113]

When the rosary emerged as a popular devotion in Germany in the late fifteenth century, the Dominican preachers most active in promoting it appealed to the affective power of incense in vernacular handbooks filled with miraculous exemplary tales (*exempla*). *Exempla* reported witnesses who "smelled a noble smoke, as if they were in an apothecary's shop," while someone devout prayed the rosary.[114] Tales also commonly identified the devotion with a "good-smelling smoke," or "censer burning full of good incense and noble herbs," all of which had the power to drive away evil spirits and turn the souls of sinners toward their "noble smell."[115] Such utterances could certainly veer into the domain of allegorical language, but they also retained grounding in practical liturgical considerations. Theorists commonly recommended the affective power of these smells to cultivate feelings of positive physical, psychological, and moral transformation, and collective identity in the Christian community.[116]

Several factors reinforced the affective potency of smell in ritual practice. The most important was the observation in the natural philosophical literature that the sense of smell in humans, while not as refined a cognitive tool as it was in other animal species, was nonetheless very efficient at making binary judgments about good and bad objects in the environment.[117] Such objects were, properly speaking, any kind of "odor dispersed through the heat of an odoriferous thing" and could be classified into two basic categories: "sweet and fetid, or delightful and horrible."[118] The soul felt profound delight or disgust in response to the odoriferous stimuli it encountered.[119] Because odors were so intimately bound up with notions of pleasure and disgust, they were eminently suited to excite human emotions and were difficult to judge rationally.[120] Contemporaneous medical discourse heightened the emotional charge associated with smelling. Aerial theories of disease transmission, well known among historians of medicine, were one expression of a larger complex of ideas in late medieval health literature deeply concerned with relationships between smells, bodies, and souls.[121] To combat corrupting foul smells, late-fifteenth-century printed health regimens prescribed the use of aromatics in the daily maintenance of the Christian body and soul, as well as toward the prevention of disease. Heinrich Steinhöwel, author of the popular *Pestilence Ordinance Booklet* (1473) thus recommended the daily use of fragrances of aloewood, incense, amber, musk, and cloves, and other plant resins and oils: "I have often said that [such] good-smelling things strengthen the heart."[122]

At the end of the fifteenth century, the humanist Neoplatonism exemplified by Marsilio Ficino made its way into German discourse and placed still more acute emphasis on the affective power of smell in ritual practice. As with the sense of hearing, the application of Ficino's teachings on spirit to the traditional Aristotelian natural philosophy was especially critical. Magnus Hundt explained:

> Comforting the spirit are things pertaining to the heart, as Avicenna describes, such as amber, gold, musk, basil, camphor, and pills of gold, incense, and myrrh. Likewise [the spirit] is nourished by inspired air and comforted by aromatic odors, like mint, wine, honey, apples, pears, warm bread, and others, as described by Marsilio Ficino, a man of our age, speaking clearly in his *De vita longa*. To those desirous to promote life in the body, honor this spirit . . . and feed everyday with sweet odors. Delight with sound and songs. And just as odor is the sweetest food for the soul, so too does bad and putrid stench infect and corrupt the spirit. In other respects, it can be useful, delightful, and honest.[123]

Hundt made clear that smell integrated biological, physical processes with aesthetic pleasure and spiritual edification. The sense traversed the lines between embodied and disembodied because of its affinity with the concept of spirit in particular. Hundt described the highest form of spirit in animated subjects (*animalibus*) as a vapor, in general "earthy and aqueous" in its humoral qualities. When entering the heart, the vapor could become "airy and fiery," while in the ventricles of the brain it became "ethereal and celestial." It served to vivify the soul and body and move its parts. Odors were especially efficacious in this domain because they were substantially similar to spirit: as vapors, they were composed of a "certain substance having lucid and clear air, classified as celestial in nature."[124] As Hundt argued, the mere act of breathing affected the lungs, heart, arteries, and brain, all of which "conform to odorous things" through inhalation. Conversely, odors also had a high potential to corrupt body and soul. Even fish, Hundt claimed, could be corrupted by odors transmitted through water, just as the smell of sulfur transmitted through the air had the power to corrupt human souls.[125]

In Hundt's view, Ficino's thinking about the spirit served as further justification for the use of aromatics in church ritual, aligning not only with the Aristotelian science but also with the scriptural definition of the soul as "a fume and breath in our nostrils, and a scintillating word, agitating our heart."[126] Others, including Hundt's contemporary Cornelius Agrippa von Nettesheim (d. 1535), were likewise influenced by Ficino and conceptualized smell in similar fashion.[127] The olfactory dimensions of the ritual environment were therefore of central import in late medieval thinking.

In the late medieval worldview, the sense of touch was ubiquitous. As Magnus Hundt and his colleague Johannes Peilicke observed in Leipzig, touch was the "sense of all senses." Following Aristotle and Albert the Great, Hundt considered touch a precondition to all animal forms of life: put simply, touch was "that which senses."[128] Peilicke concurred: "Touch is the basis of all other senses, and is identified in the instrument of each sense."[129] Such utterances referenced the fact that all sensory modalities functioned according to the passive reception of sensible species impressed into the organs of perception. Taste, smell, hearing, and vision were in effect extended, more mediated versions of touch.[130] Because of its unmediated nature, touch was widely viewed as the most reliable of senses: the media through which species traveled were subject to environmental changes, which could affect the reception of odors, sounds, or visible species.[131] Touch was also clearly the most intimate sense: there was no separation between sense organ and object at the moment of perception. As Hundt and others observed, tactile sensation relied on a system of organs distributed throughout the entire body. The *caro nervosa*—flesh "enmeshed" with nerves and diffuse below the skin and in the internal organs—received tangible species. The endpoint of all tactile experience was the heart, which was affected by the various tangible qualities it perceived.[132] In this context, one's tactile engagement with the world had profound ethical, moral, and spiritual stakes. "Goodness of touch," asserted Johannes Peilicke, "attains to a good bodily complexion, and nobility of the soul follows from good complexion."[133]

Because of these distinctive qualities, intellectuals found touch useful for thinking and talking about the emotive, prelinguistic aspects of the human experience of the divine. The same view of touch articulated in the natural philosophical tradition informed late medieval mystical traditions. Largely following the example of Bernard of Clairvaux, late medieval thinkers from Albert the Great to Gertrude of Helfta promoted the language of touch to describe immediate mystical union with God. In this respect, the Song of Songs, with its evocations of kissing and caressing between lover and bride to describe the relationship between Christian soul and God, became a key text.[134] Authors strove to distinguish these as moments of "spiritual" or "inward" touching, but the overwhelming tendency of the late Middle Ages was to blur the lines between body and soul, interior and exterior, human and divine. This was at least in part due to the fact that thinking with touch was an especially useful way to talk about how the external objects of ritual contexts produced internal, affective transformations in the souls of those who participated. As Niklaus Largier explains, the language of touch was not simply "a means to allegorize something that can not be said otherwise . . . rather, it is a technique, a practice of the use of biblical language in prayer, through which a transition from a lack of sensitivity and emotional intensity toward a state of aroused sensitivity is performed."[135]

Given its applicability in ritual contexts, touch became particularly important in Eucharistic devotions from the thirteenth century onward.[136] Under the doctrine of transubstantiation, priestly consecration transformed the profane elements of bread and wine into the actual body and blood of Christ, and so receiving Communion was effectively a practical extension of the mystic emphasis on fusing human and divine. Reception involved direct, unmediated contact with the divine.[137] This privileging of liturgical tactile piety was initially prominent in female religious communities of the fourteenth century. Following the example of leading theorists such as Gertrude of Helfta, Mechthild of Magdeburg, and Hadewijch of Brabant, male clergy, especially members of the Dominican order, appropriated and cultivated it in the later years of the century. Above all, Henry Suso's ebullient, deeply emotive Eucharistic piety relied upon appeals to touch. His autobiographical writings frequently referenced feeling Christ's "loving caress and sweetness" while fervently praying before a crucifix or contemplating the Host, and he described his experience of the divine as an "impact" or "impression" (*Einschlag*) on the soul.[138] Suso's instructions for receiving the sacrament described the Eucharist Host as a manifestation of Christ's love that penetrated the heart, and enflamed the spirit.[139] It was "to the touch the most tender, and to the heart the most loving," and a "delight" to the "dry mouth of my soul."[140] In the fifteenth century, manuals like the *Book for the Exercise of Devotion* harvested Suso's tactile piety. Eucharist devotions were analogous to Christ's "embraces and kisses," which "do not blemish, but rather purify and sanctify the soul."[141]

Whether it was immediate contact with objects of devotion or with one's fellow churchgoers, the hapticity of ritual practice affected and transformed the minds and bodies of churchgoers in positive ways. To be sure, haptic practices always threatened to enflame lust and sinful desire, but they could also work in the opposite direction. This justified the mediation of touch during the Mass prevalent in wealthier urban communities. Gabriel Biel, along with other churchmen, recommended the kissing of pax boards, relics, and *Agnus Dei* images in lieu of flesh-on-flesh kissing during the kiss of peace in the Mass because it circumvented lustful feelings. Nonetheless, learned discussions were equally concerned with "good" kisses that sparked feelings of affection and charity toward one's fellow churchgoers and encouraged thinking about the union between human and divine achieved during the Eucharist.[142] As the German translation of Durandus's *Rationale divinorum* explained, "people kiss each other at Mass" before Communion not only because Scripture and Canon Law commanded it, but also because it effected a real change in those who participated: "In the kiss, flesh is united with flesh, and spirit with spirit, and we who are joined in the flesh by our descent from Adam, will be connected by the bond of love."[143] Durandus was clear that the ritual kisses were both "spiritual" and "bodily" in nature, affecting not only "peace in our mouth but also in our heart."[144] The same principle guided understandings of the handling of the Eucharist. The consecrations, elevations, and fractions were performed carefully with both hands, which were meticulously washed prior to the rite. Proper performance was affective: in performing the gestures, the priest had "love and desire" in his will, which was "more secure and safer" than intellectual understanding of religious truth acquired by reason.[145] The same logic justified the stipulation that the Eucharist "must not be eaten like other food, but rather, discreetly, with moderation and gently; and it must be held behind the front of the teeth and softened with the tongue."[146] Chewing it like some coarse piece of daily bread was objectionable and impious, drawing dangerously close to the more sinful pleasures of the dinner table.[147]

Beyond the Mass, clergy promoted other eminently tactile practices like the rosary according to this same affective logic. Alanus de Rupe (d. 1475), one of the early promoters of the devotion, described the "old fathers" of the early church carrying rosaries "in their hands and on their belts." So long as they maintained contact with the prayer beads, their souls were fortified against the temptations of the devil; when they dropped them, the devil succeeded in driving them into the desert.[148] Elsewhere, Alanus also claimed to have witnessed people dying of the plague rescued simply by touching a rosary, and a mute man able to speak after kissing a rosary and pressing it to his neck.[149] Similar tales proliferated in Alanus's work and in other popular printed rosary handbooks of the late fifteenth and early sixteenth centuries. Technically, the a priori internal disposition of the faithful was supposed to underlay the efficacy of the rosary in such situations, but the tales seldom made this clear. Indeed, they actively promoted the opposite: haptic engagement with the device sparked internal devotion and faith. Thus, a mid-fifteenth century manuscript explaining the origins of the rosary identified a "simple layman who was in the habit of weaving garlands of roses, flowers, or herbs . . . and setting them upon a statue of the most Blessed Virgin Mary."[150] As the story went on to explain, "with this act, he sensed a great devotion," and, partaking in the "incarnate Grace through the glorious Virgin," entered a religious order.[151] The early-sixteenth-century rosary handbook of Markus von Weida (d. 1516), a Dominican preacher and contemporary of Magnus Hundt and Johannes Peilicke in Leipzig, articulated this principle in both word and image. His glosses on images of men and women kneeling and clutching rosaries before apparitions of the Virgin Mary thus described the practice as benefiting both spiritual and "bodily salvation."[152] The "most useful fruits" of this practice were the inward focusing of the heart and mind on purely religious truths, the comforting of afflictions suffered in body and soul, the enflaming of "heartfelt desire" for God, the awakening of faith, and the strengthening of hope.[153] These internal feelings were insuperable from the external objects that impinged upon the flesh.

Taste, too, was centrally important in late medieval ritual theory. As we saw in chapter 1, the first published vernacular exposition of the Mass in Germany described the Eucharist as "in its nature sweet."[154] The text's author also supplied readers with a set of Eucharist prayers, laced with syrupy sweetness. In the prayer to be spoken by the laity during the elevation, the Host was "sweet food," and "exalted desire of the heavenly court." A translation of the Communion prayer spoken by the priests addressed the Host as the "highest sweetness."[155] The author of this text was likely a diocesan priest in the Augsburg, but his utterances were broadly paradigmatic: intellectual discourse across the Holy Roman Empire in the fifteenth century regularly encouraged thinking about the Eucharist as something sweet to taste. At midcentury in the city of Mainz, an explication of the Mass addressed to the Cistercian community of the city explained that the

Eucharist "feeds the body and has a taste to the soul." The bread specifically had "all good taste and sweetness."[156] Henry Suso's Eucharist prayers, in addition to their tactile appeals, had frequent recourse to the gustatory, addressing the Host as "sweet, good-tasting bread of heaven, which contains in it all the sweetest taste according to every hearts' desire."[157] Other well-known vernacular prayers, such as those by the early German humanist Johannes von Neumarkt (d. 1380), linked the sweetness of Christ's body and blood to health and purification of both body and soul.[158] Popular images of the *Mass of St. Gregory*, such as the 1510 woodcut produced by the Nuremberg artisan Wolf Traut, included inscriptions proclaiming Christ as the Lamb of God "whose taste is sweeter than honey" (see figure 2). Popular preachers, like the Franciscan Stefan Fridolin, declared that the essence of the Eucharist was not simply gazing at its beauty, but "enjoyment of its sweetness." He explained that Christ's "holy body in the form of wheaten bread by given to the soul as food, and his precious blood as drink of wine, so that in this our time of pilgrimage and sorrow, the devout may seek out and revel in the taste of divine sweetness in the sacrament, in which exist the tastes of all sweetness."[159]

While describing ritual wine as sweet is somewhat unexceptional according to modern sensibilities, utterances about sweet Eucharist wafers may come as somewhat surprising. One could easily reduce them to purely conventional language, intended to signify higher, more abstract, theological truths. There is some basis for this interpretation: a considerable body of scholarship has suggested the ways in which the language of touch and taste generally, and the language of sweetness specifically, served a rhetorical function to reflect on moral goodness or knowledge of divine wisdom. The evidence for this interpretation stems from such early patristic authors as Origen and Augustine, to its apparent flourishing at the beginning of the late Middle ages, with the likes of Bernard of Clairvaux.[160] However, describing the experience of the divine as sweet went well beyond this narrowly defined religious sphere because sweetness also evoked natural philosophical and aesthetic discussions of taste. Learned discourse from the early Middle Ages had established some of these connections; by the late Middle Ages, it had accumulated a critical density.[161] No other term, Mary Carrruthers explains, was used more frequently "to make a positive judgment about the effects of works of art."[162] And the Eucharist was most certainly a work of art, pleasing to the eye, but also made to be eaten.[163] How one understood Eucharistic sweetness was closely tied to these discussions of taste. Like ritual touching, ritual tasting in intellectual discourse cohered under the terms stipulated by the science of the soul.

The central point in the fifteenth century was that Eucharistic sweetness affected real transformations in the souls of those who received it. These were aesthetic transformations in the Aristotelian and medieval senses of the term:

sweetness simultaneously conjured a connection between knowing and feeling and did not allow for any straightforward separation between intellectual and physical domains. Like evocations of the sense of touch, refrains on Eucharistic sweetness almost always explained its effects as igniting desire in the hearts of communicants. Suso's Eucharist prayer identified this as taking place in the will, which was "enflamed with your [God's] sweet love" at the moment of reception.[164] The reception of Eucharistic sweetness had material and immaterial effects, as other model prayers petitioned Christ to "become to me the bread that has the taste of your divine sweetness" in order to "make me healthy" and "come into my heart and cleanse it of all bodily and spiritual sins."[165] The sweetness of the Eucharist articulated a bundle of physical, intellectual, and emotional changes that were supposed to take place in the soul of the communicant, as the Franciscan Otto von Passau's *Twenty Four Elders* explained. A vernacular text popular on late-fifteenth-century printing presses, the text prepared communicants for reception by instructing them to "think on the sorrow of Jesus Christ, on whose account the most worthy sacrament is instituted and established; and with all the power of your soul you should have much divine observance with much fervent, perfect love of all the tender sweetness . . . which by divine nature is contained in this most worthy sacrament."[166]

From the standpoint of those designing, producing, and performing the Eucharist, the affective power associated with its sweetness was a necessary and useful means for laypeople to access the divine. As a widely circulated fifteenth-century tract known as the *Philosophia spiritualis* explained:

> One discovers God also in desire and in sensitive sweetness, as a very lowly simple person who does not know the Scriptures, but nonetheless recognizes God in love and in steadfast service. In a similar manner is the distinction between the recognition of the sweetness of honey through hearing words describe it, and the recognition of the sweetness itself in tasting it and in desiring for its taste.[167]

"Sensitive sweetness" as a visceral, prelinguistic experience had the added benefit of being more immediate and potentially more powerful in ritual contexts than the rational declamation of the meaning of Scripture. The words describing the sweetness of honey were not the same thing as the sweetness itself. The taste of the Eucharist was a more immediate, profound, and certain union than simply hearing about it or gazing at the Host. On similar grounds, Heinrich Herpf asserted that Christ had specifically wanted to institute the Eucharist as a meal because of its affective potential. The experience of food appealed to human emotion and thus left a deeper imprint on the memory.[168]

Late medieval natural philosophy reinforced the value of Eucharistic sweetness as prerational or prelinguistic yet at the same time more certain than intellectual or philosophical aspects of religion. Inverting the traditional sensory hierarchy that placed vision at its top, the treatise *Summa de saporibus* thus explained that "only taste is ordained above all the other senses as properly and principally the investigator of the natures of things."[169] The discretionary power of taste was partly due to its close relation to touch. Taste was a proximity sense, relying on direct contact between object and organ for its functioning; in some circles it was seen as a modified form of touch. The sense participated in its objects in a more basic, "intrinsic" matter, as the late-fifteenth century commentators explained.[170] Also like touch, the discretionary power of taste stemmed from its role in making judgments about what to let into the body and what to keep out. Flavor played the essential role in this process, helping the body distinguish healthy from harmful at a prerational, intuitive level. As Avicenna had succinctly put it, the body quickly learned "that which tastes good nourishes."[171] At the end of the fifteenth century, Magnus Hundt echoed Avicenna's position: "That which tastes good to the mouth the stomach well embraces, distributes, and digests, and is very useful for promoting well-being."[172]

In this framework, sweetness was the best of all possible flavors. The balance of humoral properties in a given object determined its flavor profile, helping the tongue determine whether or not something should pass to the stomach. Humorally, sweetness signified the perfect balance of heat and moisture and was the most desirable flavor in the human experience. Bitterness was the least desirable flavor and opposite of sweetness because it represented utter immoderation of humoral properties.[173] This view had widespread currency in contemporaneous medical and dietetic literature. The *Arzneibuch* (Medicine Book) of Ortolf of Bavaria, printed in Nuremberg in 1477, prescribed sugar-based syrups for "bad blood" accumulating in the head, along with a variety of intestinal disorders and heart palpitations. For the elderly, Ortolf recommended a daily regimen of sweetened wine.[174] Cookbooks, too, frequently prescribed wine fortified with copious amounts of sugar to sick patients "for the strengthening of the body and the reestablishment of its natural heat."[175] The printed regimen *Provision for the Body, Soul, Honor, and Well-Being of a Human*, appearing in Nuremberg in 1489, defined both bodily sickness and depression as a lack of desire or taste for food and drink, and prescribed a variety of concoctions laced with sugar, honey, and pureed fruits to restore said desire.[176] For medicinal prescriptions of the late fifteenth century, the perception of their efficacy was typically based on how their "good flavor" indicated their power to balance the humors of the afflicted body.[177]

There was an intuitive logic to the fifteenth-century theory. As modern anthropological, biological, and psychological research has shown, humans generally tend to avoid bitter tastes and pursue sweet ones. The typical evolutionary explanation given for these dispositions is that poisonous substances in nature are often bitter, while sweetness usually signifies fruit, milk, or other desirable edibles.[178] In this context, the meaning of Eucharistic sweetness went well beyond theological rhetoric. It was a metaphor, but one that entailed concrete, experiential referents in the daily lives of those who participated in the ritual. The Eucharist had to be sweet because it was by definition the best of all possible foods. Theologians explained that sacramental Communion had real powers to transform the body and soul: the body and blood of Christ, incorporated into the bodies of communicants, worked as an antidote against poisons, cured disease, energized the lethargic, delighted the poor of spirit, improved the taste of ordinary food, and of course mediated salvation.[179] By the fifteenth century, numerous preachers across the Holy Roman Empire promoted such benefits of sacramental Communion while at the same time drawing attention to its sweetness. These were widely represented positions: for example, Johannes Herolt's sermons alone were printed fifty-seven times prior to 1520.[180] As Johannes von Paltz explained (d. 1511) in his *Coelifoedina* (Heavenly Quarry), the root of these transformations was the "delight of the spirit" (*delectatio spiritualis*) felt when eating and drinking the species of Christ's body and blood: the Eucharist "gives sweetness to the soul that it touches, and indeed, the soul is preserved to esteem itself healthily, and then has spiritual delight in itself."[181] Taste, like smell, carried with it strong emotional valences in daily life. Eucharistic sweetness evoked these concrete indices and was a means of consolidating the church's ritual control over them.

This chapter has demonstrated the central place accorded to the senses in the development of learned theories of church ritual on the eve of the Reformation. It has surveyed discourse among intellectuals and shown that thinking with the senses was an essential means of explicating the power of ritual practice to affect and transform the bodies and souls of churchgoers. The discourse established that the ritual edifice of the church produced very real, highly affective transformations in the souls of those who engaged it or—more accurately—were engaged by it. The origins of this explanatory paradigm extend back to the sacramental theology of the twelfth and thirteenth centuries and drew upon both the Christian religious and Aristotelian natural philosophical traditions. By the fifteenth century, these seemingly disparate threads had become inextricably intertwined. Learned statements about the sensuous appeal of worship were part and parcel of a much more comprehensive "science of the soul." They were therefore not merely answers to questions of what rituals did; they were also broader claims about the institutional church's authority to delimit and define reality as a whole. So long as these claims went unchallenged, the late medieval church endured. For the Reformation to begin, a tear in this fabric would be necessary.

Before we get to that point, however, the discourse would continue to shape the meaning of religious experience, at least among the most learned classes. At the same time, it was apparent that important shifts at the level of what we might identify as "vernacular theology" raised new concerns. As Berndt Hamm and Caroline Walker Bynum have recently shown, the very materiality of ritual practice became "a more insistent and problematic locus of the sacred in the twelfth to sixteenth centuries" than it had been in the early medieval world.[182] From the perspectives of more ordinary sorts of people, insofar as we can approach them, the objects mobilized in church liturgy did not simply symbolize, reference, or point to divine truths in Scripture or those hidden behind the veil of the natural world; they insisted on their own "stuffness" or "thingness" and demanded explication. To what extent was learned discourse a useful way to address this challenge, and how did it inform these people's experience and understanding of the sensual in religion on the eve of the Reformation? As we will see in chapter 3, the experience of the senses in vernacular theology presented a paradoxical, sometimes dangerous challenge to the normative expectations of authorities.

3 The Senses and Religious Experience in Vernacular Theology

On January 2, 1421, a day after receiving Communion, Katharina Tucher (d. 1448) was at home, fretting over her prospects for salvation. The situation appears to have been exacerbated by her confessor, who berated her for her immature understanding of Christian doctrine, her frivolous lifestyle, and for indulging in too much wine. Katharina was nonetheless reassured of the value of her devotion and its positive effects on her soul in a series of visions that culminated with Christ's appearing before her later that evening. As Katharina wept on the floor, Christ assuaged her fears, pledging that his sanctifying grace would be imparted to her through the sacrament, and that he would "press the trunk of my cross into your heart."[1] Upon perceiving this, her anguish dissipated, the flow of tears dried up, and she felt a joyous renewal within.

Katharina described these events in a kind of spiritual diary she kept. After moving to the city of Nuremberg around 1417, she began to keep the diary, making a total of ninety-four entries over the course of the next four years. Katharina was a laywoman, attended church services regularly, and reflected on her personal religious experience in evocative, often highly sensual language. Christ's promise to "press the trunk of his cross" into her heart clearly had a sexual connotation, drawing on rhetorical conventions that extended all the way back to the biblical Song of Songs. In the European Middle Ages, theologians like Bernard of Clairvaux, and then especially religious women of the thirteenth and fourteenth centuries, built on these traditions and laid much of the groundwork for the more affective, sensualized, religious vernaculars that would permeate religious culture in the fifteenth century.[2] However, the language Katharina used in her diary also revolved around the more immediate, concrete, circumstances of her daily life. Of central import here was the matter of Katharina's relationship to the ritual life of the church.[3] When describing her participation in the Eucharist as efficacious and transformative, Katharina used language that was manifestly tactile and even paralleled the passivity associated with sensation in contemporary natural philosophy. Her entire experience of Christ in the sacrament was one of impression, profoundly affecting Katharina's emotional and moral core in the depths of her soul. In reflecting upon her own experience of the religious world she inhabited, Katharina thus drew together many of the various threads in late medieval sensory culture.

Katharina Tucher's diary offers unique insight into how laypeople understood the significance of the senses in their day-to-day religious experience. That she left behind such a document is exceptionally rare: only a handful of autobiographical writings from the fifteenth century survive, and authors seldom provide anything more than the passing reference to their experiences in church. The peculiar genre in which she chose to write, however, disguises the fact that Katharina's use of sensory language exemplified a much more widespread pattern among urban, literate laypeople in fifteenth-century Germany. In distinction from the university-educated theologians we encountered in chapter 2, these people read, wrote, and listened in the vernacular. Latin was not entirely unknown, but the primary language in which they made sense of their religion was some form of German. They borrowed ideas from learned Latinate culture, but they also went beyond them, adapting them creatively to their own purposes. Put another way, people like Katharina Tucher were practitioners of a vernacular theology in dialogue with the ideas disseminated from the universities and monasteries of the German-speaking world.[4]

This chapter traces how vernacular theology in the fifteenth century embraced religious sensuality in both theory and practice. First, I analyze the case of Katharina Tucher, bringing details from her diary into conversation with other books in her personal library, showing how her playful use of sensory language was an important means of synthesizing her religious experience and translating the complexity of lived religion into written text. Given the somewhat unusual nature of Tucher's diary, it is also important to assess whether or not she was a fair representative of the broader fifteenth century scene. The second part of this chapter takes on this problem through analysis of personal prayer books kept by people who lived in the fifteenth century. It shows that people enthusiastically embraced sensory language in their prayers, especially in prayers specifically designed to facilitate their participation in the Eucharist. I set this cultural phenomenon in its social historical context, using prosopography to show how the language of sensation circulated between monasteries and literate laypeople in the cities, between men and women, and across a variety of status groups. In this regard, this chapter follows the model set down by Virginia Reinburg for the contemporaneous French context, where she has demonstrated how prayer book owners built their own "archives of prayer."[5] Here, I would suggest more narrowly that German-speaking prayer book owners built their own vernacular archive of the senses. This archive was essential to defining and communicating the religious experiences of more ordinary sorts of people in the fifteenth century.

As with many other developments in the history of the senses in late medieval Germany, I discuss this as a phenomenon of the literate, urban world. The senses, to be sure, were an important component of the religious experience of rural people, but there is simply no evidence to permit comment on their perspectives. They left behind no firsthand accounts of their experiences, and so our understanding of the sensory history for most of late medieval Germany is incomplete.[6] People in the towns and cities, however, did, although most often only in ways that appear alien to modern eyes. Their impressions survive in manuscript sources that are rather difficult to navigate and interpret, and as a result, they have often been overlooked. This is true not only among sensory historians but in scholarship more broadly, where the fifteenth century still remains largely uncharted territory to all but a handful of specialists.[7] By engaging closely with fifteenth-century manuscript culture, this chapter contributes to all these fields and seeks to bring the place of the senses in vernacular theology into focus.

We find that, at each step, vernacular theologians understood the senses in much the same way as learned elites did, even as they went beyond and diverged from them in other respects. They supposed, with their university and monastic counterparts, that church ritual actuated a potent affective bond with churchgoers. Occasionally, this was explicitly theorized, but more often than not, people evoked it through narrative description or other poetic devices. On the other hand, vernacular theologians went beyond their learned counterparts. They were less precise, less systematic in their explications of the power of sensuous worship, but more concerned with narrating the complexity of their own religious experience. Correspondingly, their utterances were more intersensorial, even chaotic, attempting to account for things unfolding over a specific time, in a specific place. One might therefore understand the difference between learned and vernacular ways of thinking with the senses as analogous to Saussure's classical linguistic distinction between *langue* and *parole*. Learned elites had articulated the underlying principles of sacramental efficacy, whereas vernacular theologians used the principles and played language games with them, elaborating how sensuous worship worked on and interacted with the concrete circumstances of individual experience. By bringing these complicated issues to the fore, vernacular theologians offer a unique opportunity to enrich our understanding of the dynamic relationship between sensory production and sensory consumption at the heart of religious experience, in premodern and modern times alike.

This dynamic also necessarily raised the issue of power, to which we turn in the final stages of this chapter. As urban church liturgies evolved progressively more complex appeals to the senses over the course of the late Middle Ages, learned elites sought to define and limit the meaning of those appeals. Ritual, however, as Catherine Bell reminds us, is always a "strategic arena for the embodiment of power relations."[8] Religious sensuality was contested in the fifteenth century. The fact that vernacular theologians played so much with the boundaries of sensuous sacramentality raised serious questions among male scholastic and monastic thinkers. Even as they asserted that church ritual was part of the positive side of the "sensual coin" of humanity, they wondered what was going on in the souls of those who so enthusiastically embraced it and claimed their own peculiar form of religious authority from it. That so much of the vernacular theology of the senses originated in female religious communities, and often undermined norms of gender and sexuality, only added fuel to the fire. Often, this inclined church authorities to a kind of "double-externalization" of church ritual. It was not only external in practical terms as an appeal to bodily senses; it was also external to the normative center of the Christian community, which was seen as masculine, intellectual, and sensorially transcendent. Sensuous worship was a matter of "others": women, children, the intellectually and spiritually weak, and, of course, non-Christians. These kinds of people needed sensuous worship, but they failed to grasp the transcendent essence of religion. Church authorities would work with these tropes, but the problem was irresolvable. As we will see in chapter 4, it continued to resonate in the early culture of the Protestant Reformation.

Following discussion of the power dynamics embedded in sensuous sacramentality, I conclude part 1 of this study by reviewing some of the major issues raised in chapters 1, 2, and 3, bringing them into conversation with some of the guiding narratives and hypotheses that have cohered in the burgeoning field of sensory history. Here, we have occasion to think critically about religious experience in the late Middle Ages as a complex dynamic of sensory production and consumption. This challenges the often static and distorting view of late medieval religion we have in hand when we approach the problem of the Protestant Reformation as a desensualizing force in the history of Christianity. Undermining a key part of this narrative forces us to begin rethinking the meaning of this religious movement and its associations with religious and European modernity more broadly.

Katharina Tucher's diary offers a rare glimpse into how vernacular theologians made sense of religion in fifteenth-century Germany. Many details about her childhood and family background are uncertain, but it seems that Katharina was born sometime in the late fourteenth century, perhaps around 1380. She was already married and a widow by the mid-1410s. She had been the wife of one Otto Tucher of Neumarkt (in northern Bavaria), who was apparently a fairly successful cloth merchant. On the basis of her marriage and subsequent removal to Nuremberg after Otto's death, we can guess at a few other things about Katharina's background. She probably came from a similarly affluent, although non-noble, merchant family as her husband's in the same region, as intermarriage between such families was common. She certainly had some connection to Nuremberg prior to Otto's death, quite possibly through his family. Otto was a member of the Tucher family, well known as textile merchants and members of the highest patrician estate in fifteenth- and sixteenth-century Nuremberg. Otto himself was apparently barred from entering the city prior to his death, and her own biological family's connection to Nuremberg is unclear.[9] In any event, the fact that she moved from Neumarkt to Nuremberg after Otto died (a reasonably short but not insignificant distance) indicates she was securely plugged in to the urban milieu of the free imperial city. She therefore came from a wealthy station in life, and relative to many women (and men for that matter) in fifteenth-century German society, she likely enjoyed considerable power and prestige, but was not of the noble estate, nor a member of a religious order.

After her arrival in Nuremberg, some details about Katharina's life are more certain. She chose not to remarry, remaining a widow until her death in 1448. She also refused the other path commonly taken by women under similar circumstances: she did not enter a convent, at least not until much later in life. Instead, she lived with her daughter and perhaps a few other women in her own house. She attended church regularly, and immediately engaged in a life of devotion and religious study. In addition to her diary, she amassed a formidable personal library of twenty-six volumes.[10] She also had connections with the Dominican women's convent of St. Katherine in the city, where she eventually retired shortly before her death. The connection certainly aided her pursuit of knowledge and the practical devotions that engaged her in day to day life, as many of her books were either penned in St. Katherine's scriptorium or procured from abroad by the efforts of the Dominican nuns.[11]

Katharina composed her spiritual diary from 1418 to 1421, shortly after arriving in Nuremberg to begin her new life. It does not seem that she had a particular audience in mind as she did so; rather, the diary appears as a personal account of her own religious experiences during this transition. When she entered St. Katherine's shortly before her death more than two decades later, she brought the diary with her, and it became the property of the convent, along with all of her other books. The diary is an unusual document, somewhat artlessly composed as one commentator has observed.[12] Although she was certainly influenced by autobiographical traditions among female religious communities in the preceding century, Katharina made no pretense of offering any kind of coherent narrative of her life in these years. She began and ended the writing rather abruptly, and the reader is left with the general impression of Katharina lurching somewhat violently between states of fear and uncertainty about her own salvation at one extreme, and ecstatic joy at the other. The diary spanned a total of ninety-four entries, most commonly taking the form of visionary experiences in which Tucher engaged Christ or the Virgin Mary in conversation. On a few occasions, she spoke with saints. In one somewhat unusual entry, she documented her thoughts about the soul. Most of the time, however, her conversations dealt with more traditionally bounded theological issues, sometimes as abstract as the nature of the Trinity, and sometimes as concrete as the adoration of the Eucharist. Katharina related these issues to the specific circumstances she confronted in her daily life, frequently noting the times and places in which visions occurred, as well as the activities that seemed to provoke them. As such, the diary provides a fascinating window into the formation of a vernacular theologian in the fifteenth century. We see Katharina working to comprehend the relationships between what she was reading, her daily life as a widow, and the ritual edifice of the church.

At the center of this struggle was the matter of the senses. She explicitly theorized the senses in terms that bore traces of influence from the science of the soul. Specifically, she described the five senses as "faculties of the soul" and provided a basic outline of their functioning that squared with the major points of learned discourse.[13] The senses mediated between external world, body, soul, and the internal faculties, which she identified elsewhere as will, reason, understanding, heart, and thought.[14] Tucher added that, because they played such a crucial intermediary role, the five senses had to be disciplined to Christ.[15] The mechanism for achieving this end she identified quite explicitly as participation in the ritual life of the church, singling out fasting, celebrating feast days, and prayer. The *telos* of ritual practice involved not only doing God's will but also disciplining the senses in order to affect and perfect the soul of the practitioner.[16] Ritual moved the soul so that it "would desire a drop of the sweet honey of God's divinity."[17] Evaluated strictly in terms of the learned discourse on the senses, these utterances appear fairly unremarkable, although they are in all likelihood one the few, if not the only, documented instance of a layperson (male or female) without a university education making them in the fifteenth century.

Katharina, however, went well beyond the boundaries defined by intellectual discourse, making abundant and playful use of sensory language in her diary. She often embellished her relationship with Christ with intersensorial imagery to articulate a powerfully affective, sometimes erotic connection. Beyond utterances of Christ's pressing his cross into her heart, much of this language closely paralleled imagery from the biblical *Song of Songs*.[18] Jesus addressed Tucher as his "bride," promising to adorn her with beautiful clothing, shoes, a garland of pearls, and a wedding ring, surrounding her with roses, lilies, and violets, and serenading her with harps, violins, and singing.[19] Elsewhere, Tucher described walking with Christ through fragrant gardens and meadows, picking ripe fruit from trees, and making garlands of violets and white lilies.[20]

It is clear that the diary built on many rhetorical conventions from vernacular religious literature in the fourteenth century, particularly female hagiography and autohagiography.[21] Among the volumes in her library were vernacular translations of the life of Catherine of Siena, the revelations of Bridget of Sweden, a substantial collection of mystical lyrics and poetry, and Henry Suso's *Little Book of Eternal Wisdom*.[22] These materials commonly framed the relationship between human soul and divine as analogous to that between bride and bridegroom, and used strongly intersensorial language to do so. Additionally, Tucher owned several prayer books that used similar sensory language.[23] One of these included Henry Suso's Eucharist prayer, which we analyzed in chapter 2.[24] Another contained a variety of Eucharist prayers similar to Suso's: dwelling on the affective bond between communicant and Eucharist, they begged Christ to penetrate the heart and "fill the veins" with the "good taste" and "sweetness" of the Eucharist. Eucharistic sweetness mediated spiritual gifts of mercy and grace, as well as "health of the body and the soul, that I become purified in body and soul, that I might become worthy of the heavenly kingdom, and feed me so graciously with your holy Body, and quench me so sweetly in your blood, that I must be in your presence and eternally rejoice."[25] Katharina avidly consumed this way of thinking with the senses, building a library filled with such language.

What was the significance of intersensorial language in Tucher's diary? On the one hand, it was a useful way of gesturing toward the unspeakability and unintelligibility of the divine, and making it accessible to the human soul, if in an only partial and imperfect manner. On these grounds, it was, as Gordon Rudy suggests, a rhetorical strategy for mixing or "breaking" sensory tropes:

> What is mixed or "broken" are the distinctions between the five senses (or perhaps "classes" of sensation) that people seem to regard a "given" or "natural." . . . Understood as a rhetorical technique, we can fruitfully compare synaesthetic rhetoric to negative dialectic or apophatic language. If we can say that broken metaphors are built on contradiction and paradox, it is perhaps not too much to say that like apophatic language, synaesthetic language "unsays" itself.[26]

On the other hand, we would be presenting an incomplete picture if we left intersensoriality as merely a rhetorical technique, confined largely to intellectual trends within the Christian tradition and absent any meaningful information about personal experience of religion.[27] On this interpretation, Katharina Tucher would simply have been parroting things she had heard or read before. There is no question that her diary exhibits the influence of many items from her personal library, but it is also clear that she was attempting to translate the raw, pre-linguistic expansiveness of her own religious experience into the narrow confines of language. Here, rhetorical conventions collided with more practical referents, especially the concrete reality of the ritual environment, conjoined with Aristotelian natural philosophical imperative to think with and about the affective bond this environment was supposed to establish with churchgoers.[28] Intersensorial language evoked all of these elements as they unfolded across time and place, describing the movement of the external object from the field of perception, through its bodily engagement with Katharina, to its penetration into her internal faculties, and its permanent impression on her soul. In this regard, the full weight of late medieval sensory culture was brought to bear on Katharina's attempt to narrate her religious experience.

Tucher made clear in many of her entries that she was engaged in this narrative project. She commonly noted that she received visions while "attending services," occasionally even identifying the particular church where she was. Often, these were popular feast days when it was common for the devout to receive Communion.[29] At these times, she almost certainly had one of her prayer books with her and had read from it as the priest administered the sacrament. The sensory language she used in her diary evoked the affective change she perceived through her participation in the ritual. In the entry for Pentecost in 1418, Christ instructed her to receive the sacrament "on this day and every Pentecost," because it was especially beneficial: "Know that I grant more grace in the sacrament on Pentecost than at other times."[30] On St. Sebald's Day in 1418, Christ commanded Tucher to "receive your lord . . . do not let him go, so that he might have a dwelling in you; caress yourself with him, fall on your knees, lift your hands up to him and unite yourself with him."[31] Tucher also related drinking blood from Christ's side wound in several entries, lingering on the blood's tactile, gustatory, and even olfactory qualities. In one entry, Christ commanded Tucher to "drink from my heart," the blood that was "warm and not cold."[32] In another, he commanded her to "approach his open side," from which flowed "all fragrance, taste, and sweetness."[33] Tucher thus wove together the sensory production and consumption of late medieval religion, leaving behind a remarkable record of the religious experience of a relatively ordinary churchgoer in fifteenth-century Germany. Unlike the accounts of learned elites, which sought to pin down, dissect, and explicate the various components of sensuous experience, Tucher's vernacular theology played with its complexity, leaving a dynamic narrative of her engagement with the ritual edifice of the church.

Because of the diary she left behind, we know a considerable amount about how Katharina Tucher thought with and about the senses as they related to her own religious experiences. In the broader context of fifteenth-century vernacular theology, this makes her somewhat unique. Her case was exceptional in other respects as well. Her personal library of twenty-six volumes was huge, much larger even than many clergymen's collections in the fifteenth century.[34] This doubtless was connected with her rather unusual situation as a wealthy widow living in Nuremberg, one of the great cultural centers in the German-speaking world at the time. She had the time, financial resources, and educational capital needed not only to read and study but also to write down and develop her own theology of the senses. All this argues against Katharina as a good representative of how people thought with the senses in the context of their religious experiences in the fifteenth century. However, although few people could claim a personal library of comparable size, many owned prayer books very much like those Katharina brought with her into church. The prayers that people inscribed in their books suggest that many thought with and about the senses in much the same way as Katharina did.

As with Katharina's diary, we can read the prayers people collected and used in their daily lives as part of a broader "harvest" of intellectual and cultural developments of the preceding two and a half centuries, weaving together threads of Aristotelian natural philosophy, mysticism, and nonreligious literary traditions, especially courtly culture.[35] The resulting tapestry clearly depicted the sensual coin of humanity: the five senses were the "gates" through which "the soul reaches outward creation, and outward things reach the soul," as one woman's devotional from the early sixteenth century put it.[36] This openness to the world inclined the senses toward sin, but also salvation. Prayer books tended to emphasize the latter. The senses were "useful and necessary for external things," as noted in the late-fifteenth-century prayer book of Katharina Kannengiesser of Cologne. Further, their very nature as God-given instruments meant that they had a specifically ritual purpose: in daily life, but especially in church, they were to be exercised in order both "to serve and to honor" God.[37]

Although divine gifts, the senses were simultaneously a fact of biological life, and prayer books often characterized them according to the vocabulary of Aristotelian natural philosophy, describing them as "faculties" or "powers" of the soul. In the prayer book of Margarita Vornam, a Dominican nun in the city of Nuremberg in the late fifteenth century, for example, a prayer meant to prepare her for receiving the Eucharist implored Christ to take control of all her faculties, "instruct my senses, and order my desire."[38] The prayer book of Jakob Käbitz (ca. 1457) approached the matter similarly, describing reception of the Eucharist in the first instance as a bodily phenomenon: "My body becomes full of virtue with bodily practice in praise of you."[39] Käbitz's prayers commonly deployed the language of sensory impression to describe the dynamic interaction between ritual object and churchgoer, explicitly identifying the Eucharist as a seal, pressed into the heart and soul.[40] The prayer books facilitated and reflected upon this bond in a variety of ways.

To cultivate the positive potential of the senses, prayer books as material objects oriented people's attention to the structured ritual environment in a variety of ways. Typically composed in small formats and equipped with enamel or leather page markers for quick reference to specific prayers, they emphasized portability and ease of use.[41] They all contained prayers to be read by an individual, who more often than not spoke them aloud. Particular verses were often keyed to specific ritual gestures or objects. Communion or Eucharist prayers, for example, were identified with headings such as "before the sacrament," "before the Lord's Supper," "before reception," "during the Elevation," "during the transubstantiation," or "after reception." Alongside these headings, instructions regularly indicated bodily gestures to be performed at particular points in liturgical practice. Good Eucharist prayer, according to a prayer book associated with Caritas Pirckheimer (d. 1532), abbess of the Poor Clares of Nuremberg, involved kneeling before the Eucharist while speaking "sincerely and joyfully," with a "devoted soul."[42]

The liturgical prayers themselves deployed sensory language to evoke the profoundly affective relationship between ritual object and churchgoer, by which the soul could become joyful, devoted, and purified. Most typically, they used intersensorial language to do so, appealing to two or more sensory modalities simultaneously. This pattern was especially prevalent in Communion or Eucharist prayers. A late-fifteenth-century Dominican woman's prayer book from the Moselle valley thus described the Host as "food of my mind and my sick soul."[43] The mind, soul, and body constituted a unity in these prayers, and the power of the Eucharist to feed and heal was closely associated with its sensory aspects:

> O heavenly bread, you are earnest food of angels: come [to] me and purify the heart of all its blemishes of sin. O sweet heavenly bread, make me healed of all pain from sin, from which my heart feels no sweetness . . . O light-shining bread that has in you all pleasure and all taste of sweetness. You are food to us at all times and in you my heart must never break. My heart must thus eat you so that my soul is filled with your sweetness.[44]

The Moselle prayer book identifies several tropes that recur in manuscripts throughout the fifteenth century. Sweetness was commonly applied to the bread of the Eucharist; additionally, but somewhat less commonly, it described voice, song, music, smells, kisses, or caresses. Clarity or shining light was another common way of describing the Eucharistic potency. Although absent from the Moselle manuscript, the tactile experience of heat was also frequently evoked. Whatever sensory modalities prayer books deployed, they reinforced the power of ritual to affect transformations of mind, soul, and body, from healing physical pain and sickness to washing away sin, inciting feelings of love and devotion, as well as mystical union with the divine.

Throughout the fifteenth and early sixteenth centuries, individuals made creative use of these patterns. A schoolmaster named Lentzen Hanns entered a series of Eucharist prayers for use during Holy Week into his manuscript in the late fifteenth century. One such prayer, for recitation on Maundy Thursday, evoked the tactile, visual, and gustatory simultaneously:

> O sweet Lord Jesus, my insincere, cold heart desires today to be united to you, therefore enflame it with the fire of your love, enlighten my blindness with your true presence, for you are the beautiful brilliance of brotherly clarity . . . my comfort, my love, my sweetness and all that is good . . . in enjoyment of this heavenly food, transubstantiate me into you.[45]

Similarly, Margete Bromse of Lübeck (northern Germany) kept a prayer book in the first decades of the sixteenth century that included Eucharist prayers begging Christ to "feed me with the sweet food of your blessed, holy body and blood."[46] Another called the Host "sweetest of all bread, you feed the people with your holy body . . . make my heart healthy that I may assume the love of your sweetness."[47] Still other prayers associated the love felt after receiving the Host with the fragrance of rose blossoms.[48] In a prayer for recitation during the Elevation ritual, the Nuremberg patrician Wilhelm Rümlin (d. 1449) identified the Eucharist as a "good-smelling, sweet sacrifice."[49] Other prayers in his manuscript invoked intersensoriality to reinforce the affective transformation of the ritual experience. A prayer attributed to "a Carthusian" thanked God for "feeding the hungry spiritually with all goodness of this sweetest of all breads" but continued, blurring the lines between spiritual and physical sensing:

> You are sweet to taste, desirable to sensation (*Empfindlichkeit*), a sweet check on our sorrow, protect us, visit us, renew us with deep devotion and love, and shield us from all harmful unpleasantness to body and soul. O Jesus Christ, beautiful lamb, fountain and love of all virtue in the world . . . look upon us with mercy and powerfully satisfy us with your holy body, and soak us in your holy, salvific, most noble, rose red blood, washing us of all sins and impurity.[50]

The prayer book associated with Caritas Pirckheimer, mentioned above, similarly defied categorical division of spiritual and sensual reality, addressing the Eucharist as "love and desire of my heart," "sweetness of my mind," "flame and fervor of my heart, light of my eyes, clarity of understanding," and at the same time "the fulfillment of my senses, a sweet sound in my ear, a honey-sweet taste in my throat, a lovely sight to my eyes."[51] Likewise, nun's prayer books from the middle Rhine region around Mainz commonly characterized the Eucharist as "heavenly bread of divine sweetness" and "an ornament of angels, a sweet song in the ears, a wonderful honey in the mouth, a heavenly assurance in the heart . . . fountain of truth, light of the mind that meets all joys and all desires, satisfies the mind . . . those who taste you hunger more, and those who drink you thirst more."[52]

As in the case of Katharina Tucher, we need question what the intersensorial language found in prayer books tells us about the religious experience of more ordinary sorts of people in the fifteenth century. Here, we seem to lack any kind of descriptive, autobiographical account along the lines of Tucher's diary, and so we are left with an even more extreme case of purely rhetorical language, which at best might be interpreted as normative, and imposed from above. To be sure, in many cases, prayer books presented their owners with a kind of emotional and aesthetic "script," outlining a proposal for how people should feel about their participation in worship in a given moment.[53] As an artifact of late medieval religion, the prayer book had a deeper history in the interactions between wealthy, typically noble lay patrons and monasteries or convents, going back to the twelfth century.[54] The exchange was especially fruitful between female patrons and female religious communities in this earlier period. Much of the sensory language found in the prayer books originates from these patterns of exchange.

By the fifteenth century, however, prayer book culture had gained more widespread currency among literate, urban segments of the lay population. At this point, we can detect a greater degree of agency on the part of owners, suggesting that the use of sensory language in prayer books was a meaningful choice taken by a burgeoning culture of vernacular theologians. People actively choose to include, or exclude, the prayers they found most useful in the context of their own experience. The prayer book was a living document in the hands of its owner, accompanying him or her in daily life. People added to their manuscripts over the course of a lifetime. From the perspective of owners and users, such additions could seem almost like a kind of journal or diary entry, albeit one in which language conventions played a more obvious role than we often imagine in modern forms of private life writing. Nonetheless, owners made choices about which prayers to include in their books, exercising a circumscribed form of agency and playing games with the sensory language they had at their disposal. This was a fairly widespread phenomenon, moving from monastic to lay urban communities and crossing gender boundaries across fifteenth-century Germany. Additionally, while many of the men and women who owned prayer books remained anonymous, and increasing number of owners, patrons, or donors identified themselves by name in the pages of the manuscripts, suggesting an increased sense of individual ownership over prayer book content.[55]

The collective biography of prayer book owners provides critical social historical background to the development of a vernacular theology of the senses in late medieval Germany.[56] To this end, I have assembled a sample of fifty-four manuscripts identifiable with an individual (see table 3). Analysis suggests several salient issues. Above all, prayer book ownership in fifteenth-century Germany was characterized by a high degree of fluidity, with manuscripts changing hands

Table 3: Collective Biography: Late Medieval Prayer Book Owners (Sequenced Chronologically)

MS Shelfmark	Date	Owner Name	Owner Gender	Owner Estate	Owner Profession	Geographic Location
TbA, Hs. 529	ca. 1400	"Widow of Lüneburg'	Female	?	Housewife; nun in widowhood	St. John's Parish, Lüneburg
NSB, Cent IV 36	1400–1425	Anna Kochin	Female	?	Dominican Nun	St. Katherine's Convent, Nuremberg
NSB, Cent VII, 8	ca. 1415–1447	Katharina and Barbara Ruczin	Female	?	Dominican Nun; Dominican nun	Nuremberg
NSB, Cent VI, 43o	ca. 1415–1448	Katharina Tucher	Female	Urban Professional	Merchant's wife; nun in widowhood	Nuremberg
NSB, Cent VI, 91	ca. 1415–1448	Katharina Tucher	Female	Urban Professional	Merchant's wife; nun in widowhood	Nuremberg
NSB, Will II, 19 8°	ca. 1415–1448	Katharina Tucher	Female	Urban Professional	Merchant's wife; nun in widowhood	Nuremberg
MSWB, Hs. II 283	1420	Konrad Rumpf	Male	?	Benedictine monk	St. Stephan Convent, Würzburg
BSB, Cgm. 29	1426	Elisabeth Ebran	Female	Lesser Nobility	Lesser nobility	Regensburg-Munich
LkAN, Fen. IV 90 12°	1429	Jacob and Kordalla Hübner	Male-Female	Urban Patrician	Merchant(?)	Nuremberg
NSB, Cent VII, 24	ca. 1425–1450	Wilhelm Rümlin	Male	Urban Patrician	Merchant(?)	Nuremberg
NSB, Cent VII, 34	ca. 1425–1450	Barbara Gewichtmacherin, Katharina von Mühlheim	Female	?	Dominican Nuns	Schönensteinbach Convent (Strasbourg): St. Katherine's Convent (Nuremberg)
MSWB, Hs. I 221	ca. 1425–1450	Friedrich zum Eselwecke	Male	?	Lay brother (Mainz Carthusians)	Mainz
NSB, Cent VII, 62	ca. 1425–1450	Felicitas von Watt	Female	Urban Professional	Merchant's wife(?); nun	St. Katherine's Convent, Nuremberg
Berlin Staatsbibliothek, Mgo. 628	ca. 1425–1450	Ennelin Meygerin	Female	?	Dominican Nun	St. Katherine's Convent, Nuremberg
NSB, Cent VI, 82	ca. 1425–1455	Klara Nützlin	Female	Urban Patrician	Dominican Nun	St. Katherine's Convent, Nuremberg
NSB, Cent VII, 60	ca. 1425–1466	Brigitta Schenkin	Female	?	Dominican Nun	St. Katherine's Convent, Nuremberg
NSB, Will 7, 1447	1425–1466	Klara Ridlerin	Female	?	Dominican Nun	St. Katherine's Convent, Nuremberg

continued

Table 3: *Continued*

MS Shelfmark	Date	Owner Name	Owner Gender	Owner Estate	Owner Profession	Geographic Location
FBeA, Hs. 11	1441–1443	Dominican Nun	Female	?	Dominican Nun	Freiburg im Breisgau
BSB, Cgm. 255	1448	Konrad von Egloffstein	Male	Nobility	Chamberlain to Albrecht IV of Bavaria	Bavaria (Munich)
NSB Cent VI, 43p	ca. 1450	Konrad Schelhorn	Male	?	?	Nuremberg
NSB Cent VI, 85	ca. 1450	Barbara Prucklerin	Female	?	Housewife	Nuremberg
NSB Cent VI, 43n	ca. 1450–1495	Ursula Hoschlin	Female	?	Dominican Nun	St. Katherine's Convent, Nuremberg
HU, Cpg. 640	1456	Hannsen Beyss	Male	Urban Professional	Weaver	Augsburg
BSB, Cgm. 4483	1457	Jakob Käbitz	Male	Urban Professional	Son of bureaucrat; poet and songwriter	Wemding, Bavaria
KeDD, Cod. 1503	1453-ca.1500	Katharina Kannengiesser	Female	Urban Professional	Housewife	Cologne
GNM, HS 1734	1461–63; 1475–77	Brother Augustine	Male	?	Monk	Swabia/Bavaria
FHHS, Ms 23	1462	Nicholas Muffel	Male	Urban Patrician	Senator	Nuremberg
HAAB, Oct. 76	1466	Lorenz Orreum	Male	?	?	Prague
NSB, Cent VII, 67	1471–1503	Gertraut Tetzlin	Female	?	Dominican Nun	St. Katherine's Convent, Nuremberg
GNM, Hs 22403	1472	Hilgen van den Byrcken	Female	?	?	Lower Rhine (near Cologne)
NSB, Cent V, App. 81	ca. 1475	Margarita Vornam	Female	?	Dominican Nun	St. Katherine's Convent, Nuremberg
HAAB, Q. 59	1475–1490	Margarete von Rodemacher	Female	Countess	Countess	Rodemachern (Rhineland/Elsass)
NSB, Cent VII, 7	1475–1532	Anna Rümlin	Female	Urban Patrician	Dominican Nun	St. Katherine's Convent, Nuremberg
FBAugustiner, Inv. Nr. 11741	1477–1479	Dorothea of Strassburg	Female	?	Dominican Nun(?)	Diocese of Strassburg
HU, Cpg. 645	1483	Lentzen Hanns	Male	Urban Professional	School Master	Southwest Germany/Switzerland

MS Shelfmark	Date	Owner Name	Owner Gender	Owner Estate	Owner Profession	Geographic Location
FBU, Hs. 79	1487–1498	Helena Roererin and Hans Haffner	Female-Male	Urban Professional	Nun and Layman	Constance
MWSB, Hs. I 82	1490–91	Johannes Steinbach	Male	?	Prior, Mainz Carthusians	Mainz
Tübingen Universitätsbibliothek, Md. 123	1496/97	Hillaria Heigin and Wife of Heinrich Linck	Female	?	Housewife	Swabia/Franconia
FHHS, Ms 52	1498	Leonhart Schielin	Male	Urban Professional	Artist/Scribe	Augsburg
FBStadtA, B1, Nr. 126	1500	Ursula von Stoffeln	Female	Nobility	Dominican Prioress	Basel and Freiburg
Rostock Universitätsbibliothek, Mss.theol.14	1500–1515	Margarete Bromse	Female	Urban Professional	Housewife; daughter of city councilman	Lübeck
FBU, Hs. 213	1504	Elisabeta Bontin	Female	Urban Professional	Housewife	Oberschaffshausen (Black Forest)
FBeA, Hs. 13	1506	Dominican Nun	Female	?	?	Lake Constance
GNM, Hs 1733	1506–1573	Anna von Eberstein	Female	?	Nun	Southwest Germany
FBU, Hs. 477	1507–1518	"Housewife of Freiburg"	Female	Urban Professional	Housewife	Freiburg im Breisgau
FMU, Ms. Germ. oct. 3	1508	Claus Humbracht	Male	Urban Patrician	Linen Merchant	Frankfurt am Main
BSB, Cgm. 165	1510	Elisabeth Roebin	Female	?	Dominican Nun	St. Katherine's Convent, Nuremberg
MSWB, Hs. I 422	1511	Anna Kamberger	Female	?	Nun	Rhine-Main
GNM, Hs 1737	1515	Ulrich Montfort and Evan von Schwarzenberrg	Male-Female	Lesser Nobility	Lesser nobility	Montfort (Swabia/Bavaria)
BSB, Cgm. 91110	1515–1525	Jakob and Anna Sattler	Male-Female	?	Merchant?	Nuremberg
GNM, Hs 158088	1519	Bernhard Gruber	Male	?	Benedictine monk	St. Egidien's Convent, Nuremberg
FHHS, Ms. 442	1543	"Nun of Hechingen"	Female	?	Nun	Swabia/Southwest Germany
FBU, Hs. 209	1551	Balthasar Mayr	Male	?	Pastor	Dürrheim (Württemberg)
HAStK 7020 72	1575–1580	Heinricus Lennep	Male	?	?	Lower Rhine

frequently and moving between laity and religious, male and female, and various socioeconomic statuses. These patterns were widespread in urban communities, but the geographic heartland of prayer book production and consumption lay in southern German-speaking lands. In this largely fluid context, prayer book owners exercised limited but significant degrees of individual agency when making use of sensory language in their prayer books. Sometimes they copied prayers word for word from models like Henry Suso. At other times they made more creative use of sensory language, adapting ideas from one author and blending them with their own personal aesthetic choices. In still other cases, people chose not to use sensory language at all.

Religious orders in the fifteenth century exerted profound influence on prayer book ownership and, correspondingly, the place of the senses in vernacular theology.[57] About half of the manuscripts in the sample here identified members of religious orders as owners. The percentage would likely be higher if the sample included the many manuscripts that identified a religious community rather than an individual, or if it were possible to identify the many anonymous manuscripts that survive. Excluding these, however, 48.1 percent of the manuscripts in our sample unambiguously identified a lay owner. Closer scrutiny of the sample reveals that the most common reason for ambiguity was that ownership of prayer books frequently changed hands, passing from religious to laity, or from laity to religious. There were several variations on this pattern. Most often, laywomen owned prayer books prior to taking vows and joining a religious order. Anna Kochin (d. 1447) and Ursula Hoschlin (d. 1495), for example, owned prayer books prior to entering the Dominican women's convent of St. Katherine in Nuremberg.[58] These women lived most of their lives as wives and mothers, only entering religious life in widowhood. After entering the convent, women often kept their prayer books until death, after which the texts became the property of the convent or a designated heir. When Katharina Ruczin died in St. Katherine's of Nuremberg in 1447, her prayer book went to her biological sister Barbara. Barbara also became a nun in St. Katherine's and kept the manuscript until her own death in 1472, when it devolved to the convent library.[59]

In other instances, lay members of religious orders—those who had not taken religious vows but nonetheless remained attached to particular order and participated in a portion of its liturgical life—also kept their own prayer books, as did Friedrich zum Eselwecke, a lay brother of the Carthusians in Mainz.[60] Prayer books were also donated directly to convent libraries by members of the laity with the means to do so: Barbara Prucklerin, a "housewife" of Nuremberg, donated a manuscript to St. Katherine's around 1450.[61] Gifting prayers books could also operate in the opposite direction when wealthy laypeople patronized religious houses to produce prayer books for their own personal use. Inheritance and trade on secondhand markets removed manuscripts still further from the monastery or convent. The Swabian count Ulrich VII of Montfort, for example, received a richly illustrated, professionally scribed prayer book as a gift in the early sixteenth century. After his death in 1520, his daughter Eva inherited the manuscript, carefully maintained it, and ensured that it remained a family possession.[62]

As this last example suggests, prayer books also traversed gender boundaries. Almost one third (27.8 percent) of the sample identified male ownership. This figure is significant, as a considerable body of scholarship has suggested that the sensual, embodied language characteristic of these manuscripts was largely restricted to female piety in the late Middle Ages.[63] Without question, the origins of these patterns lay with female religious communities in the thirteenth and fourteenth centuries. By the fifteenth century, however, both women and men found such language broadly useful for devotional purposes.[64] It was common for religious men, in their roles as spiritual advisors or confessors, to write or commission prayer books for women, lay and religious alike. A curate named Hausch, for example, produced two such manuscripts for Dominican women in Freiburg im Breisgau and Konstanz at the end of the fifteenth century.[65] It was also quite common for female convents to produce prayer books, as well as other forms of spiritual literature, for male patrons.[66] Further, many prayer books were jointly owned and used by married couples. The richly illustrated manuscript of Jakob and Anna Sattler, produced in the second decade of the sixteenth century, is an especially striking example of this pattern of ownership.[67] In addition to inheritance, trade on secondhand markets moved prayer book manuscripts from male to female hands, or female to male hands. In Konstanz, for example, a manuscript owned by the nun Helena Rorerin in the 1480s was acquired by a layman called Hans Haffner in 1498.[68] This last pattern is especially important when considering how socially widespread prayer book ownership was: for people of somewhat lesser means, commissioning a manuscript directly from a religious house was a less likely scenario than acquiring one in the manner Haffner did in 1498. Some bear the marks of this gender fluidity: a late-fifteenth-century manuscript originating in Freiburg im Breisgau contains several prayers in which feminine pronouns have been written over the original male pronouns.[69]

Prayer book owners in fifteenth-century Germany represented a variety of professions, economic profiles, and levels of wealth. Priors, prioresses, nuns, monks, and lay brothers and sisters were of course common, but so too were members of the lower nobility. The manuscript of Elisabeth Ebran, daughter of a knight from the region between Regensburg and Munich, was especially important: several surviving manuscripts suggest that all or parts of it served as models for other prayer books. The prayer book of Konrad von Egolffstein, chamberlain to

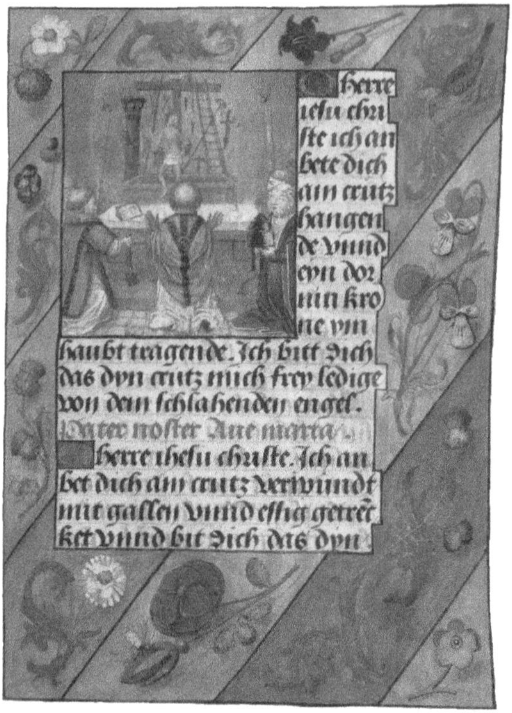

Figure 4: "Mass of St. Gregory, Prayer Book of Claus Humbracht (1508)." Ms.germ.oct. 3 (fol. 21r). Universitätsbibliothek Johann Christian Senckenberg, Frankfurt am Main.

Duke Albrecht IV of Bavaria (1447–1508), was one such manuscript, and several copies were made in the convent of St. Katherine's in Nuremberg.[70] To the west, and of a slightly more elevated social status, the countess and book collector Margareta of Rodemacher (d. 1490) kept a prayer book with exceptional miniature illustrations, to which she appended a brief family chronicle later in her life.[71] More numerous and arguably more significant were prayer book owners from the urban professional and artisanal classes. Claus Humbracht, a linen merchant from Frankfurt, commissioned an ornately illustrated prayer book in 1508 that rivaled Rodemacher's (see figure 4).[72] The wives of merchants were also enthusiastic consumers of prayer books, as the case of Katharina Tucher makes clear. Prayer books were also popular among urban bureaucrats: Margarete Bromse, whose prayer book was quoted above, was the daughter of a city councilman in the northern city Lübeck.[73] Similarly, Jakob Käbitz was the son of an official responsible for managing the grain supply in the town of Wemding (Bavaria).[74] Professionals and artisans were also enthusiastic consumers of prayer books. The Augsburg weaver Hannsen Beyss carefully kept a manuscript (ca. 1456), replete with prayers for a variety of liturgical occasions.[75] Katharina Kannengiesser's prayer book accompanied her as she rose through the social ranks of the city of Cologne. Apparently from an artisanal background, Kannengiesser later married into the city's ruling class, becoming the mayor's wife in the late fifteenth century.[76] Finally, the aforementioned schoolmaster Lentzen Hanns (d. 1541) hailed from the region around Freiburg im Breisgau, acquired a prayer book in 1483, and carried it while traveling to different jobs throughout southwestern Germany and Switzerland.[77] Beyond these specific examples, numerous manuscripts identified their female owners as "house wives," strongly suggesting an urban, artisanal social profile.[78]

Prayer book ownership also shared a common geography. Prayer book production and consumption was largely a southern German, urban affair, and the sample here reflects this: if we assume the river Main as an approximate border between southern and northern regions (a common way to approximate the divide), then 88.8 percent of the manuscripts in our sample qualify as southern. This geographical distribution was largely the effect of the Observant Reform movement, which centered in southern German towns and had somewhat limited impacts in less urbanized northern Germany. Seeking to improve religious life through stricter discipline and better education, cloistered nuns and monks systematically went to work copying and circulating manuscripts, while monasteries and convents sought external donors to supplement the expansion of their libraries.[79] Nowhere was the impact more profound than in the Dominican women's convent of St. Katherine in Nuremberg, which expanded its manuscript library from thirty-six manuscripts in 1428, prior to the introduction of reform, to nearly six hundred by the end of the century.[80] The significance of this cultural work extended well beyond the walls of convents and monasteries. Laypersons with the necessary economic and cultural capital enthusiastically participated, financing, donating, and consuming much of what these religious communities produced.[81] From these southern urban centers, prayer book culture traveled north along the Rhine river to Cologne; to a lesser extent, it permeated northern German towns like Bremen, Münster, and Lübeck, reaching as far east as Prague.[82]

Regardless of their particular urban setting, when using their prayer books, owners responded to and made use of some common cultural paradigms. Learned discourse on sensible sacramentality was of course important, but it was typically mediated to increasingly wide social circles through the dissemination of fourteenth-century vernacular mysticism. Particularly through the initiatives of Dominican convents and monasteries touched by Observant Reform, more people gained direct access to the writings of luminaries of the mystical tradition like Henry Suso, Catherine of Siena (d. 1380), Johannes Tauler (d. 1361), Margaret Ebner (d. 1351), and Meister Eckhart (d. 1328). Of the surviving manuscript copies of texts from Eckhart, Suso, and Tauler, 80 percent were produced in the fifteenth century.[83] Suso was in all likelihood the most widely read author of the fifteenth century, his practical devotional handbook, the *Little*

Book of Eternal Wisdom, probably the most-read single text. Likewise, Catherine of Siena's biography was translated into German around 1400 and endured as a "best-seller" of manuscript culture for the remainder of the century.[84] Beyond complete works of individual authors, a wide array of popular lyrics, poetry, letters, sermons, dialogues, hagiography, and images mediated their ideas to lay audiences in fragmentary form.[85]

The fact that people frequently collected this material in their prayer books suggests that they found the language useful and meaningful for their own purposes. On one level, prayer books were normative, didactic sources that originated with those tasked with defining and controlling religious meaning. Critically, however, they simultaneously opened up space in which ordinary people could exercise a limited degree of agency to respond creatively to make sense of their own experience. To borrow Virginia Reinburg's helpful explanation, as an individualized "archive," the prayer book "framed religious practice for its users."[86] German vernacular prayer books, like French books of hours, were "the product of many hands," including not only the scribes, artists, and religious advisors engaged in their design and execution, but also the lay patrons who commissioned and used them. The collaboration produced "a prayer book in which texts and images were woven together in a compelling work of the devotional imagination."[87] The prayer book did not emerge from the scriptorium as a completed, self-contained object: in the hands of owners, each prayer book remained a dynamic archive of individual and communal devotional life. People added new prayers they found meaningful, rebound them with other works, or sewed in pilgrim badges and other images.[88] Lentzen Hanns, who took his prayer book with him as he moved from job to job in southwestern Germany and Switzerland, added a variety of prayers over the course of his life. Because of his itinerant lifestyle, he found it useful to include several prayers for "when you want to travel over land" or water.[89] The Augsburg weaver Hannsen Beyss added his Eucharist prayers in 1490.[90] Over the course of the next four years, he added a collection of legendary tales on the miraculous powers of the Eucharist, as well as explanations of the various kinds of symbolism in the tales.[91]

In this domain of circumscribed agency, prayer book owners also manipulated the sensory language they encountered. Prayer books of course contained heavy doses of conventional language, but the content of individual exemplars varied significantly. Collecting and archiving prayers provided owners "multiple personal scripts for prayer. The scripts could be—indeed, by definition were—modified by the books' owners, who used, read, and looked at their books in wildly different ways."[92] Particularly striking in this regard is the way in which people made use of Henry Suso's work: of the sample taken here, 24.1 percent specifically included Suso's Eucharist prayer, referenced in chapter 2. An additional 7.4 percent contained other excerpts from the *Little Book of Eternal*

Wisdom. The creative use of Suso and other authorities manifested in other ways as well. Eucharist prayers in the manuscript of Lorenz Orreum of Prague (ca. 1466), for example, borrowed heavily from Suso's language of affective devotion, beginning with an address to the Eucharist as "eternal wisdom" and "food to my thirsty soul" and ending with an overture to the "sweet, good-tasting bread of heaven [to] come today powerfully into my soul, strengthen it against all your enemies, [and] light in me the light of Christian faith."[93] Others made use of imagery of sucking blood from the wound in Christ's side, a trope associated with Catherine of Siena.[94] Eucharist prayers in an anonymous manuscript in the city of Münster reflected on the sweetness, good smell, and cool, satisfying mildness of Christ's body and blood, while pleading that "I might suck from your wounded side the yield of the spirit and the wine of life."[95]

Some prayer books exhibited even more idiomatic sensory language that nonetheless bore a close relationship to the intersensorial patterns we've encountered above. The mid-fifteenth-century manuscript associated with Jakob Käbitz, for example, included a series of somewhat unusual, and by comparison highly literary, Eucharist prayers addressed to the "body of God." In addition to the common ascriptions of its taste as "sweetness over all honey," prayers reflected on receiving the Host as "a powerful thaw of all grace . . . whereby fragrance flows through the very arid earth of the heart of humanity, so that it is revitalized in virtue."[96] Reception of course retained all the physical and metaphysical benefits typically associated with it, imbuing body and soul with strength and power, enlightening conscience, and saving the communicant from the blindness of sin.[97]

Finally, while most prayer books included some form of Eucharist prayers, not all deployed sensory language so enthusiastically. The weaver Hannsen Beyss, for example, added several Eucharist prayers to his manuscript in the late fifteenth century but typically described "enjoying" the Eucharist not as a sweet taste, feeling, or smell, but as "most worthy divinity."[98] At other points, the prayers identified the Eucharist as the "font of all divinity and sweetness," but on balance, the manuscript avoided sensory language, replacing it with more abstract concepts like "mildness," "divinity," "goodness," "worthiness," or "holiness."[99] The early-sixteenth-century manuscript of the housewife Elisabeta Bontin of Oberschaffshausen favored similar vocabulary and avoided the language of sweetness altogether.[100] To be sure, the subdued sensory language in the prayer books of Beyss and Bontin was rather exceptional, but it nonetheless underscores the point that individual owners exercised a degree of agency in how they consumed late medieval sensory culture. While agency here should not be confused with intention, the social history of prayer book ownership suggests, in broad strokes, that something was at stake in sensory language on the eve of the Reformation. People made use of it because they found it to be a meaningful way of articulating their own religious experience. They borrowed it, played with it, or, in some cases, ignored it. Like Katharina Tucher, the moves they made in this domain reflected their development as vernacular theologians. They built upon what the institutional church provided them, but they manipulated it in new and creative ways that spoke to their immediate circumstances.

Perhaps somewhat paradoxically, many of the same church authorities that had promoted the positive, salvific side of the sensual coin of humanity were also deeply troubled when they confronted its manipulation by vernacular theologians like Katharina Tucher. The coin had two sides, after all, and simple people, even those who could read and write in the vernacular, could easily be led down the path of sin. This tension produced what I called earlier a kind of "double-externalization" of church ritual. Not only external in its sensuous appeal to the body, church ritual also became alienated from what many male church authorities imagined to be the normative center of the Christian community.

In some instances, the drive to externalize ritual led male church authorities toward a stronger gendering of the senses, consolidating associations between dangerous sensuality and femininity. Whatever their meaning to those who claimed to experience them, visions and auditions like those reported in Katharina Tucher's diary represented a challenge to the institutional authority of the church in the eyes of many clergymen, especially those caught up in the zeal of the Observant Reform movement. In the previous two centuries, claiming to have received visions or direct inspiration from God afforded women a degree of religious authority unseen in the western church since the apostolic age. The institutional church had even attempted to coopt it for the purposes of improving popular religious life from time to time. Even as it did so, however, the church was becoming increasingly preoccupied with the problem of heresy, and the apparent individualism of these forms of piety among the laity raised many questions in the minds of clergymen. If women could claim to receive direct visions or auditions from God, weren't they short-circuiting the sacramental authority of the church? Somewhat paradoxically, clergymen were able to ignore the fact that a good deal of these reported experiences were grounded in the ritual life of the church in the most basic ways: above all, the Eucharist served as the central focus of devotion and the catalyst for most of the sensory culture of the late Middle Ages. Perhaps even more troubling was a related question of religious epistemology: Were these women experiencing divine inspiration, or demonic illusion? As Nancy Caciola has demonstrated, church authorities by the fifteenth century tended to be more convinced it was the latter. According to prevailing cultural norms, female bodies were simply physiologically more susceptible to infiltration by demons. These concerns culminated with the publication of Heinrich Kraemer and Jakob Sprenger's *Malleus maleficarum* in 1486, and the great age of witchcraft persecutions in the next century. The female visionary of the late Middle Ages had been reborn in the witch of the early modern era.[101]

In the German-speaking world, these issues weighed heavily on the minds of leading reformers and led to a concomitant gendering of religious sensuality more broadly. As noted in chapter 2, the revelations of Bridget of Sweden came under intense suspicion at the Council of Basel in the 1430s. Spiritual letters to female monastic communities in the fifteenth century, written by male authorities, took an increasingly cautious approach the ritual life and material culture of the church, and the language of sensation commonly deployed to explicate it. In a letter titled "On True Devotion," Eberhard Mardach (d. 1430), prior of St. Katherine's convent in Nuremberg in the late 1420s, warned against confusing the divine with human sensuality. Addressing the many women who had come, Mardach noted: "[You claim] in your devotion, you have and feel such sensible sweetness and such good smell in your mouths, nose, and bodies, such that it is unspeakable," and he used this as evidence to argue that the senses were easily coopted by the devil and were ultimately something to be transcended.[102] Others framed the issue in less extreme terms, viewing the language of sensation found in devotional materials like prayer books as a form of eroticism. On balance, it tended to stir up fleshly desire rather than devout charity in the hearts of churchgoers, leading them into sin.[103] By the end of the century, the gendering of the senses as feminine had become much more widespread, particularly in learned culture. Other qualities commonly associated with the female sex, such as frivolity, foolishness, and attachment to worldly things, attached themselves more consistently to representations of the five senses.[104]

Along a somewhat different trajectory, a second intellectual response to the popular reception of sensual religion cohered somewhat later in the fifteenth century, taking an anthropological view and stressing the indifference of sensuality in religious practice. In some respects, this was a harvest of the sacramentality of Hugh of St. Victor, who had taken an anthropological view of religious practice already in the twelfth century. By the late fifteenth and early sixteenth centuries, however, new concerns motivated discussions of ritual practice. The early violent expansion of European power into Africa, Asia, and the Americas confronted churchmen with an expanding array of new civilizations and cultures far removed from the familiar system of beliefs and practices that prevailed at home. Non-Christian religions brought thinkers to face to face with the problems of superstition and idolatry with increasing urgency. If so many heretofore unknown peoples were worshipping the sensual and material in lieu of the true essence of divine, they were certainly damned. But how could a merciful God have condemned so many people to such a fate? The solution, developed with particular force among early humanists influenced by Italian Neoplatonism, was known as *prisca theologia*—original theology, or more commonly, "natural religion." The theory of *prisca theologia* held that all religions had a common origin in prehistory, when humanity enjoyed a more direct relationship with the true God. All humans had begun by worshipping the same God and, due to the natural limits imposed by the human body and soul, had developed a cult of sensual practice to do so. As people spread across the earth, civilizations rose, fell, and were separated by great amounts of time and space: the natural outcome of this was the evolution of religious cults and the diversification of appeals to the senses. This diversity, however, was less important than the essential fact that all religions had originated in worship of the one true God. An element of this lingered in all religions and rendered all outward forms of religious practice ultimately *adiaphora*, or matters of indifference in the broadest philosophical sense.[105]

This view of religious practice justified surprising conclusions among many of the same intellectuals who made strong arguments for the positive role that the senses could play in religion. In his role as a reforming bishop concerned with the uniformity and probity of religious practice in his diocese, Nicholas Cusanus advocated the salvific side of the sensual coin. In his philosophical dialogues, however, Cusanus took a broad view in which Christianity was located on a spectrum with other religions of the world, even polytheistic ones: "The entire diversity lay in rites rather than in the worship of one God. From all the writings, which had been collected into one, it was learned that since the very beginning all have always presupposed God and worshipped Him in all their religious practices."[106] This led Cusanus to the radical conclusion that *all* external practices of Christianity, even the celebration of the Eucharist, were technically *adiaphora*.[107] Other like-minded humanists, such as Hartmann Schedel and Conrad Celtis in Nuremberg, and Conrad Mutianus in Erfurt, adopted Cusanus's position. It even gained traction in a number of the earliest published pseudo-ethnographic works of the sixteenth century.[108]

Not all took this route, however. On the eve of the Reformation, in the hands of more reform-minded humanists like Erasmus, *adiaphora* became more dangerous. In the interest of intellectual clarity and consistency, Erasmus made a less subtle, although hierarchically clearer, distinction between profane senses and sacred spirit than had often prevailed in the fifteenth century. Just as in biblical hermeneutics, where the external letter of the text could distract from or distort its true spiritual meaning, people's misguided attachment to outward ceremonies threatened to turn them into something other than true Christians. At best, they might be coarse simpletons, perhaps with a vague inclination toward paganism. At worst, they were responsible for bringing about their own perdition, to the delight of the devil.[109] Ritual and its sensuousness had become an object of intense debate and, by the early sixteenth century, seemed to be migrating away from what at least some thinkers considered to be the normative core of the Christian community.

For their own part, vernacular theologians like Katharina Tucher and the various prayer book owners we have encountered here were largely content to ignore these increasingly negative views of religious sensuality. Both men and women continued to embrace the senses with great enthusiasm in the first decades of the sixteenth century, much as they had since they began to "harvest" its potential a century earlier. Among the learned elites tasked with controlling the meaning of ritual, however, the sinful side of the sensual coin was growing in prominence. The externalization of sensuous worship and its separation from the normative core of Christianity remained persistent tropes when Protestantism emerged on the scene. The notion that attachment to the sensuous world was a problem specific to the female sex, or non-Christians, strengthened associations between sin and the senses and motivated reform-minded individuals to imagine and identify with its opposite. These men came to see themselves as true Christians, besieged by the overbearing sensuousness of traditional worship. Impulses set in motion during the fifteenth century therefore resonated into the sixteenth century, shaking the foundations of late medieval Christianity until giving way the cultural earthquake that was the Reformation movement in the early 1520s. Even if they ultimately did not live up to their own expansive visions for leveling traditional Christianity, their construction of a narrative of the Reformation as a desensualizing moment in the history of the religion came to define their worldview and has the shaped how people talk about the break between medieval and modern worlds ever since.

Before we turn to this matter, however, it is necessary to draw some conclusions from part 1 of this study. Here, we have dealt with religion in late medieval Germany as a matter of sensory production and sensory consumption. It is worth returning to what these concepts mean in order to take a broad view of where this particular work fits into some of the major narratives of sensory history. Production refers quite simply to the objects, practices, and environments that appeal to, and occupy the attention of, the human senses at a given historical moment.[110] When discussing the late Middle Ages, we have often been accustomed to think about sensory production in a few different ways. With respect to worship in particular, the common refrain has been that "fifteenth-century European Christianity was aesthetically vibrant," rich in the array of things it held out to churchgoers for consumption.[111] Additionally, we have often seen this rich sensory production as working according to a strongly visualist logic. The entire assemblage of sensuous things associated with the Mass, or ritual practice more broadly, were intentionally placed to promote a kind of spectacle or "visual theophany," as Charles Zika once put it.[112] The internal dynamics of these claims have never really been tested up to this point but rather have been taken as articles of faith, for lack of a better term, by specialists in late medieval and Reformation religion, and even to some extent by those dedicated to moving the field of sensory history forward.

As we have seen here, however, it is simply inaccurate to assert late medieval ritual production subordinated nonvisual modalities to the sense of sight, and it is not enough to say that religious life was rich in aesthetic appeal. The only guiding rules of sensory production were concrete and practical, grounded in local political economies: What kinds of stuff did a church have on hand? Was a school attached to the church to furnish it with a choir? Was there money to repair broken liturgical vessels? How was our liturgy supposed to be distinct from that of our neighbors? Answers to these types of questions lay at the heart of the matter, making the reality of late medieval sensory production not nearly so coherent as we are usually given to think. It is not necessarily a problem to emphasize late medieval ritual as an aesthetically rich or vibrant environment. In a certain sense, this is something of a truism, as rituals are almost by definition aesthetically rich environments.[113] It is, however, problematic that the tendency has been to make the upper limits of what could be achieved in practice stand in for all of late medieval worship. The maximal has thus almost always become the "bare minimum." In truth, however, the sensory production of religion was highly varied from one place to the next, with a major line of division prevailing between urban and rural spaces. Over the course of the late Middle Ages, as cities grew in wealth and as civic officials arrogated to themselves more control over local ritual life, liturgies often evolved to approximate something resembling the upper limits of sensory worship we commonly imagine. However, this was an expensive and organizationally complex production and was, simply put, beyond the means of most communities. Instead, substitution, abbreviation, and improvisation were the rules of sensory production. People made do with the resources they had on hand. Instead of burning incense imported from the Arabian Peninsula, they might use an essential oil derived from local herbs. Or they might not use anything, in which case they confronted more acutely the bodily odors of their fellow churchgoers, famously so noxious to the delicate sensibilities of churchmen like Thomas Aquinas.[114] To be clear, this is not to imply that rural worship was "less sensual" than its wealthy urban counterpart. Monophonic congregational singing was just as "aural" as polyphonic choral music accompanied by an organ. It was, however, significantly different, and failure to appreciate this difference runs the risk of reinforcing some of the same stereotypes about this period, and the more distant past in general, that scholars often claim to be challenging. Assertions about the rich aesthetic appeal of late medieval religion, without qualification, can be read quite easily as an indication that it was *more* sensual than that which came later, even when this is not the intention. Attending to the political economy of sensory production hews closer to reality and inhibits the development of such a narrative.

So much for sensory production in late medieval Germany. What about consumption, or the historically and culturally specific ways people take in their sensory environments? Time and place shape the senses people attend to, even, in some cases, setting the limits of what is or isn't perceivable. They also condition judgments about specific objects of the senses: what is pleasing or painful, delightful or disgusting, is an effect of the peculiar, historically situated, sensory ideology to which one ascribes.[115] Sensuous experience of the world is therefore not purely physical but rather a matter of how the objective world of sensory production aligns with the cultural contexts defining sensory consumption. How has scholarship addressed this relationship in the late Middle Ages? Mostly, a harmonious interpretation has emerged: ecclesiastical authorities promoted the idea that sensuous engagement with church ritual, especially the Eucharist, could move people and in so doing yield rich benefits, physically, psychologically, and spiritually. For the most part, people embraced this idea. The most exceptional example of how this impacted the religious lives of ordinary people has been the supposed popularity of sacramental gazing, which came to define people's experience of the Mass in the fifteenth century.[116]

For the most part, this interpretive turn has been a welcome corrective to the well-worn narratives of the decadence and decline of the late medieval church. The idea that the institutional church was irredeemably corrupt and was incapable of engaging ordinary people in anything more than the most superficial ways in the fifteenth century has effectively served as a kind of preface to the Reformation in popular histories of the period and has even been somewhat surprisingly resilient among certain academic circles.[117] There are some areas where a more dynamic historical view could nonetheless benefit and nuance what has become, for the most part, a scholarly consensus. It is certainly important to take into account the subject positions of those who left behind records discussing the consumption of sensuous worship. Among learned elites, the promotion of a theory of sensuous sacramentality was essential to consolidating their status as ritual experts. They promoted the affective bond established between churchgoers and sacraments, especially the Mass, through its multimodal sensory appeal. The power of these appeals, not restricted to the sense of sight, to shape people's souls intellectually, emotionally, and morally was a statement defining the reality of sensory consumption, but it was also essential to the construction of the clergy's primary pastoral role as sacramental ministers. In each case, learned discourse sought to define and carefully control what it meant to sense the ritual environment offered up to churchgoers. More ordinary sorts of people consumed religion in this environment, and when they did, they enthusiastically embraced the senses. This does not mean, however, that their embrace was fully consonant with the expectations of learned elites. The fifteenth century saw a flourishing of vernacular theologians who developed their own meanings from the sensory culture they encountered. They made playful use of this culture, but this shouldn't be seen as a sign of diminished sophistication. Such play with custom and convention, as Clifford Geertz reminded us long ago, can be profoundly and disarmingly deep.[118] For vernacular theologians, the senses were a useful way to narrate their own individual, albeit historically situated, experiences of religion. These experiences certainly bear strong traces of the dominant tropes of learned discourse, but they also could break with and rearrange them in creative, if somewhat limited, ways.

The more dynamic, historicized vision of sensory production and consumption in late medieval Germany advanced here has aimed at prohibiting the construction of oversimplifying narratives of change over time often attributed to this era and cited in discussions of the "origins" of the Reformation. The reality of lived religion at this time was bewilderingly complex, and what we have examined here represents only a small portion of this complexity. Nonetheless, we can at least now say that we have the beginnings of a hermeneutics of suspicion from which we can approach Protestantism's relationship to this world. We have a feel for some of the major sensory contours of late medieval religious life and, through that familiarity, can recognize that any attempts to describe it as intensely sensual, decadent, and inexorably giving way to a necessarily less sensual, purified form of Christianity in the sixteenth century have an ideological flavor to them. This ideology has remained, in one form or another, an important part of how we conceive of the story of Christianity and of modernity more broadly. It too has its own history, and in part 2 of this study we examine its origins and impact in the sixteenth century.

4 The Reformation of the Senses in Early Evangelical Culture

In the early sixteenth century, the place of the senses in religion was deeply ambiguous, subject to wide variations, contradictions, and disputes. The church was still somehow managing to hold together this assemblage of divergent impulses, but an articulate, activist minority, centered in the cities of the German-speaking world, increasingly vocalized the need to resolve the paradox of the senses in religion. Prior to the 1520s, the most visible exponents of this position were reformers and humanists like Erasmus of Rotterdam, but the first people to call themselves Protestants became part of this milieu. Convinced by the humanist call for closer engagement with the text of the Gospels (*Evangelium*) and more widespread preaching that disparaged religious sensuality, initially these people simply called themselves "evangelical" Christians. However, they very soon began to see their relationship to the sensory world of the late medieval church in terms of a rupture more fundamental than someone like Erasmus had ever envisioned.

Recent scholarship emphasizing significant continuity between late medieval and Reformation-era Christianity has overlooked this most central aspect of the history of the senses.[1] While there were strong continuities in many domains of belief and practice, the early Protestants did not always perceive that to be the case. Indeed, the first Protestants recognized themselves in a mythology that framed their new religion as utterly different from what their parents and ancestors had practiced. It was less sensual, less concerned with "mere ritual" or "empty ceremony" and more oriented toward the properly interior, spiritual, and disembodied domains of "true religion." Peter Reychart, a furrier swept up in the ebullient pulse of the evangelical movement of the early 1520s, put the matter simply and effectively: in the old faith, people had worshipped "according to fleshly sense," whereas in the brave new evangelical world, true Christians' devotional focus was internal, withdrawing from the senses and unfolding purely "according to the spirit."[2] This narrative I call the reformation of the senses. The reformation of the senses was a story early Protestants told themselves about themselves. It did not provide an empirical description of reality, but it did provide a lens through which people viewed, experienced, and understood that reality.

Those who narrated the reformation of the senses painted in broad, unambiguous strokes, making both evangelical Christianity and its late medieval precursors seem much more coherent than either actually were. Late medieval religion had been purely superficial, consumed utterly by the production of an overwhelming sensory spectacle. The Reformation brought with it a comprehensive transformation of this scene—a perfect "stripping of the altars," to borrow Eamon Duffy's felicitous expression.[3] Although usually regarded as liturgically moderate, or even conservative, Martin Luther was hardly averse to telling this story. Already in 1520, in his famous *Babylonian Captivity of the Church*, Luther condemned a variety of extraneous things that had accumulated in the practice of the Mass since the thirteenth century—"such things as vestments, ornaments, chants, prayers, organs, candles, and the whole pageantry of outward things."[4] The obvious implication was that a new, purified form of Christianity would come to its senses by ridding itself of these innovations. Luther made this still more explicit in a sermon he preached on the Mass that same year. "If we wish to keep and understand the mass properly," he exhorted, "we must let go of everything that the eyes and senses might present and mark out in this business, be it clothing, chiming, song, ornament, prayer, carrying, elevating, laying, or whatever else might be done in the mass."[5]

The reformation of the senses, as a narrative, insisted on difference between this ensemble of sensuous things and early evangelical religion. The story was constitutive of early nascent Protestant identity. It is important to keep in mind that, before reformers took any tangible action to change late medieval practice, they told themselves the story of sensory reformation. It was the first act of iconoclasm, and it unfolded in the rhetoric and imaginative landscape of would-be reformers well before we can speak of Lutherans, Calvinists, Anabaptists, or any other denomination as coherent and distinct in any meaningful sense. Before these movements coalesced, the reformation of the senses had been accomplished, at least culturally and narratologically.

This chapter takes up that transformation, tracing the emergence of sensory reformation in vernacular discourse of the early 1520s. It shows that Luther was far from alone in his storytelling. His call was echoed, amplified, and transcended within a few short years. It is important that those who elaborated the myth of sensory reformation could point back to Luther and claim a certain kind of solidarity with the Wittenberg monk, while simultaneously speaking to broader cultural concerns. Early evangelicals transformed traditional Christianity into an undifferentiated, hypersensual thing by consistently foregrounding the various objects and practices that could appeal to the senses, and they forged negative associations between this assemblage and women and non-Christian cultures. Late medieval worship was feminine and foreign—completely opposed to the virile, German Christianity they liked to talk about. Evangelicals completed the narrative of sensory reformation by contrasting the chaotic hyperaesthesia of traditional Christianity with proper evangelical devotion to the Word. This was a profound rupture with the late Middle Ages, and one that took place principally in the urban centers of the German-speaking world, reflecting the imaginations and ideological needs of a highly educated, mostly male constituency. Despite its narrow origins, the early evangelical dominance of communication technology—namely, the printing press—spread the story of sensory reformation to other segments of society. Although it was just a story, the reformation of the senses had profound implications for the religious realities these people inhabited, shaping how they understood themselves as well as religious outsiders.

The reformation of the senses began well before the various Protestant denominations differentiated themselves from one another and coalesced around distinctive, well-defined doctrines of belief and practice. Many reformers in the fifteenth century had of course regarded the religious provision for sensuality with unease and suspicion. By the second decade of the sixteenth century, more people knew that traditional Christianity was preoccupied with sensuality, and that this preoccupation was a dangerous thing. Johann von Staupitz (1465/68–1524), famous as one of Luther's teachers, often condemned popular devotion to "outward ceremony" and claimed that the essence of Christianity was that which "none of the senses can feel, but it is felt by the faith."[6] Staupitz's rejection of religious sensuality had its origins in a reassertion of St. Augustine's strong distinction between interior, metaphorical or "spiritual" senses, and exterior, bodily senses—something that had often been blurred in the religious culture of the late Middle Ages.[7] Like his intellectual hero, Staupitz clearly assigned primary importance to the former and tended to disparage the latter. The distinction was highly useful rhetorically for the purposes of defining true Christianity, and he regularly deployed it in his sermons.[8] In other respects, Staupitz reflected a broader cultural pattern, dimensions of which could be traced to the mysticism of male Dominicans like Meister Eckhart, who, in contrast to someone like Henry Suso, much more clearly emphasized the human-divine bond as both asocial and asensual.[9] It also resonated with the humanist critique, made so often but perhaps most eloquently by Erasmus of Rotterdam: Christianity's overbearing ceremoniousness focused on the purely external while neglecting the underlying philosophical meaning of the Gospels, which of course was a matter of disembodied, intellectual introspection.[10]

These kinds of criticisms of late medieval piety circulated widely in the spoken and printed word in the first decades of the sixteenth century. Staupitz traveled extensively throughout the German-speaking world, preaching in Tübingen, Salzburg, Nuremberg, and Munich, among other places. He spoke to the concerns of urban, educated circles of fairly powerful men: civic authorities, administrators, and members of the clergy, as well as academics, intellectuals, and artisans.[11] Serving briefly as a professor of biblical theology at the university of Wittenberg, he directly influenced some of the first leaders of the Reformation, including Martin Luther and his colleague, Andreas Bodenstein von Karlstadt (1477/86–1541).[12] In Nuremberg, common interest in both Staupitz and Erasmus brought together famous intellectuals and artists, including Willibald Pirckheimer (1470–1530) and Albrecht Dürer (1471–1528), with officials concerned with improving moral and religious life in the city, including the city treasurer Hieronymus Ebner (1477–1532), city-council clerk Lazarus Spengler (1479–1534), and the Wittenberg-trained legal counsel Christoph Scheurl (1481–1542), as well as clergy like Wenceslaus Linck (1483–1547), the former prior of the Augustinian Order in Wittenberg, whom Staupitz dispatched as a preacher to Nuremberg in early 1517.[13] Similar associations appeared in cities all over Germany at the same time, laying the groundwork for the evangelical reform movements that would first take root in the 1520s. These associations functioned as semiformal institutional avenues by which ideas could travel.[14] Of course, ideas flowed through other, less formal channels as well: sixteenth-century Germany was still a predominately oral culture. From the pulpit, the notion that the church was overly preoccupied with sensual, bodily devotion wound its way into public discourse in the streets, taverns, and the privacy of the home.[15]

Whatever its mode of transmission, criticism of sensuous worship gained a much wider currency on the urban scene during the first decades of the sixteenth century than it ever had in the fifteenth. In Nuremberg, three years after Staupitz had graced the city with a series of Advent sermons, Wenceslaus Linck reminded congregations that the "lustfulness of the flesh" and "desire of the eyes" cultivated in contemporary church practice constantly hindered the heart from feeling true faith and "love of God." The Word of Scripture, by contrast, constituted the only sure path to salvation.[16] In the same year, Lazarus Spengler made a similar argument but cast attention on more specific practices. Criticizing the clergy for confusing poor, simple Christians and disquieting their consciences, he condemned the church's "external ceremonies," including praying many Psalters, "babbling the rosary, performing many pilgrimages and fasts, great churches, lighting lights, [and] comforting poor souls with holy water."[17] The sensory pandemonium evoked by this list of practices stood in sharp contrast to the divine simplicity of the Word. The former represented "flesh" and the law of the Old Testament, the latter pure spirit and grace.[18]

The Nuremberg circle was perhaps somewhat precocious, but public opinion in many German cities was soon to follow suit. As Martin Luther's dispute with the Church of Rome expanded into public discourse, those who identified as fellow evangelicals took their message to the printing presses in an unprecedented fashion. Most of their publications appeared as short vernacular pamphlets—"cheap, crude, and effective," as Robert Scribner once characterized them.[19] Between 1500 and 1530 an estimated ten thousand pamphlet editions appeared in Germany. Of these pamphlets, 75 percent were produced in the years 1520–1526 alone, the majority by evangelicals.[20] Specialists often refer to this short period of exceptionally intense polemical debate and publishing activity as the "wild growth" (*Wildwuchs*) years of the Reformation. During this heady period, there was a good deal of inconsistency, divergence, and confusion in how early evangelicals understood the significance of various elements of Luther's message. Doctrinal differences between denominations that would eventually come to be known as Lutherans, reformed (or sometimes Zwinglians, after the Swiss reformer Huldrych Zwingli), and others had yet to crystallize. All could nonetheless agree on their opposition to a wide array of beliefs and practices in the traditional Church of Rome.[21]

In the midst of the excitement and confusion, the story of sensory reformation took more definitive shape. The story appeared in many genres, from dialogues and polemical essays to popular plays and poetry. Regardless of genre, the story of sensory reformation took a common form, similar to Lazarus Spengler's 1519 critique: long lists of substantives, identifying objects and practices of traditional Christianity, strung together to evoke the benighted state of Christendom, dissolved by the new evangelical faith's central focus on "the Word." The shoemaker Hans Sachs (1494–1576), also of Nuremberg, has left us one of the most extensive and evocative examples of how early evangelicals told the story of sensory reformation in his 1523 poem, *The Wittenberg Nightingale*. In the poem, the nightingale represented Martin Luther, whose brilliant Gospel song dispelled the darkness of traditional Christianity under the tyrannical yoke of the papacy. At the vanguard of the Church of Rome's assault was the ritual environment it held out to poor, honest Christians. Sachs chose simply to list, in rhymed verse, the objects and practices most closely associated with this environment. "Day and night," the church "blared" with

> vigils, fasting, long prayers, with flagellations, laying cross-wise, with kneeling, bowing, bending, stooping, with ringing bells, blasting organs . . . with relics, carrying banners, with censing and with baptizing bells, with filling lamps, selling grace, with blessings of church, wax, salt, and water, and similar things . . . with

> sacrifice and with burning little candles, with pilgrimage and worshipping saints, fasting in the evening, feasting in the day . . . with confraternities and rosaries . . . with kissing paxes, viewing relics, with decorating the altar at great cost, altarpieces . . . velvet vestments, golden chalices, with monstrances and silver images, in convents collecting rent and interest, all of this the pope calls divine worship.[22]

Sachs's rhythmic, repetitive listing of these objects and practices echoed and amplified Spengler's shorter list and clearly drew from Luther's writings, especially the *Babylonian Captivity*. It proved a powerful rhetorical device in the early years of the Reformation, reflecting the oral culture in which these new religious messages emerged and took shape. Carrying the "liturgical *gravitas* of a hymn or chant or creed," as Peter Matheson points out, the aesthetic of early reformation rhetoric reinforced the emotional impact of the evangelical message and likely aided in the process of its memorization.[23]

It also had the effect of reifying the sensory elements of late medieval religion: eliding the complexities of their production and consumption, the *Wittenberg Nightingale* established a powerful, easily comprehensible narrative of change over time. The late medieval church *was* the litany of objects chained together in Sachs's poem, and its relation to churchgoers was one of overwhelming sensuality, or hyperaesthesia.[24] By contrast, evangelical Christianity emanated from the measured tone and brilliant clarity of Martin Luther's words, which themselves sprang from the very Word of Scripture. Sachs ensured that no one would mistake the contrariety between old and new: throughout the poem, the Church of Rome was tied not only to tyranny but also to a whole legion of hellish wolves and demons. The devil himself, and Antichrist, stood behind the sensory production of late medieval Christendom.

Such binary, apocalyptic imagery was common in the polemical disputes of the early 1520s. It reflected the moral certainty with which early evangelicals confronted the problem of church reform, as well as a much more deeply rooted culture that tended to emphasize "polarity, duality, antithesis, and contrariety" to understand and describe all manner of "natural, intellectual, and social phenomena."[25] In the cosmological struggle between light and dark, good and evil, God and the devil, people consistently identified sensory production and consumption at the frontlines. Other hyperaesthetic litanies, similar to Sachs's, abound in the pamphlet literature of the Reformation's wild growth period, deployed metaphorically for the Church of Rome. Given the sheer volume of evangelical publishing in this era, it would be difficult to identify all examples, but a small sample of materials from the years 1518 through 1525 underscores the fact that the rhetoric was widespread: of two hundred pamphlets identifiable with 102 different individual authors, a full third contain litanies similar to that of Sachs's, of varying lengths.[26] Some, like Sachs, wove litanies into rhymed verse. Others spent more time expounding their significance in prose, while still others rather artlessly listed objects in long chains. Closer examination of a few examples makes clear the power that such imagery held in the imaginations of early reformers, lay and clerical alike.

One of the most prolific polemicists to tell this story of sensory reformation was Johann Eberlin von Günzburg, formerly a Franciscan who had been a strict adherent of the Observant Reform movement most of his life. In 1520 he encountered Luther's writings, left the Franciscan order, and arrived in Wittenberg by 1522. From there he traveled and preached in Ulm, Basel, Rheinfelden, Rottenburg, Erfurt, and other towns, leaving nascent reform movements in his wake before landing a more permanent position as preacher in Rotenburg ob der Tauber in 1525. Like many other evangelical preachers and polemicists, Eberlin had frequently referred to traditional Christianity as sensuous "jugglery" (*Gauckelwerck*) in his sermons from these years. While preaching in Erfurt in 1524, he clarified what he meant, satirizing popular devotion to the sensuous dimensions of church practice:

> Look at this house [church]: how wide, how tall—a steeple like a mountain keep! What long windows, how well plastered, how diverse the choir and church, what exquisite colored Venetian glasswork, what beautiful pictures painted on the wall. How much iron and lead used in the steeple and entire house—even more than the straw in a peasant's house! What beautiful stalls in the choir, for chattering, fat priests . . . additionally, exquisite stone at many altars, beautiful cloths upon them, and beautiful golden altarpieces, tin and brass candelabra . . . so many rods, banners, skirting, exquisite doors . . . one must have mass books, song books, crucifixes, monstrances of silver, oil canisters, little houses for the sacrament, baptismal fonts, and fully ornamented clothes, choir robes, and albs of fine linen, velvet, silk, damask, et cetera . . . one must have altar candles, angels for the altar to hold the candles, much oil for the lamps, and wax for the candles . . . silver and golden chalices and patens, velvet corporal cloths, pearl paxes, linen for corporals . . . and many cloths, jugs, basins . . . we must have a sacristan, a pastor, sexton, choir boys, et cetera, and many bells.[27]

Other clergy like Günzburg, who became entangled in the evangelical movement, also began to see traditional Christianity as a litany of hyperaesthetic abuses. Matthäus Hitzschold, a former Benedictine prior preaching in Mühlhausen (Thuringia) in 1522, disparaged "babbling out special masses and vigils, altars, altarpieces, candles, founding chapels and other things."[28] Erasmus Alberus, a student of Luther's at Wittenberg, published a pamphlet in 1523 in which he contrasted "true Christian faith" with the Church of Rome, embodied in "ceremonies, indulgence, fasting, feasting, bells, censing, organs, singing many hours, long prime, terce, sext, nones, and other things."[29] Theobald Billican, working to reform the churches of Nördlingen in 1524, preached against the complex ritual practice of the Mass, singling out anointing with oil, dividing the Eucharist Host into three pieces, special blessings, and other "wondrous customs," as well as "priests' gowns," and "chests with mass vestments, albs, and chasubles of all manner of colors" that filled the sacristies of churches in Nördlingen and across the German-speaking world.[30] One would do well to refrain not only from these practices, argued Martin Bryßgauer, but indeed, from "all outward pomp, [and] devotion, which is a work of the body." Bryßgauer, preaching in southwestern Germany, complemented Billican's litany by adding "bending the knees, stooping, fasting, pipes, organs, burning wax, and ringing bells."[31] Johann Sonnentaller concurred, complaining of the church:

> They have tonsures, cowls, they wear long robes, their religious clothing is of many specialized colors; they are anointed with oil, they have their white choir robes, they hold Masses, sing high and read quietly, they kneel down and get back up, they play organs, sound bells, bless candles, fumigate incense, sprinkle water, carry crosses, banners, golden chalices and silver monstrances.[32]

Similar litanies punctuated the sermons of early evangelicals such as Leo Jud in Zürich, Gallus Korn in Nuremberg, Martin Reinhart in Jena, Michael Keller in Augsburg, and Philipp Melhofer in Eriskirch.[33] Urbanus Rhegius, a well-known, humanistically trained preacher active in Augsburg in the early 1520s, and later a leading reformer of the Duchy of Lüneburg, offered up three litanies in his sermons during this period.[34] Jakob Strauß, who had preached in the service of the early Reformation in almost every corner of the Holy Roman Empire by 1525, condemned enthusiasm for "gold, silver, velvet, silk, ringing, lights, shrieking" as well as "keeping relics with gold, silver, precious stone" and "singing, praying, piping, organs, burning candles" and other similar practices.[35] "When you come to mass," he argued, "it is not necessary for you to pay attention to these manifold abuses," nor "anything else done there that is other than what Christ instituted."[36]

As with Staupitz before them, the work of these preachers permeated the consciousness of a significant portion of the ruling classes in the urban milieu. A year after the publication of Luther's *Babylonian Captivity*, the Swiss physician Joachim von Watt produced an extensive list of complaints similar to Sachs's *Nightingale*. Written just prior to his attempt to reform the churches in the city of St. Gallen, where he had recently succeeded his father as a member of the city council, von Watt's 1521 *On the Old and New God, Faith, and Doctrine* construed the overwhelming sensuality of ritual as a metaphor for late medieval Christianity. Watt's description of the Mass consisted of: lords in fur mantles, white choir shirts, green silk cords, ostentatious waving of hands, kissing the cloth on the altar, as well as the Gospel-text, ludicrous bowing, singing in five-part harmony, weeping, howling "like cats in heat," blasts from organs and wind instruments, marching about with silk banners and crucifixes, burning candles, silver censers, parading with an ornate Gospel-book, ornamented in gold, silver, and jewels, and ringing bells.[37] Building on the logic of contrariety, such an assemblage, in von Watt's estimation, represented the absolute inverse of evangelical Christianity, and any true reformation would require stripping worship of all such practices. For von Watt, this point offered the first means of confessional differentiation: one of the first to use the term "Lutherans," von Watt saw the movement emanating from the city of Wittenberg as an important plot point but not as the true resolution of the story. This would only be achieved with a more robust iconoclasm that would come to be associated with the Swiss Reformation under the leadership of Ulrich Zwingli.[38] The first cracks in the façade of evangelical Christianity were already beginning to emerge in this violent rhetoric, to be actualized only in the later 1520s.

Joachim von Watt and the various preachers roaming from town to town in the service of evangelical reform were among the educated elite in the German-speaking world, and they actively sought to shape opinion with their rhetoric. A measure of their success in this project is apparent in the enthusiastic embrace of the narrative of sensory reformation by less educated, urban laymen. Mostly, these were artisans and tradesmen, like Hans Sachs, but also lesser-known figures like Hans Greiffenberger, a painter from Nuremberg. Greiffenberger viewed the Church of Rome as an agglomeration of "pharisaical, dissembling, trifling works" assembled by the devil and Antichrist. Motivated by this apocalyptic vision, Greiffenberger began to preach on street corners, where he took up the story of sensory reformation. He condemned the "howling, burning lights, and works of juggling," the "clothed and crowned images" that filled church interiors, as well as the sartorial concern of priests over whether they wore "black or blue cowls, and white or brown mantles." Although the church extolled such things as good works, they were, in reality, simply "filth," and "matter not at all before God."[39] Johannes Herbst, a citizen of the town of Schwabach, not far from Nuremberg, criticized the church's doctrine that good works merited salvation, identifying "fasting, praying, going on pilgrimage, burning lights, founding anniversaries, vigils, vespers, singing Mass, building churches and altars, having vestments made, ringing bells, and other things."[40] Utz Rychssner, a weaver from Augsburg, decried the entire ritual edifice of traditional Christianity as "lying and compromising the Word of God, through which we are saved," threading litanies into his polemics to condemn fasting, feasting, special blessings, the burning of candles, the use of chrism oil for anointing, the opulence of priests and church interiors, bedecked in fine velvets, silks, silver and gold liturgical furniture, as well as "many other works of juggling."[41]

On some occasions, the story even infiltrated the countryside. Hans Schwalb, who was perhaps the son of a peasant but nonetheless had learned to read and write, put his skills into the service of introducing evangelical Christianity into the regions around Erfurt. In 1521 he disparagingly compared Christ's modest entrance into Jerusalem on a donkey to the pomp of papal processions, in which the Pope often appeared with his cardinals and priests, arrayed "with golden pieces, with purple velvet, silk vestments, and with a great war-horse." The vanity of such practices extended from the greatest heights of the church in Rome, down to the parishes, where Schwalb called for the removal of "precious cloth, [and] beautiful tapestries." Moreover, the priests there "do not teach, or preach. They keep useless choirboys who fill the church with blaring and shrieking, and do not know what they sing . . . then precious bells and organs come into the church, and they say it is the ornamentation of God, by which one praises God."[42]

How can we be certain that these litanies were self-conscious evocations of the "hyperaesthesia" of traditional Christianity, as I have suggested? The activity of simply listing the objects and practices could (and did) make connections to a whole variety of economic, social, cultural, and theological problems in the late medieval church. However, polemicists were quite clear that sensuality lay at the heart of the matter. Luther had, of course, already come to the point in 1520, exhorting his audience to let go of all that came before the senses in the daily practice of the Mass.[43] Other early evangelicals were also unequivocal. After his expulsion from the city of Ulm in 1522 for subversive preaching, Heinrich von Kettenbach, a former Franciscan monk, published pseudo-autobiographical dialogue in which he, as a representative of evangelical Christianity, attempted to dissuade an elderly woman of the city of Ulm from her attachment to the practices of traditional Christianity. Despite Kettenbach's admonitions, the woman remained firm in her devotion to collecting rosaries, praying with them in church, lighting candles, gazing at icons, clutching small gold and silver figures, and listening to sung Masses. Such things, she claimed, affected her heart with "joy and devotion."[44] Kettenbach despaired of converting the woman, exclaiming, "Oh sensuousness!"[45] In such utterances, Kettenbach disclosed the powerful hold sensuous worship could have on the minds and bodies of churchgoers, underscoring the urgency of the early evangelical call to reform.

A variety of associations shaped the meaning of late medieval religion in the minds of the early evangelicals. Above all, public discourse forged connections between sensuous worship, femininity, and foreignness. As such, the early evangelical movement built upon tropes common to the "double-externalization" of worship already underway in some circles in the fifteenth century, discussed here in chapter 3. These associations distanced traditional Christianity from what evangelicals imagined to be the normative core of true religion. They were ideological, to be sure, but they resonated with concrete concerns over male power and authority in the contemporary urban German scene.

As Kettenbach's dialogue suggests, the sensuousness of traditional Christianity was deeply gendered in the minds of early evangelicals. Viewed from a rhetorical standpoint, this was one strategy deployed by evangelicals in a broader attempt to distance what they imagined to be the new evangelical Christianity from its antecedent form and to associate it more closely with the worldviews of the educated and ruling classes in German cities. Throughout the dialogue, Kettenbach made his female interlocutor, whom he addressed as "little old mother," appear foolish and childish in her devotion. "You religious women," he wrote, "desire praise of your conduct and your superstition, which is without foundation in Scripture and is against God."[46] Kettenbach was hardly alone in this assessment, and condemnations of devotion to traditional worship often associated it with innate predispositions of children, fools, and "old hags" toward sensuous baubles.[47] As Urbanus Rhegius explained, such "womanly, foolish and shrewish [*altvettelisch*—literally 'old haggish']" inclinations could captivate the conscience and threatened to make "knaves of people."[48]

The story of sensory reformation also articulated male anxieties over maintaining control over female sexuality. Joachim von Watt compared traditional cantors to the sound made by "hens when they wish to lay," as well as the howling of "cats in heat."[49] Perhaps most famously, the popular image of the *Papal Ass*, interpreted by Philipp Melanchthon in 1523 for a popular audience, demonstrated that the entire church of Rome was completely dominated by its "womanly belly and breast," ever inclined to pleasures of eating, drinking, sex, and all manner of desire pertaining to luxurious living. Melanchthon painted in broad strokes, applying this criticism to all clergy from the Pope to the cardinals, bishops, priests, down to the lowliest students and "other similar whores."[50] Most commonly, evangelicals feminized the church and its ritual practice as a harem of courtesans or, less imaginatively, as the "Whore of Babylon."[51] Luther, of course, had laid the groundwork for this imagery in the *Babylonian Captivity* and in other writings and sermons. Other images of transgressive female sexuality permeated early evangelical polemic: particularly potent were the frequent references to illicit affairs between monks and married women, and their socially disruptive, emasculating effects.[52]

There were several reasons that evangelicals gendered traditional religion as female in the peculiar way they did. Perhaps most obviously, it was a narrative written by men. The sample of pamphlets analyzed here includes contributions by all known females who publicly supported the early evangelical cause: none of them considered the matter of sensuous worship, nor did they gender traditional religion as feminine in order to disparage it.[53] The story of sensory reformation drew much of its ideological force from a patriarchal worldview that insisted on the innate moral and intellectual weakness of the female sex and the need to discipline and contain natural feminine inclinations toward bodily sinfulness (sexual or otherwise) within the well-ordered confines of the private, male-led household. This ideology came into especially sharp focus in the urban centers of the late fifteenth and early sixteenth centuries, and it goes to the very heart of the Reformation movement itself.[54] The ability of evangelicals to align their religious message with a politics of women's orderly submission to marriage and paternal authority over the household "was the key to its successful implementation and establishment" across the urban German-speaking world.[55] The polemics of the early 1520s harnessed the contemporaneous but separate tendency to feminize sensuality generally to broader views about social order and its normative organization around male power and authority.[56] For anxious patriarchs inclined toward the evangelical message, the narrative of desensualization became an important rhetorical and psychological means of distinguishing their new religion from the social and moral disorder that had prevailed in the previous generation.[57]

Complementing this gendering of the sensual in traditional religious practice was a tendency to exoticize it, or establish associations with external, non-Christian cultures. The Augsburg preacher Konrad Adler put it bluntly in sermons given in 1523: the church of Rome was no different than Turks, Jews, Tartars and other "heathens" in its devotion to the flesh. The true Christian community, by contrast, was infused by the Word of the Gospel in spirit and "in hands, in mouth, eyes, tongue, [and] ears."[58] Here, Adler invoked a broader cultural shift that confronted sixteenth-century German Christians with the religious practices of other, non-Christian civilizations, and oriented early evangelical religious discourse around stark distinctions between idolatrous and non-idolatrous cultures.[59] Although Germans were largely absent from the early expansion of Europe into the wider world, they were nonetheless avid cultural participants in the colonial enterprise, eagerly consuming narrative and pseudo-ethnographical accounts that appeared in a steady stream from the late fifteenth century through the first half of the sixteenth century. Production and consumption of these materials was centered in cities and was often closely associated with humanist culture.[60]

These developments shaped the early evangelical social imagination in a variety of ways, above all reinforcing the need to define true Christian religion as unambiguously as possible, in terms of contrariety and opposition to all external, "foreign" cults. This was especially clear in the contrasts regularly established between proper Christian practice and the "fleshly ceremonies" of the Jews. The fasting, dietary restrictions, and hygienic rituals of contemporary Judaism served as an especially effective foil to the "pure Word" of the Gospel:

they were directed at the body and had many clear parallels with traditional Christian worship.[61] The various sacrificial practices of the historical Jews of the Old Testament served a similar purpose. Not only did they reference the late medieval theology of the Mass as a sacrifice, universally an abomination in the eyes of evangelicals, but they also evoked its practice. The imagery of burnt offerings and incense served as a powerful reminder that the Church of Rome was filled with lingering vestiges of idolatrous Jewish ceremony.[62]

Although traditional Christian practice most commonly drew such comparisons with Judaism, parallels with other religions, including Islam and vaguely defined "heathens," also appeared in the rhetoric of the early 1520s.[63] Perhaps most famously, one of the first editions of Andreas Karlstadt's pamphlet *On the Abolition of Images* (1522) was published with a title page bordered by imagery of "new world" cannibals.[64] The lay pamphleteer Cuntz von Oberndorf saw members of the Church of Rome as "Turks," and though they claimed to be Christians, it was clear that their "lives and customs" were Turkish.[65] The humanist Joachim von Watt deployed creative but rather suspect etymological analysis to the word "ceremony" in order to connect his litany of abuses to paganism, contending that the word derived from the ancient Roman goddess of agriculture Ceres, who demanded sacrificial offerings closely resembling the material culture of late medieval Christendom.[66] Heinrich Kettenbach simply advanced the syllogism that heathen kings by definition ruled over men's bodies, while true Christian kings ruled over men's souls; therefore, the Pope was a heathen king, and the Church of Rome a heathen institution.[67] One of the most powerful and repeated tropes in the rhetoric of the 1520s was the comparison between the Church of Rome and the priesthood of Baal that frequently confronted and tempted the ancient Israelites with idolatry, as detailed in the Old Testament Books of Kings.[68] With its fetish of gold and silver altar ornamentation, burnt offerings, and rich priestly vestments, the priesthood of Baal had clearly been a demonic cult and, as such, drew especially effective parallels to traditional Christian practice in preaching of men like Wenceslaus Linck. Linck, who had experienced firsthand the elaborate ritual of wealthy urban communities like Nuremberg, saw the corrupting power of such extensive appeals to sense and flesh. "Without the Word of God," he preached, "going about with [such] ceremonies and human innovations is serving the idol Baal, or the belly."[69]

Mounting concern over idolatry changed the nature of sensuous ritual in the minds of early reformers. The somewhat permissive attitude toward diverse cultic practice, characteristic of fifteenth-century humanists like Nicholas Cusanus, was largely displaced by an intense preoccupation with distinguishing between "true" and "false" religion. As such, no external practice could ever really be completely indifferent, and most things classified as *adiaphora* tended to slip into the category of idolatry in the heated atmosphere of the early Reformation.

Unreformed religion was largely idolatrous religion, and more nuanced readings of it were avoided, regardless of what appear today as manifest contradictions and empirical inaccuracies. This was as true of the distant Mayans and Ottomans as it was of the more familiar Jews and Papists in reformers' midst.[70]

In this context, evangelicals encouraged one another to identify with the great iconoclastic kings of the Old Testament, above all Josiah and Hezekiah, when imagining their relationship to traditional Christianity. It is not surprising to find this trope among well-known iconoclasts like Huldrych Zwingli and the Anabaptist Ludwig Hätzer, but during the *Wildwuchs* years, it became an important component of the imaginative world of the evangelical community more generally and was promoted by supposedly more moderate reformers like Stephan Agricola and Georg Spalatin, who eventually came to identify as "Lutherans."[71] Spalatin, as secretary to Frederick the Wise, Elector of Saxony, proved especially important in this regard. In 1525, at the end of the wild-growth period, Spalatin published a pamphlet, *On the Removal of Ceremonies and Unfounded Abuses in Divine Worship*, in which he singled out the traditional performance of the Mass at Nuremberg as especially offensive and encouraged reformers to approach such practice as both Josiah and Hezekiah had in the Old Testament.[72]

Early evangelical concern with the foreignness of traditional worship also worked in tandem with criticisms of Aristotelian natural philosophy. In 1520 Luther had called for rejecting it as a basis for the educational system: "My advice would be that the books of Aristotle, the Physics, the Metaphysics, Of the Soul, Ethics, which have hitherto been considered the best, be altogether abolished, together with all others that profess to treat of nature."[73] In its place, he recommended the reinstitution of the Word, which the "blind heathen master" had obscured and distorted for so long. This was the proper and sufficient basis of all Christian knowledge, and the only elements from the Aristotelian corpus that might be worth retaining were grammar, logic, and rhetoric, but only to be put into the service of communicating the Word. Philipp Melanchthon made similarly comprehensive criticisms in sermons and lectures given in Wittenberg in the early 1520s.[74] These were not entirely original positions of course, as humanists like Erasmus had long excoriated Aristotelian learning and advocated for similar reforms of the educational system. Many nonetheless perceived the criticisms as novel and distinctive to the new evangelical movement, and the opposition to Aristotelian natural philosophy became a keynote in early evangelical discourse, alongside criticism of sensuous worship. The reformation of the senses therefore represented a systematic attack on late medieval religion, disparaging its actual practice while undermining the theoretical system that justified it.

In this regard, recourse to Aristotelian natural philosophy instead of Scripture was a sure sign of a bad preacher.[75] As the early evangelicals saw it, this was not incidental, reflecting the behavior of a few "bad seeds." Rather, it grew out of a much deeper structural problem of "foreign" influence in the German educational system more broadly. In a 1522 dialogue, the layman Balthasar Stanberger thus criticized the prominence of Albert the Great in Germany's universities, calling him a "heathen master" because of his role in introducing Aristotelian natural philosophy into curricula.[76] Similarly, Johannes Lonicer, who had studied with both Luther and Melanchthon at Wittenberg, cited Aristotelianism as one of the causes of false belief and practice and, following his teachers, called for systematic educational reform. He defended Luther's criticisms of Aristotelianism's role in the "most shameful customs of the universities," which corrupted the youth through "teaching and instruction with heathen, unchristian writings."[77] Johannes Fritzhans concurred, adding that the late medieval recourse to Aristotelianism had lent the ritual practices of the church a false sheen of intellectual rigor. The only solution was for people to heed God, who would "return to us purely and clearly [his] holy Word."[78] Fritzhans took things one step further, gendering late medieval theologians' reliance on Aristotle as both feminine and childish in contrast to a properly masculine mastery of the Word, "clearly and purely preached, administered, and expounded just as if it had gone up clearly and purely from the mouth of God."[79] According to Joachim von Watt, Aristotle was not only a godless, idolatrous heathen; he was no different than other "Arabs" and "sodomites" like Averroes, and as such, he refused normative gender roles defined by God and nature, and typified in the patriarchal household at the center of early evangelical culture.[80] This philosophical system, in conjunction with the "appearance of sanctity" promoted by church ritual, had been the means by which papal tyranny had infiltrated the German-speaking lands, "corrupting body, soul, honor, and wealth."[81] Lamenting this fallen state of affairs, Heinrich Kettenbach appealed specifically to German nobles to "see how you all have become knaves to womanly, sodomitical fools . . . impoverished and corrupted."[82]

Early evangelicals' concerns with the foreign enmeshed with concrete, political-economic power struggles in the specific to the German-speaking world in the early sixteenth century. The same ships that carried news of faraway cultures and peoples also delivered cargoes of exotic goods, closely associated with indulgence, luxury, and, above all, sensuality. In the late medieval imagination, the exotic origins of such things had often mobilized positive physical and spiritual associations: spices especially were good for bodily and spiritual health, and often their geographic origins in the east linked them with biblically inflected visions of paradise.[83] By the early sixteenth century, however, the growing presence of spices, silks, novel foods, and other luxuries, as well as the growing power of the merchants who delivered them, came under closer critical scrutiny, particularly among intellectual classes. Increasingly, these goods were regarded simultaneously as physical, moral, and economic threats to particular German bodies and what was imagined to be a common German body-politic. Again, this was primarily an urban concern: it was in the cities that the merchants who imported spices had a defined social status, and it was in the cities that financing was available to undertake international commercial enterprises.[84] The chief dividing line drawn by humanists and evangelical polemicists like Ulrich von Hutten was between a common "German" domestic space and the foreign, outside world, writ large. The consumption of sensuous luxuries, but especially foreign spices, was dangerous because it "created a direct, physical link between the native (body) and the foreign (ingested substance), ideally suited to represent the possibilities and dangers of bringing the foreign home. Their expense and their use as status symbols allowed spices to stand in for any number of other foreign luxury goods that provoked the wrath of moralists."[85]

The concern over international commerce reached its peak in the urban German scene between 1521 and 1530, coinciding with the emergence of the evangelical movement. The idea that merchants were parasites on the local community, draining it of its intrinsic, native wealth in exchange for worthless foreign goods, found wide purchase.[86] At the same time, real economic changes charged these ideas with a new sense of urgency. In the largest cities of the German-speaking world, the greatest disparities in wealth emerged between the wealthy merchant and entrepreneurial classes and the middling laborers and producers not engaged in international commerce.[87] Imperial ordinances, such as the *Polizeiordnung* of 1521, as well as deliberations at imperial assemblies, such as the Diet of Nuremberg in 1522–23, forcefully condemned the spice trade as a monopoly that gouged customers with exorbitant prices and yielded massive, unseemly profits for merchants, who put their own self-interest ahead of concern for the common economic good.[88] Beyond presenting an external economic threat, spices were seen as a decadent luxury that could "threaten the essence of Germanness," associated with values of simplicity, modesty, and hardiness.[89] When discussion of the spice trade turned specifically to consumption, the issue of defining boundaries between German domesticity and foreignness became more acute. The formal similarities with contemporaneous evangelical imagery of traditional Christianity were striking. The *Polizeiordnung* of 1521, for example, identified spices as a bad kind of cultural and economic exchange for Germans, along with "golden cloth, velvet, damask, goldwork, pearls and ostrich feathers" used for "lavish magnificence of clothing and jewelry."[90] The ordinance went on to explain that these were bad imports because "all must be brought and bought from foreign lands . . . this lavish magnificence does not come from our ancestors in the German nation, but the custom has only been introduced in recent years."[91]

The imagined contrasts between German simplicity and foreign luxury formed an important context to the polemics of the early reformation years and lent them an additional emotional charge. As Philip Broadhead notes, Hans Sachs had frequent recourse to it and explicitly yoked the abuses of the foreign Church of Rome to the economic hardships of his friends and fellow artisans in Nuremberg.[92] Already in 1519, Ulrich von Hutten had played on the contrast to lodge a broader criticism of the clergy. In a moralizing tale on the deleterious effects of luxurious living, he described a prelate recently returned to Germany from Rome. While in the eternal city, "he had learned from a Cardinal how to live a soft life," and thereafter he could only drink wine and eat pheasants "seasoned with pepper, cinnamon, ginger and cloves."[93] In the early 1520s, Hutten emerged as a vocal supporter of Luther, who was similarly concerned with the moral, physical, and economic threats presented by international commerce, and similarly drew parallels to Germans' relationship to the Church of Rome. Both often described this relationship as one of tyranny: since the thirteenth century, the Papacy in Rome had exercised increasingly "tyrannical" levels of control over the sacramental system to cultivate magnificent spectacle and the appearance of sanctity. The Papacy thus appeared as a foreign power, deceiving and taking advantage of "poor," "simple" German Christian folk. Luther's view of the matter verged on the dystopian and evoked a nearly totalitarian level of societal control. "All things," he claimed, "are regulated by the chief knaves of Rome, even the offices of sextons and bell-ringers in all churches."[94]

Of course, this vision of centralized control over ritual practice flew in the face of reality. As we saw in chapter 1, the matter of producing sensuous worship was polycentric, rife with variation, and reflected the limitations of local economies. However, this was immaterial in the *Wildwuchs* years: the coherence of the image of a foreign Pope tyrannically imposing spectacular church rituals that were physically, morally, and economically corrosive to the essential simplicity of Germanness was just too useful to abandon in the early evangelical movement.[95] Many evangelicals appear to have been persuaded by Luther's vision. As Leo Jud put it, "The papists coerce all people to pray at such and such time, to such and such an extent, for so long, however it pleases them. They coerce all people to pray, sing, read, live, fast, eat, indeed, to believe what and how the Roman Antichrist the pope prays, sings, reads, lives, fasts, eats, believes."[96] Johann Günzburg made the crudely materialist thrust of this foreign coercion even more apparent. The whole purpose of all traditional Christian worship was to exploit the German "nation" specifically and drain it of all its wealth. The church was run by "merchants," who required Germans to pay for the incense, vestments, blessings, bells, chalices, and all manner of liturgical furniture, thereby transforming Christianity into a series of vulgar economic transactions.[97] The foreign power of Rome had always had the upper hand, and as a result, it was hardly surprising to Günzburg that there was no money left in Germany by the 1520s.[98] The broader political economic context of the early sixteenth century thus reinforced the efficacy of the story of sensory reformation and the emergent evangelical view of traditional Christianity.

The associations conjured in the early evangelical discourse lent it an almost dreamlike quality. This, however, does not mean it didn't have a profound impact in the real world. Indeed, it is often precisely this oneiric quality that makes storytelling such a powerful ideological tool.[99] In their story, which they repeated over and over again, early evangelicals consolidated connections between sensuous worship, femininity, and foreign cultures, and in doing so, they "de-Christianized" the late medieval church. It was effectively a kind of orientalism *avant la lettre*, albeit one that usually evoked time rather than space to establish a privileged distinction between the evangelical observer and his object of concern. This was ideologically necessary: we should not forget that the initiators of the Reformation were, after all, late medieval Christians.[100] In order for a movement to cohere, people first had to imagine an unbridgeable gap between themselves and the religious world they inhabited. Storytelling allowed them to make that imaginative leap. The rhetoric of sensory reformation laid claim to a certain degree of pseudo-ethnographic authority, purporting to describe an external culture but building that description as a kind of inverted image of socially dominant—or at the very least preferable—values and beliefs. Traditional Christianity was antithetical to the gendered worldview of the men charged with maintaining civic order in the urban communes of the German-speaking world. It existed somewhere beyond the walls of these cities as an external threat.

Up to this point, we have largely focused our attention on the first half of the story of sensory reformation. The narrative, however, necessarily articulated a dynamic of change over time and found its resolution in the singular emphasis on the "pure" and "clear" administration of the Word.[101] Balthasar Hubmaier, a Swiss pastor preaching in 1525, put the matter simply and concisely: after an extended litany dwelling on particular objects and practices, he declared all ceremonies of traditional Christianity "outside the Word of God."[102] Hubmaier, one of the intellectual architects of the Anabaptist movement and widely regarded as an exemplar of the most radical wing of the Reformation, was hardly in the minority in the early 1520s.[103] Luther himself, observing the contrast between the "pomp" of the traditional practice of the Eucharist and the simple meal according to the Word of Scripture, had envisioned a radical ritual reform already in 1520, proclaiming, "We must turn our eyes and hearts simply to the institution of Christ alone" and establish a "totally different kind of ceremony."[104] This was as true of trained clergy like Luther and Hubmaier as it was of laymen like Hans Sachs.

But why was it reasonable for early evangelicals to make this contrast in the first place, and what did it mean, precisely? Put another way, why was the Word as an object of devotion a sufficient replacement for the extraordinarily complex array of objects, practices, and beliefs that had evolved in late medieval religious life? Modern attempts to answer these questions by Reformation historians share a common intellectual genealogy with sensory history. Largely building on the great divide theory elaborated by McLuhan and Ong in the 1960s, two schools have emerged, taking rather contradictory positions. One the one hand, Protestantism has been seen as part of a broader shift away from a predominantly oral-aural culture toward an overwhelmingly ocular-centric one, expressing the "typographical revolution" inaugurated by the printing press.[105] Somewhat paradoxically, others have cited the same Reformation emphasis on the Word as evidence of precisely the opposite development: that a great divide had emerged, but that the new Protestant culture was one of the ear, displacing the traditional medieval Catholic valorization of the eye.[106]

More recent analyses by Reformation scholars have made it difficult to accept these variations on the great divide theory in all but the most qualified sense.[107] The Word could, and did, absorb a whole assemblage of meanings that stood in tension, if not outright contradiction, with one another. The Word was the Word of Scripture, written by hand or pressed by machinery onto a page. Huldrych Zwingli put it simply in 1522: "The foundation of our religion is the written word, the Scripture of God."[108] The visible clarity and certainty of the Word, laid bare on the page, reassured the early evangelical mind that the new religion was built on a firm foundation. It reflected a culture, originating to a large extent in the humanist celebration of the word, in which acts of writing, reading, annotating, or even merely carrying a book could take on semi-devotional significance.[109] In many Lutheran churches, painting and etching passages of Scripture into walls and altars became an adequate replacement for much of the traditional ornamentation in these spaces.[110] Luther's subtle redefinition of sacramentality also reflected intensified focus on a visual Word. Rejecting the broad late medieval classification of sacraments as sensible signs or things, Luther returned to a narrower view: invoking Augustine, he called them specifically "*visible* words." By this, he meant that the Word "becomes attached to, and therefore perceptible in, an act or a thing" constituting the sacrament.[111] The Word of Scripture also provided a narrative account of events that visually modeled sacramental practice and demanded rigorous imitation in contemporary Christian worship. Although their sacramental theologies ultimately diverged, both Luther and Zwingli insisted in the early 1520s that the visible performance of the Eucharist was to mirror the events of the Last Supper as closely as possible.[112]

It was also self-evident that the Word was an aural object. Luther believed that he remained faithful to the teachings of Augustine (and Paul) in his understanding that "the ear, not the eye, was the Christian sense," and that the Word was simply "to be heard, a promise to be received in faith, not a text to be pored over."[113] Preaching on behalf of Luther in 1523, Johannes Fritzhans explained, "Faith comes from that which one hears and grasps of the Word of God."[114] Following this position to its most extreme logical conclusion, the preacher Martin Bryßgauer argued that the most effective way to receive the Eucharist was not the oral or visual modes of Communion so popular in the later Middle Ages, but rather aurally "through the Word, or through faith in the Word."[115] Correspondingly, polemics of the early 1520s disclose a strong concern with the pitch, tone, clarity, and volume of evangelical pastors' voices, contrasted with the immoderate "shrieking," "blaring," "crying," and high voices of chanting priests one encountered in traditional services. In tandem with this, evangelicals frequently and pointedly claimed that the sensory chaos of traditional Christianity prevented parishioners from hearing the Word.[116] Traditional church ritual was nothing more than "diabolical voluptuousness," according to Hans Schwalb, intentionally designed to divert people away from the Word: amid the cacophony of the traditional Mass, he explained, "no one can hear.[117] For this reason, Urbanus Rhegius remarked, "The devil loves the pomp,"[118] and, especially in the case of the Eucharist, "would gladly suffer all manner of external reverence toward the sacrament."[119] Others made similar arguments opposing the "jugglery," "ostentation," and "pomp" of traditional ritual to the audible Word.[120] According to Johannes Bugenhagen, one of Luther's most important surrogates in northern Germany, the simplification of ritual practice was critical because it cleared space to listen and "hear rightly." With respect to the Mass, the aural Word inhered in sacramental practice in a manner analogous to its visual aspects articulated by Luther: acts of eating and drinking were meaningless without a proper understanding of the words of Scripture, which depended on "good hearing."[121]

There was a fairly prosaic reason for the evangelical conception of the Word as something both visible and audible: most people could not read, so they accessed the Word aurally, through their local preacher, who presumably could read. Luther thus often called preachers "living books" in the midst of their flocks, just as essential to the dissemination of the Word as any of his writings.[122] Sixteenth-century pedagogy responded to this reality pragmatically, observing that optimal learning occurred through a balanced ratio of hearing and seeing.[123] As Albrecht Dürer wrote in 1510, vision was "the noblest of all senses" but could not be separated from hearing, for people "grasp something even better when it is both heard and seen."[124] Dürer, one of the most famous representatives of the German renaissance and later a supporter of the evangelical cause, was broadly representative of the core of both humanist and early Reformation pedagogy. Education in churches, homes, and schools was principally a matter of blending communal and individual listening to sermons and lectures, singing, praying, recitation, and observing liturgical practice.[125]

Viewed from the standpoint of late medieval sacramentality, the sensible dimensions of the evangelical Word represented an intensification of patterns, rather than any kind of major break. As such, the Reformation fetish of the Word was of a piece with a much broader drive in late medieval religion toward an idealized "normative center."[126] The major development came with the office of preaching eclipsing the primary function of late medieval priests as sacramental administers. The religious sensorium thus appeared to collapse into hearing and vision while retaining the underlying principles of traditional, affective piety. This is most apparent in the emphasis on the emotional impact of the Word on its viewers-hearers.[127] It articulated, as John Bossy has described it, "the classical understanding of *fides* [faith] as the feeling of conviction which the orator was supposed to arouse in this audience."[128] Correspondingly, the emotional impact of hearing the Word, and its implications for the moral formation of the soul, took on particular significance. As Luther pointed out, "We never read that the Holy Spirit was given to any one when he did works, but always when men have heard the Gospel of Christ and the mercy of God. From this same Word and from no other source must come faith."[129] Lazarus Spengler of Nuremberg concurred: those who truly believed in God "hear his Word and his voice . . . the Word of God alone must speak to the heart."[130] This concern with the emotional impact of language and its power to affect faith influenced Luther's translation of the New Testament in 1521–22: he often listened to people speaking in town squares and marketplaces and attempted to capture the natural musicality of ordinary German language when he returned to his translation.[131] In the minds of many other early evangelicals, both the visual and aural efficacy of the Word served as a viable alternative to the broadly sensual sacramentality of late medieval Christendom, infested as it was with all manner of "idols." In contrast to such external things, it alone truly penetrated into the heart and moved the soul.[132] Viewed from this perspective, the reformation of the senses represented a shift in the terms used to define ritual specialists' authority over religion. Mastery of the aural-visual Word, rather than the sacramental complex, was the defining feature of this authority.

While the early Reformation fetish of the Word may have de facto intensified or compressed preexisting late medieval patterns of sensuous devotion, it is important to register that the evangelical community perceived a much more comprehensive rupture taking place. The same evangelicals who extolled the power of the visible and audible Word simultaneously rejected utterly the notion that it could be anything but a completely disembodied, internal, and spiritual thing. It had to be, because, as Johannes Fritzhans explained, it "came purely and plainly from the mouth of God," a transcendent being beyond all sense.[133] Martin Bryßgauer concurred, hastening to point out that, while hearing the Word was an efficacious substitute for oral or visual Communion, "true enjoyment" of the sacrament was "purely and totally spiritual."[134] Wenceslaus Linck, preaching on behalf of Luther in the Thuringian town of Altenburg from 1522 to 1524, frequently admonished his parishioners to abolish "all unfounded, external worship" accumulated by the church and "turn to the internal, spiritual, divine essence of the Gospel."[135] Johannes Oecolampadius, a humanist and leading voice of reform in the city of Basel, derided the "many devout exercises and ceremonies" filling churches because they had no bearing on the relationship between the Word of Scripture and the conscience of the individual Christian, which was a purely spiritual matter.[136] Christ, he pointed out, "had demanded nothing of us regarding ceremonial customs, without doubt because he commanded higher things to us."[137] Inverting traditional paradigms of affective piety, he argued that pure, spiritual faith in the Word directly cultivated a disposition in the soul by which "we are touched by him [Christ], and by his mercy we become healthy . . . there is no evil spirit that he cannot drive out with his touch."[138] Oecolampadius, like many of his contemporaries, used language of embodiment and sensuality, but circumvented the meanings assigned to this language under late medieval theories of sacramentality. The complex interaction between body, soul, and external objects of perception was removed from the equation. Rather, the language of sensuality invoked to describe the relation between Word and human soul often referred to "spiritual sensation," analogous to the concept developed by Johann von Staupitz and other preachers who applied a more self-consciously Augustinian view of the relation between body and soul.

The evangelical Word therefore may have been something audible or visible from time to time, but what mattered most in the minds of early evangelicals was that it transcended utterly the sensuality embedded in the late medieval system of religious belief and practice. The narrative logic demanded this view: if the church in the medieval past had been hyperaesthetic and fleshly, the evangelical movement brought Christianity into a new era of devotion to purely spiritual things. Captivated by the grand sweep of its narrative, many followed the story of sensory reformation to its logical conclusions, moving to implement radical reforms that would seemingly have transformed Christianity beyond all recognition. In Nuremberg, for example, the painter Hans Greiffenberger, along with a schoolteacher called Hans Denck, were brought to trial before the city council in late 1524 and early 1525 for subversive preaching. They had apparently developed a significant following among artisans in the city, including three young artists who would eventually rise to prominence: the brothers Sebald and Barthel Beham, and Georg Pencz. From testimonies given at the trial, this cadre of "godless painters," as they were called, made a radical argument against religious sensuality of any kind. The only true source of spiritual nourishment was the "invisible Word"; the bread and wine of the Eucharist, and even the very *written* Word of Scripture were mere externalities. That Andreas Osiander, preacher in the church of St. Lorenz and the leading evangelical voice in the city, felt compelled to preach against this radical vision of reform suggests that it had gained considerable traction among many ordinary townsfolk of Nuremberg.[139] This should not have been all that surprising, as it was intellectually consistent with the rhetoric of the early 1520s. The godless painters' timing, however, was infelicitous: by 1524, members of the city council, with the support of Osiander and other evangelical clergy, were already beginning to turn to the problem of establishing an evangelical church in actual practice. The vision was obviously impractical in this domain, and found few sympathetic ears among authorities. The Nuremberg city council quickly and unceremoniously exiled Denck and Greiffenberger in early 1525, just prior to introducing official reforms in accordance with what they considered the more moderate "Lutheran" position.[140]

In Wittenberg, the story produced more tangible results but, like the case of Nuremberg, ended with a widening rift between magisterial, moderate reformers and more radical sects. In mid-1521, after Luther had been placed under imperial ban at the Diet of Worms, his patron and territorial lord, Frederick the Wise (d. 1525), elector of Saxony, took him into hiding at the Wartburg Castle. During his absence, leadership of the evangelical movement in Wittenberg devolved onto his colleagues in the university and religious orders. The most outspoken of these colleagues were Andreas Karlstadt and the former Augustinian monk Gabriel Zwilling. Both men were particularly vexed by the traditional uses of images and preached ardently against them while Luther was away. At Christmas in 1521, Karlstadt administered an evangelical Mass. Altars were cleared of ornamentation, and the sacrament was distributed in both kinds, the laity enjoying both bread and wine. The Christmas Mass seems to have inspired more radical attempts at reform. In early January, Zwilling led the destruction of some images and altars in the Augustinian cloister, captivating the attention of the city. It was at this point that the city council moved to stem any further destruction of church property, issuing an ordinance mandating that "the images and altars in the church should also be removed, in order to avoid idolatry, for three altars without images are enough."[141] From the perspective of the growing iconoclastic faction in town, the problem with this decree was that it did not set a date for the sanctioned removal of church furniture. Karlstadt and Zwilling therefore continued to agitate for action on the part of the city council, appealing to the public in their sermons. It was at this point that Karlstadt published his famous pamphlet, *On the Abolition of Images*. In conjunction with the formal decree already issued by the city council, this agitation seems to have led to the first significant instance of iconoclastic violence of the Reformation.[142] Sometime between January 27 and February 5, a mob of Wittenberg citizens stormed the city church, destroying a considerable amount of the property ornamenting its altars.[143]

More specific detail on what precisely was destroyed in these riots is unfortunately lost, but if Karlstadt is in any way indicative of the mood in the city, the problem was not simply the images themselves but indeed the entire ecology of worship to which they were linked. In this respect, the iconoclasts were enacting the narrative of sensory reformation. The images were "oil-idols" (*Ölgötzen*), evoking the fragrant chrism oil used in anointing ceremonies. They appeared to people arrayed with rich silk, velvet, and damask clothing, crowns and jewelry of gold, silver, and precious gemstones. People came into the churches to offer wine, bread, candles, precious fragrances, and prayers, kneeling, bowing, or laying prostrate before the images.[144] In characterizing these devotions, Karlstadt also told the story of King Hezekiah, who had destroyed the bronze serpent when people began to offer incense to it—yet another evocation of olfactory experience. Idolatry was a serious sin and, as such, a theological problem, but there was an underlying anthropological argument here as well. Karlstadt acknowledged the power of such sensible practices to move the soul, and that even a committed iconoclast like himself had to struggle against habitual dispositions ingrained after years of immersion in traditional Christian ritual. Reflecting on his own childhood, he evoked the awe, love, and fear associated with these experiences and admitted "how firmly and deeply images are seated in my heart," even as he fulminated against them.[145] The whole ritual edifice of the church was potentially so dangerous because humans were by nature disposed to become attached to the objects that entered their perceptual field through the windows of their five senses. Removal of such things was therefore necessary because the churches were "houses in which God alone should be heard, appealed to, and worshipped."[146] The evangelical Word, here understood aurally, thus stood against the sensuous ritual of traditional Christianity, but Karlstadt was uncertain of its power to overcome idolatrous attachment to other sensibles. Although the events of 1521–22 are often interpreted as narrowly concerned with visual piety, the stakes were much more broadly sensorial. Idolatrous worship, as a theological and anthropological problem, involved the full range of sensuous experience.

When the smoke had cleared, the city council issued another ordinance reiterating that such actions were the prerogative not of ordinary folk but solely of authorities, "who, prepared, suited, and fit, are alone entrusted with that task, and no one should lay a hand on anything unless he has been ordered to do so."[147] Afterward, some of those who participated were arrested and forced to pay a fine. When Luther returned later in March 1522, he lent his own charismatic authority to the ordinances of the city council, sharply condemning the violence of Karlstadt and his faction, and praising the secular magistrates as true guarantors of orderly reform.[148] The divisions established in this moment, between radical and magisterial branches of the Reformation, would remain permanent and continue to resonate in the sensory culture of sixteenth-century Germany, as we will see in the coming chapters.

Despite this widening divergence after 1525, the radical and mainstream wings of the Reformation had first recognized themselves in the story of sensory reformation. The story had cohered in the immediate context of the early sixteenth century and spoke to the concerns of a largely urban, educated, male elite. To be sure, this represented a tiny minority of the population, but it was a minority that had outsized access to the levers of political power and more or less controlled cultural production across the German-speaking world. With respect to the latter, the printing press was of undeniable importance. The disparity between Catholic and evangelical publishing between 1520 and 1525 was such that the evangelical message circulated virtually unopposed. It took years, and in some cases decades, for Catholic controversialists to develop a response.[149] The affordability of the pamphlet form was also an important factor contributing to the circulation of the evangelical message. A single pamphlet might cost an artisan between three and four hours of labor—comparable to the cost of a hen, a kilogram of beef, or a pound of wax.[150] By comparison, the limited numbers of Catholic responses often circulated in larger format books, in Latin, and were many tens, if not hundreds, of times more expensive than evangelical pamphlets. People actually bought evangelical pamphlets, and seemingly in large numbers.[151] In 1524, for example, the Leipzig city council felt compelled to petition the city's territorial overlord, duke George the Bearded of Saxony, to rescind a prohibition on printing evangelical works because of the heavy losses the printing industry in the city had suffered. The printers were in danger of losing "all their livelihood" because of the ban on works that "one would gladly sell and for which there is demand." By contrast, the Catholic material they were allowed to print "is desired by no one and cannot even be given away."[152]

Even if people didn't buy the evangelical pamphlets, the sheer volume of material in circulation very likely created the impression of an unstoppable movement in opinion. During the *Wildwuchs*, perhaps as many as ten million copies of between six thousand and seventy-five hundred separate editions of pamphlets appeared in small formats, in German.[153] Population numbers are of course difficult to come by for the sixteenth century, but according to the best estimates, there were only about ten million people in all of Germany in 1520.

Only about 16 percent of this population lived in urban centers, where virtually all pamphlets were produced, and where most circulated. In other words, roughly six evangelical pamphlets were published for every person living in German cities at the time.[154] Strictly according to these metrics, it seems clear that people were immersed in evangelical culture and were repeatedly, aggressively exposed to its dominant narratives. Of course, this doesn't account for the diffusion of the early reformation message as a multistage, multimedia process, involving literate elites transmitting information from print into oral culture and its wider circulation. At least some people who could not read purchased pamphlets and asked literate neighbors, friends, and relatives to explain or read them. Both in print and through the spoken, heard, or preached word, the story of sensory reformation, so frequently told in these materials, would have been a constant presence in people's daily lives. Through repetitive engagement with it, the narrative became a self-evident truth about the history of Christianity in the sixteenth century.

The period after 1525 marked a new chapter in the history of the senses in Reformation Germany. As secular and ecclesiastical leaders began the arduous work of practical reform in the late 1520s and into the 1530s and 1540s, the narrative of sensory reformation became somewhat less pronounced in evangelical polemic. This does not mean it disappeared completely: it certainly manifested in visual rhetoric like Erhard Schön's 1532 woodcut, *God's Lament over the Fate of His Vineyard* (see figure 1 in the Introduction), with which we began this study. In the middle decades of the sixteenth century, the workshops of other well-known Protestant artists, such as Lucas Cranach the Younger, continued to churn out similar imagery.[155] At the same time, the few examples of autobiographical writing we have for this period demonstrate that elements of the narrative were being internalized. In the late 1540s, reflecting on his experiences of in Strasbourg in the early 1520s, the Swabian chronicler Dionysius Dreytwein could only recall how the preachers Martin Bucer and Wolfgang Capito had followed the example of Luther, preaching the pure Gospel "against monks, nuns, and priests, [and] how their ceremonies were of absolutely no use."[156] In the city of Ulm, the shoemaker Sebastian Fischer's notes on the sermons of Johannes Oecolampadius, Martin Bucer, and other reformers recited elements of the story in even greater detail. Fischer had heard evangelical preaching on many occasions and had summarized his impressions in a series of articles that neatly recited the elements of sensory reformation, stating clearly at the outset that the only true worship was hearing sermons and the Word of the Gospel, and the feeling of faith this kindled in the heart. He contrasted this to traditional worship, which he described as being devoted to images, idols, fasting, praying, eating special foods, wearing special cloths, living in convents, going to Mass, and engaging in consecration ceremonies. These things were idolatrous and corrosive to the souls of churchgoers. As Fischer explained, it was according to these articles that worship had been reformed in Ulm and the Mass "done away with."[157] The story of sensory reformation had insinuated itself into early evangelical culture.

The narrative also had wider purchase throughout the sixteenth century, becoming an example of what the anthropologist Mary Douglass once identified as "implicit knowledge" or meaning.[158] Over time, the idea that late medieval Christianity was fundamentally sensual and that evangelical Christianity represented its antithesis became a widespread assumption—a backdrop to the cultural scene that didn't necessarily require explicit argumentation to survive. Perhaps the most impressive evidence of the story's success in this regard is the fact that many Catholics seem to have accepted it by the mid-sixteenth century. Writing in the 1530s, Joachim von Pflummern, master of the formerly Catholic church of Biberach, thus lamented the utter transformation of ritual life in the town. His narrative, often cited by historians since the nineteenth century as one of the few "unmediated" pictures of religious life before the Reformation, unfolded as an extended elegy of all the objects and practices that the Reformation had supposedly done away with. It reads like nothing so much as a massive expansion of the story of sensory reformation. Incense, rosaries, paxes, icons, organ music, polyphonic singing, elaborate processions with vessels for carrying the sacred Eucharist, luxurious vestments, along with many other things, presented the church of his youth as a sensuous edifice that inspired profound emotion, wonder, and devotion. There was more than a little nostalgia embedded in this narrative of a lost sensory past. Pflummern thus spoke in melancholic tones "of the five senses, which we had in the old, true, Christian faith."[159] The humanist Georg Witzel, a contemporary of Pflummern's, articulated the same ideas in his extensive liturgical histories, which implicitly accepted the story of sensory reformation.[160] Witzel's major project was to contravene an important part of that story: that the extensive appeals to the senses in church ritual had been relatively recent developments in the history of the church, innovations begun by the papacy only within the previous three hundred years or so. In both Latin and the vernacular, at mid-century Witzel's writings set out to establish the antiquity of church ceremonies such as the elevation of the Eucharist, choral singing, the use of images, candles, vestments, reliquaries, incense, rosaries, and other liturgical furniture, as well as the myriad processions and seasonal blessings. By demonstrating the antiquity of these ceremonies, Witzel hoped to convince people of the need to restore them to the church, so that it would "be seen as an image of wondrous beauty, in order that it may win the heartfelt love of those who regard it."[161]

The reformation of the senses had been accomplished in a relatively short time, but what did that mean, and why was it important? Often, sensory historians have discussed this period as one of general continuity with the late Middle

Ages. To be sure, there were some significant continuities. When putting sensory reformation into practice, evangelicals fell far short of the radical vision they had entertained in the early 1520s, retaining many of the ceremonies they had once excoriated as tools of the devil and Antichrist. The evangelical movement also never successfully replaced the traditional Aristotelian understanding of how sensuous engagement with the world acted upon and affected the human soul. As dominant in the sixteenth century as it had been in the fifteenth, this would remain an important context framing the meaning of religious ritual for Catholics and Protestants alike. We turn more attention to these problems in the next two chapters.

These continuities notwithstanding, the story early reformers told in the 1520s had cultivated a feeling that something really had changed. In a few short years, largely by virtue of its dominant command of communication technologies, the evangelical movement had disseminated a foundational myth by which it identified itself and justified its own existence. The myth told a dynamic story that overwhelmed with its moral clarity and made the traditional provision for sensuousness in religion the axis about which history turned. It was a short story, and easily comprehensible: in the medieval church, sensuous ceremonies had ruined Christianity, transforming it into something else entirely, but by stripping the altars, evangelical religion had restored the Word, and the true faith. The Reformation was manifestly a desensualizing force in the history of Christianity. This became a feature of the imaginative landscape of the sixteenth century, ordering complicated and confusing events into a coherent and ideologically satisfying whole. The gendered and ethnic animus of the narrative lent an additional emotional charge, authorizing the feeling that evangelicals were reclaiming power and privilege that was rightfully theirs but had been usurped by external threats. Certainly, isolated elements of this story had circulated prior to the reformation, but it was only in the early 1520s that they fully cohered into a story so easy to grasp and so easy to repeat. Over and over again, people recited the narrative until it became true. A rift had emerged between the old and the new, and the distance between evangelical and traditional Christianity began to appear commensurate with that between heaven and hell.

5 Implementing the Reformation of the Senses in Practice

The reformation of the senses was important not only because it narrated a particular worldview but also because it provided a prescription for right action in the world. It told evangelicals what their relationship to the material basis of worship ought to be, and demanded a response. The first and most radical of these responses was developed by the likes of Andreas Bodenstein von Karlstadt in Wittenberg, and then later by spiritualists like Hans Greiffenberger in Nuremberg, detailed in chapter 4. The story enacted by people like Karlstadt held powerful sway in the evangelical mind, but it proved impractical as actual liturgical policy in the long run: no one could dispute the superiority of immaterial, spiritual goods, but if the new religion was to survive and flourish, evangelicals would have to engage with the world of the flesh and senses. Accordingly, the radical solution throughout the sixteenth century was disparaged as the pipe dream of radical fanatics, from Karlstadt to Caspar Schwenckfeld. Already in 1525, Martin Luther criticized such fanatics for ignoring the obvious fact that the soul mediated between external world and interior spiritual reality by way of its senses, and that the external forms of worship provided by the church were therefore necessary.[1]

The reformed tradition that emerged in Switzerland and southwestern Germany developed its own response to the narrative: state-sanctioned iconoclasm. This was not the riotous violence that one often imagines but rather a carefully calculated move, demonstrating administrative efficiency and disciplined professionalism. In Zürich, beginning on June 20, 1524, a committee of carpenters, masons, smiths, and other workers appointed by the city council entered the churches. Locked inside, they began an orderly dismantling of every statue, altar, and fixture within the churches. Even the choir stalls were removed. And, of course, they stripped the sacristies and altars of all liturgical furnishings. Once this was done, each item was disposed of. Masons broke down the stone objects, the wooden items were burned, and objects of precious metals were melted down. The walls of the churches were then whitewashed. The entire project took thirteen days, and when completed on the third of July, "scarcely a statue, a painting, a crucifix, a votive lamp, a reliquary, a shrine, or image or decoration of any sort was to be seen anywhere in the Zurich churches."[2] Throughout the late 1520s and into the 1530s, many churches across Switzerland and southwestern Germany followed this model of liturgical reform. There, the imperative to curb and control potential outbursts of iconoclastic violence and the disorderly destruction of church property resulted in a liturgical policy that, if evaluated in the terms set by the story of sensory reformation, was coherent, consistent, and successful. Benefiting from the cooperation between newly evangelical clergy and secular magistrates, and arguably enjoying at least some popular support, what this new policy actually achieved in practical terms was fairly dramatic and especially influential in the domain of visual culture, as more than a generation of scholarship attests.[3] This was as close as sixteenth-century reformers came to actualizing the dream of the reformation of the senses.

For many of those living in the German-speaking world, these radical and reformed responses had little to do with their day-to-day experience of sensuous worship. Most of the new evangelical communities in the Holy Roman Empire ultimately followed the model of reform laid down in Wittenberg, where it is less appropriate to speak of a clearly envisaged and systematically executed liturgical policy.[4] The reality was rather a patchwork of improvised, ad hoc solutions to problems that periodically emerged over the course of the sixteenth century, typically deferring to local interests with specific claims on the material culture of traditional worship. Thus, the process of realizing the story of sensory reformation in practice was far less straightforward in these communities, even as they continued to invoke and identify with the story. Like their counterparts in the south, the Lutherans of central and northern Germany were chiefly concerned with introducing practical reforms in a manner that preserved civic and religious order.[5] Also like the reformed communities, Lutherans continued to identify strongly with the narrative of sensory reformation, which often disposed them negatively to the worship of traditional Christianity. Unlike the south, however, the material impact was often far less dramatic.

One example at the outset suffices to drive home these points. In 1561, Johannes Pfarrkirchner, pastor to the small village of Hüll in Nuremberg's rural hinterland, reported "terrible, horrible, idolatrous abuses" in his parish to the Nuremberg city council. He described the abuses in terms reminiscent of the old story of sensory reformation: people went "about the altar with crosses, banners, lamps, idols, pilgrimages, offering money, wax candles, human hair . . . and kneeling before and worshipping the images."[6] Most of the idolatrous devotion was focused on one particular image of the Virgin Mary. The locals had crowned the image, placed wreaths on it, and decorated it with all manner of clothing and ornamentation.[7] Pfarrkirchner further complained that parishioners regularly violated the Sabbath, refusing to listen when he preached, and impeding orderly Lutheran ceremonial practice.[8] Pfarrkirchner identified with the iconoclastic king Hezekiah of the Old Testament, reminding the city council that such impieties demanded drastic responses:

> Wherefore it should be permitted to the magistracy to take care and execute, in order that impious dogma and idolatries be removed from the church, as demonstrated by the example of Hezekiah, king of Judah, who, through the priests, took care to restore the true cults of God, and to destroy and burn all idolatrous altars and other examples, etc.[9]

After investigating the matter, the city council found Pfarrkirchner to be an exemplary pastor and concurred that the situation in Hüll was grave.[10] The council recommended that, in addition to the sacristan keeping the church locked up, the image of the Virgin that excited such idolatrous devotion be removed and replaced with a crucifix. Pfarrkirchner was encouraged to re-double his efforts as a preacher and reminded to wear a vestment when administering the Eucharist so as to inspire proper reverence toward the true object to devotion.[11] Despite authorities' desire to resolve the issue, the image remained in situ, a popular destination of both Lutheran and Catholic regional pilgrimage well into the twentieth century.[12]

Evaluated in light of sensory reformation as a prescriptive norm, the handling of this case seemed indirect, ineffectual, and somewhat paradoxical—all the more so because of how serious the authorities perceived the threat of idolatry in Hüll to be. This was not an isolated incident. Similar practices in Hüll had been marked out by authorities in Nuremberg as idolatrous since the mid-1530s, when the city council first ordered the sacristan of the parish church to keep the church locked up during the week and to refuse any offerings from pilgrims or local parishioners.[13] Lutheran liturgical policy throughout the sixteenth century encouraged people like Johannes Pfarrkirchner to identify with the story of sensory reformation, even as other factors militated against its unproblematic implementation in practice. Attempts at implementing ritual change therefore lacked the coherence apparent in what we today think of as more radical strains of Protestantism. This is not to say important changes did not occur. In a village like Hüll, effecting appreciable change was often beyond the administrative capacities of the sixteenth-century Lutheran church, even when it had the backing of secular authorities. In Nuremberg proper, as well as in other urban locales, however, some important changes did occur to the sensory landscape Lutherans encountered.

While more broadly representative of the early evangelical movements' relationship to the material culture of traditional Christianity, and therefore more relevant to peoples' actual sensuous experience of religion in the sixteenth century, it is this third, less coherent approach to reforming worship that is less understood. If there is any consensus on the matter, it is largely one of continuity with traditional Christianity. Ernst Walter Zeeden long ago pointed to the lingering "Catholic traditions" in early Lutheran churches, and since then a growing body of scholarship has confirmed and expanded upon how Lutheranism tended to preserve significant portions of traditional devotional life, particularly in the domain of visual culture.[14] And yet, the story was not solely one of continuity. Particularly if one considers the problem from a more intersensorial perspective, there were *some* significant changes. The appeal of the Lutheran church went beyond vision, but precisely how it did remains somewhat obscure, in part due to the relative scholarly neglect of how Lutheran authorities attempted to manage church property more broadly.[15] Church artwork was profoundly important, but so too were other aspects of the material culture of liturgy. It was precisely the practical use of this material culture that the story of sensory reformation held up as an object of scorn, demanding a response from authorities.

This chapter addresses this problem, first outlining the origins of Lutheran liturgical policy in the early to mid-sixteenth century, and then assessing its practical impact on the traditional elements of sensuous worship. As in chapter 1, central focus remains on the rite of the Mass, or Lord's Supper, as most sixteenth-century evangelicals preferred to call it. Building on previous scholarship, as well as primary research into ecclesiastical ordinances, inspection reports, and church inventories, I demonstrate important continuities with the sensory culture of the late medieval past, alongside some surprising, often overlooked ruptures. Most of these ruptures took place in urban locations, where there were simply more things to deal with and, in some cases, get rid of. Changes here often took place over long periods and were not necessarily permanent: things removed in one generation might be restored in the next. This was an oblique form of iconoclasm, far less dramatic than that which took place in the reformed communities to the south. Whether intentionally or not, it nonetheless partially aligned with the dominant Protestant narrative of sensory reformation. The rural parish churches, by contrast, were far less dynamic, and although documentation for these locations is sparse, church inventories suggest that sensuous worship changed very little from the late Middle Ages: there was simply not much to do away with. Setting this rather incoherent liturgical policy alongside the hypercoherent narrative of early evangelical rhetoric draws our attention to the fundamentally paradoxical nature of reforming the senses in practice.

As the Lutheran church emerged in the sixteenth century, it developed two institutions to manage both the form of worship and its material culture and thereby respond to the story of sensory reformation. These were church ordinances and ecclesiastical visitations.[16] The former entailed publishing a practical guide for church life that outlined liturgical practice, the responsibilities of local secular and ecclesiastical authorities, and the rudiments of evangelical doctrine. The ordinances therefore built on the tradition of prescriptive liturgical literature widespread in the late Middle Ages.[17] The ecclesiastical visitation was also a disciplinary practice with roots in the medieval church, but it emerged a few years after the first evangelical church ordinances. The practice of bishops touring a circuit of the parish churches in their jurisdiction to inspect and assess the state of religious life was fairly well known in Germany on the eve of the Reformation.[18] Bishops, or more often their representatives, usually known as visitors, were commonly concerned with a variety of issues, including the pastoral fitness of rural clerics, how congregations related to the ritual provisions and norms of the church, and whether or not any significant conflicts or divisions between church and laity existed in liturgical, doctrinal, or other matters. Visitors would note their impressions of local parishes and report them back to episcopal authorities. In turn, the bishop might issue decrees on necessary changes or improvements.[19] Taken together, ordinances and visitations formed the basis of sixteenth-century Lutheran liturgical policy, such as it was. Both institutions had medieval origins, but the history of their early development in the 1520s helps explain the rather paradoxical relationship between the cultural narrative of sensory reformation and actual Lutheran ritual practice.

The first evangelical church ordinances appeared in early 1522 in response to iconoclastic riots that had broken out in the city of Wittenberg at the end of the previous year. In terms of the development of a distinctively Lutheran liturgical policy, the most important fact to take away from the events of 1521–22 is that a controversy over worship was ultimately put to rest rather obliquely with a political-economic solution. The ordinances affirmed the authority of the city council to manage the material culture of worship, vaguely in the service of preventing idolatry, but said nothing directly about specific practices. This allowed evangelicals to continue telling the story of sensory reformation even as it left open the door for the continuation of more traditional modes of managing church property. This was an equitable solution for the multiple parties involved, who represented a spectrum of radical, moderate, and traditional interests in the city.

At the supposedly radical end of the spectrum, Andreas Karlstadt had advocated the *removal* of offending elements of traditional worship and was ultimately indifferent about the methods for achieving this objective. An orderly, state-sanctioned dismantling of the church's ritual edifice along the lines of what would later happen in Zürich was just as good as a violent, popular surge of destruction from below.[20] Moreover, hostility toward traditional sensuous worship was not simply a preserve of the radical fringe at this moment in Wittenberg. Karlstadt narrated the story of sensory reformation alongside his evangelical colleagues, many of whom would eventually establish themselves as moderate, magisterial reformers. Although the city council lent its authority to the ordinance, its drafting was almost certainly influenced by an advisory committee of theologians from the university, appointed with the approval of the elector. Among this committee were both Karlstadt and the young Philip Melanchthon. While the subsequent historical narrative often portrays these two as polar opposites, in this instance they worked closely in concert. Melanchthon's later tendencies toward conservative diplomacy sometimes mask the fact that he personally was quite hostile to many aspects of traditional worship. At the time of this incident, he was enthusiastically attending the former Augustinian Gabriel Zwilling's iconoclastic sermons, and he probably shared a good deal more in common with Karlstadt than we are sometimes given to think. Together, these two men steered the policy in an iconoclastic direction.[21] This allowed theologians to tell themselves the story of sensory reformation. A significant portion of the liturgical furniture was, after all, removed from the church with the apparent intention of preventing idolatry.

At the same time, the matter involved the political and economic interests of the local secular ruling class as well. The solution had to be negotiated in this context, and thus the oblique iconoclasm that occurred in Wittenberg was ultimately "sanctioned from above."[22] In addition to the committee from the university, the city council was aided and advised by representatives of Frederick the Wise, who also had strong political, economic, and authentically religious interests in maintaining as much of the material culture of traditional piety as possible. His vast collection of relics and sacred vessels, displayed in his castle church within the city walls and advertised in print, had become a popular and lucrative regional pilgrimage destination and a point of personal pride.[23] While the ordinance passed by the city council only applied to the parish church, it was desirable as a preemptive measure in the eyes of the elector. If authorities had permitted the popular violence against church property to continue, it might have spread to the castle church. Further, orderly removal by authorities preserved the property intact and left open the possibility that it might be returned to the church at a later date, an eventuality that might well have been pleasing to the elector, whose own religious sensibilities remained somewhat ambiguous.[24] Beyond this, the ordinance accorded with late medieval practice and policy at the parish level. As in Wittenberg, so too across the Holy Roman Empire: the ruling class represented by the city council had historically viewed the management and disposal of church property in the parish church as their prerogative and privilege. The ordinances preserved this state of affairs.

It is tempting to speculate that liturgical policy in the emergent Lutheran church may have developed in a rather different direction had Luther been present in Wittenberg during the riots. Before 1522 he had, after all, often criticized sensuous elements of traditional worship just as harshly as Karlstadt had.[25] As it stood, however, he was absent during the critical events. Whereas Zwingli had been present in Zürich, actively steering secular magistrates toward a more coherent (and radical) policy, Luther inherited a framework of divergent interests when he returned to Wittenberg in March 1522.[26] In any event, it is difficult to overstate the significance of this context to later Lutheran attempts to implement the reformation of the senses in practice. Over the next four years, Luther built on the outcome of the iconoclastic riot, preaching, drafting his own ordinances, and providing recommendations to the evangelical communities in Wittenberg and elsewhere. In doing so, he began to articulate a slightly more defined policy that would shape ritual practice more broadly. Like the ordinance that had emerged from the earlier controversies, Luther's policy triangulated between the various interests involved in the early Reformation and, as such, was necessarily vague and seemingly contradictory in many of its prescriptions. Nonetheless, it is possible to identify a few of its most salient features.

Many of the prescriptive materials Luther composed in the mid-1520s continued to resonate with the evangelical story of sensory reformation. Often, he narrated the tale in prefaces as a kind of justification for what appeared to be new ritual norms. His first attempt to draft a general order for divine services, written at the request of the city council of Leisnig (Saxony) in early 1523, thus began by identifying the chief concern of the newly evangelical churches as supporting the office of preaching, in order that people might hear the pure, unadulterated Word of God. Because the whole panoply of late medieval church practices had submerged the Word, the first order of business was to clear out these abuses.[27] Similarly, at the end of 1523, in his first ordinance specifically outlining the new form of the Mass, Luther began by explaining that he had been moved to action "in order first that I might turn people's hearts away from impious beliefs about ceremonies" so that room might be cleared in their souls for the Gospel, that they might be saved from the Satanic threats they confronted in the world and protected from eternal perdition.[28] He further evoked sensory reformation here, comparing the churches with "those altars and signs of Baal, and other gods," and the many abominable sacrifices performed by pagan peoples.[29] In the context of the early 1520s such rhetoric forced audiences to identify with the biblical iconoclasts Hezekiah, Josiah, and others detailed in the Book of Kings. Of paramount importance was ensuring that the evangelical community had access to the pure and unadulterated Word. All matters of worship, including the form of the rituals employed and the material culture that structured the ritual environment, were to be subordinated to this concern, at least in theory.

At the same time, Luther was concerned to differentiate the true evangelical stance from that of fanatics like Karlstadt on the one hand and the Church of

Rome on the other. The former, in Luther's estimation, were "fanatics" who despite their rhetoric actually failed to detach themselves from the sensuous world: far from elevating themselves to the spiritual realm, iconoclasts everywhere had simply fetishized traditional worship and remained just as mired in the senses and flesh as the Church of Rome.[30] Especially after the Peasants' War of 1524–25, Luther and the Wittenberg reformers also tended to associate religiously motivated attacks on church property with much more far-reaching threats to the social order as a whole, and they took a reactionary stance aligned with the secular rulers of the German-speaking world.[31] Conversely, slavish adherence to a rigidly formulated liturgical ordinance handed down from above threatened to return evangelicals to the superficial, sensuous devotion of traditional Christianity. Local authorities should exercise discretion in determining their liturgical affairs but be on guard against any potential abuses, superstitions, or idolatry, just as Hezekiah had done before the Bronze Serpent. The ordinance was, after all, "an outward thing" in itself, and as such it could serve to the good, but also lead to abuse. The late medieval church had fetishized this outward thing. In such cases, the existence of a liturgical ordinance was "otherwise worthless and serve[d] no purpose."[32]

The need to thread the needle between fanatics like Karlstadt and defenders of traditional Christianity began to make the story of sensory reformation, in Luther's telling, more ambiguous. It did not necessarily end with the wanton destruction of all church property or even an orderly, state-sanctioned "total transformation" on the model he had envisioned just a few years earlier.[33] In an ideal world, the story could perhaps end that way, but ultimately Luther took a pragmatic tack and became skeptical about the radical separation of the sensible and spiritual worlds advocated by the likes of Karlstadt. Luther observed that God *perforce* engaged humanity both internally and externally and that, for the most part, the external, sensible world served as the cutting edge of the human-divine relationship. "God," he emphasized, "has determined to give the inward to no one except through the outward"—namely, the orally transmitted Word and the material signs of the sacraments of baptism and the Eucharist.[34] A more metaphorical reading of the story of sensory reformation was therefore in order: it really stood for *subjective* detachment from the ritual edifice of the church. Luther was not enthusiastic about much of traditional ceremony and acknowledged the superstitious and idolatrous abuses it could arouse, but he thought that the destruction or removal of offending objects from churches failed to address the real problem, which was the internal, affective attachment one felt toward such things. This bond could only be broken if "torn out of the heart through God's Word," for when such things were removed from the heart, "they can do no harm when seen with the eyes."[35]

Luther here reworked the narrative of sensory reformation but held the same anthropological assumptions as his late medieval counterparts, as well as Zwingli and Karlstadt, all of whom granted that sensuous engagement with the church affected how people felt internally and related morally to their surroundings. Where his radical counterparts tended to emphasize the negative effects of this engagement, Luther was more of an optimist, but mainly with respect to the Word as an object of perception. Pressing itself into souls of parishioners, the visible or audible Word could serve as a bulwark against the potentially dangerous sensuous elements of worship.[36]

By 1525, Luther also began to classify large portions of the material culture and liturgical forms that had constituted traditional worship as *adiaphora*, or matters of indifference to the core questions of faith and salvation. The best-known example was, of course, images, well documented in the growing scholarship on Lutheran visual piety.[37] The category could nonetheless apply to virtually any practice deemed "external" and was thus not restricted to appeals to sight.[38] Luther's prescriptive writings from the mid-1520s identified a variety of traditional objects and practices as adiaphora, including the elevation rite during the Mass, the burning of incense, the lighting of candles, church music of any kind, the use of vestments, altar linens and other ornamentation, bells, and the various genuflections performed by ministers at the altar during the celebration of the Eucharist.[39] Adiaphora could be tolerated if they served a didactic purpose, teaching and strengthening the weak of faith and spirit, and if there was no evidence that they gave rise to idolatrous or superstitious abuses. They were, however, not essential for true Christian worship. Luther considered this the most scripturally justified position: beyond the words of Christ and minimal details on his gestures described in the accounts of the Last Supper, as well as a sparse description of baptism, the New Testament of the Christian Bible provided very little in the way of positive ritual prescriptions. It was also vague about what types of things should be prohibited.[40] While the Old Testament provided copious details on the ceremonies of ancient Judaism, Luther denied that any of this could be considered binding for Christians. The new covenant between humanity and God established by Christ had made such things obsolete.[41] What mattered was not the presence of particular practices or things in churches but instead how people responded to their ritual environment.[42]

The formal classification of so much of the ritual environment as indifferent was a useful theological complement to a practical reality that already existed on the ground, reinforcing local authorities' traditional claims to determine and maintain their own distinctive liturgical cultures. With respect to the celebration of the Eucharist, Luther delegated broad authority to local elites to determine virtually all of its external practices, with the exception of a few necessary things and unambiguous prohibitions. The words spoken by Christ, as well as the manner in which he distributed the bread and wine, as detailed in the scriptural account of the Last Supper, were the sine qua non of Eucharistic practice.[43] Ministers were to cleave to this example in their own performance of the rite. Luther explicitly forbade the entire Offertory portion of the Mass, which immediately preceded the benedictions and consecrations of the elements, or "canon," as it had been called in the late medieval church (see table 2 in chapter 1). This was mainly because the words, gestures, and objects manipulated during the Offertory reflected the understanding of the Mass as a sacrificial offering made by humanity to God, a categorical impossibility and theological abomination from the perspective of evangelical theology.[44] In its place, he instituted a sermon, requiring hymns be sung both before and after. Luther also prohibited the ritual fraction of the Host prior to its distribution, although the theological reasons for doing so were less clear.[45] The traditional kiss of peace and the use of pax boards during this portion of the Mass were also suppressed by Luther and his followers in the early 1520s. Instead, they mandated a sung or spoken prayer known as the *Pax domini*.[46] Beyond these strictures, Luther granted wide latitude to local communities to determine the form of their Eucharistic practice, and church ritual more broadly.[47]

Similarly, these same authorities were to enjoy significant independence in the day-to-day management of the liturgical furniture and church spaces so essential to the production of sensuous worship. Luther enshrined this principle in recommendations he gave to the city council of Leisnig in 1523, which established the idea of a communal chest. The communal chest was a repository for all local church property. The most valuable were the permanent, or renewable, forms of wealth tied up in endowments, land, rents, and rights to impose tithes, fees, and taxes.[48] More important for our purposes, however, were the smaller, more mobile forms of wealth, most notably those things falling into the category of liturgical furniture, or *kleinod*, as it was usually called. Luther was clear that managing such property was essential to cultivating true worship, which consisted of honoring of God and maintaining bonds of charity between Christians in the community under the guidance of a capable pastor who regularly preached the Word and administered the sacraments. To this end, all liturgical furniture was to be carefully examined, evaluated, inventoried, and then placed in a chest.[49] Such things were technically superfluous and thus a relatively fungible form of wealth: gold and silver objects could be melted down and readily converted to cash, while luxurious textiles could easily be sold in a variety of markets. Presumably, some liturgical furniture would be kept in use—for example, chalices would seem to have been necessary for Eucharistic practice. Luther, however, neglected to provide any specific instruction on the number and kinds of liturgical equipment that might remain in churches or the kinds of things that ought to be relegated to the communal chest. Instead, he left it to local communities to make these determinations.[50]

Consonant with the paradoxes of Luther's early liturgical policies, Philip Melanchthon drafted an *Instruction* for secular and ecclesiastical authorities conducting the first visitations of Electoral Saxony's rural parishes in 1528. The instructions invoked elements of the old story of sensory reformation, suggesting that evangelical practice, in contrast to the old religion, was simpler, less sensual, and more spiritual. Most of the traditional feast days dedicated to various saints were eliminated from the liturgical calendar, and sacramental practice, it was determined, should cleave more closely to the simple models provided in the Scriptures.[51] However, rigid obedience to liturgical ordinances simply fetishized the sensual as the old religion had done, while any threat of iconoclastic violence did the same, in addition to threatening the orderly progress of reform, and the divinely sanctioned social order more broadly. The only resolution was to cast church ceremonies as adiaphora. Melanchthon, like Luther, usually avoided specifics, though his instructions did identify church music, fasting, feasting, abstention from particular foods, and the various (though imprecisely defined) "ceremonies" that composed the Mass as matters of indifference.[52] So long as local secular and ecclesiastical authorities could determine that such ceremonies were "not against God or reason," they should be permitted, and the ideal of ritual uniformity should be abandoned.[53] Melanchthon reiterated the same points two years later in the *Augsburg Confession*.[54]

The one issue bearing on sensuous worship that Melanchthon failed to address explicitly in the 1528 *Instruction*, the management of liturgical furniture, came up in documents associated with the visitation, including a formal proclamation announcing the visitation, issued by then-elector John the Constant, and an ordinance issued at the end of the year.[55] Exchanges between Luther and Melanchthon leading up to 1528 visitation affirmed the policy set in the early 1523 communal chest ordinance: the community should exercise discretion over the kinds of liturgical furniture they kept or converted into more fungible forms of wealth.[56] Both reaffirmed the initial policy of delegating management of church property to local officials and recommended that the sale and purchase of any such property be done with the intent of supporting the preaching of the Word and the proper administration of the sacraments.

The basic contours of something approaching a Lutheran liturgical policy were more or less set by the late 1520s. The result was an ambivalent framework for implementing reforms of worship. Above all, the policy emphasized flexibility but was vague in its positive prescriptions: most of the ritual life of the church was, theologically speaking, a matter of indifference, and local authorities were thus free to determine a wide range of its material content and practical forms. However, the narrative of sensory reformation presented a countervailing impulse to these policy recommendations. When confronting the ritual edifice of the church, this policy inclined people to think of themselves as little Hezekiahs or Josiahs. Luther had done much to set liturgical policy, such as it was, but it is important to keep in mind that he was building upon the framework established while he was absent from Wittenberg in 1521–22 and subsequently responding to circumstances as they emerged. In spite of this, and in spite of the general scorn with which they regarded the ideal of ceremonial uniformity, the Wittenbergers would come to recommend the policy as a model to other communities.

In combination with the charismatic authority of Luther, the carefully crafted public image of reform in Wittenberg throughout the 1520s had significant impact on the liturgical policies of Lutheran churches across northern and central Germany. Before the middle of the 1520s, early ordinances and prescriptive materials generally failed to articulate the formal theological principle of ritual adiaphora and instead framed the issue of ritual reform in starker terms more familiar to the narratives circulating in early evangelical public discourse. For example, the ordinance for the newly evangelical churches of Elbogen, published in 1523, exhibited no hint of the doctrine of adiaphora while simultaneously asserting that it took Wittenberg and Luther as models for church practice. The story of sensory reformation as a means of differentiating between old and new religions provided the main commentary on ritual practice and its meaning.[57] Similarly, in a draft order for the Mass he completed in 1524, Lazarus Spengler of Nuremberg continued to frame the need for new practice in terms of the popular evangelical narrative, minimizing discussion of ritual indifference. Instead, various ceremonies of traditional Christianity commonly cited in the narrative of sensory reformation stood opposed to the pure administration of the Word, which Spengler sought to facilitate through a spatial reorganization of the Nuremberg churches.[58] Similar contrasts were established in early ordinances and articles issued by ecclesiastical authorities in Nuremberg's parish churches, in Worms and in Strasbourg in 1524–25. The idea that the old "external and godless ceremonies" of Rome had submerged the Word justified the need for practical reform and obscured the matter of adiaphora.[59] The general feeling was that much of traditional practice, particularly that relating to the Mass, had to be eliminated in order to make space for a simplified form of evangelical worship.[60] Notably, the provision for confiscating liturgical furniture and relocating it in a communal chest was absent from these early prescriptive materials as well.

From the late 1520s, however, these patterns underwent considerable transformation. The notion that most external ceremonies were a matter of indifference and could be retained or discarded as local circumstances required became a commonplace. One of the earliest attempts to classify external ceremony as merely indifferent appeared in the 1525 ordinance published for the duchy of Prussia. With respect to the Mass specifically, ecclesiastical authorities suggested that practice should conform to the examples given in Scripture and recommended retaining the traditional elevation, but otherwise granted wide discretion to local ministers in the use of vestments, lights, and musical embellishments during the ritual.[61] Two years later, Johannes Brenz, a fierce supporter of Luther and the leading reformer in the territory of Württemberg, published an order for the Mass that made very similar recommendations for the city of Schwäbisch-Hall.[62] Brenz's ordinance would prove a useful model for other nearby cities, including Heilbronn and Reutlingen, and would influence the course of practical reform throughout the territory of Württemberg in the 1530s.[63] In Wittenberg, Johannes Bugenhagen drafted several ordinances for some of the largest and most important northern German towns. Starting with Braunschweig in 1528, Bugenhagen declared that external ceremonies were by definition matters of indifference and that local churches should best determine the utility of such things. In his ordinance, he mentioned specifically candles, banners, chrism oil, and images, and acknowledged that they might be retained under the principle of Christian liberty, so long as they served a didactic purpose.[64] In the 1530s and 1540s, the Braunschweig ordinance became the model for disciplining efforts in Hamburg, Lübeck, as well as the parish churches in the duchy of Pomerania.[65]

Between 1528 and 1533, Lutheran theologians in the city of Nuremberg collaborated with secular and ecclesiastical authorities in the neighboring territory of Brandenburg-Ansbach in a series of ordinances and visitations of the various rural parishes in the region.[66] There, most of the ceremonies of traditional Christianity were dismissed as "childish and unnecessary," falling under the superseded Mosaic law of the Old Testament.[67] Authorities were usually content to leave this category only vaguely defined, but they occasionally mentioned specifics, including vestments, images, and church music.[68] The final product of this multiyear project was the 1533 ordinance for the churches of Nuremberg and Brandenburg-Ansbach, which became the touchstone of liturgical reform in much of Bavaria, as well as other territories in the north, such as Mecklenburg, in the middle decades of the sixteenth century.[69] Ordinances and visitation protocols for other territories in the 1540s, including the duchies of Wolfenbüttel, Göttingen-Calenberg, Lüneburg, and the Brandenburg march, came to articulate the same policy of adiaphora.[70] By the second half of the sixteenth century, it was entrenched in Lutheran liturgical culture throughout the German-speaking world.[71]

There were a few exceptions to the policy of ritual indifference, particularly with respect to the performance the Mass. The special seasonal blessings and processions that often wound their way into Masses in the late medieval church were proscribed as superstitious vestiges of paganism. Thus, in a 1526 recommendation on ceremonies to the city council of Nuremberg, Osiander derided such things as "jugglery" and, potentially, instruments of diabolical delusion.[72] All Lutheran communities rejected out of hand the sacrificial theology associated with the late medieval Mass and accordingly removed the Offertory portion of the rite from their services. As well, all instituted a sermon at the end of the liturgy of the Word.[73] Further, all agreed that the words of consecration spoken by the officiating pastor must conform to those dictated in the scriptural account of the Last Supper. Many of the gestures of the ministers were matters of indifference, but the fraction of the Host was not one of them. Ordinances followed Luther's early rejection of this rite, and it became a hallmark of Lutheran practice, especially in the second half of the sixteenth century.[74] Immediately preceding Communion, the vast majority of ordinances also included an exhortation to communicants, explaining the significance of the moment and encouraging all who were prepared to receive the sacrament to approach the altar. This was either sung or spoken by the officiating priest.[75] There was also universal agreement that congregants should receive Communion in both kinds, and pastors who withheld the wine were censured.[76]

After the mid-1520s, it also became increasingly common to establish rules for managing church wealth, including the liturgical furniture so central to ritual practice. Outside of Wittenberg, the first attempt to do so took place in the nearby city of Magdeburg in 1524. There, city officials mandated that all church property be remitted to a communal chest to support the new religion.[77] The prescription lacked specifics, failing to mention the matter of liturgical furniture or what particular dimensions of the new religion the communal chest would support.[78] Later ordinances and visitation protocols across central and northern Germany, however, filled in the details. In 1528, ordinances for the Saxon parishes of Zahna and Torgau stipulated that the communal chest was to fund the pastor, church ministers, the sick, the poor, and the local school. All possessions were directed into the chest for this purpose, including any superfluous liturgical furniture. In Zahna this meant that churches "should keep the three best Mass vestments and a chalice for daily use. The other regalia and church devices should be sold and the money put into the communal chest."[79] In Torgau the allowance was slightly different, amounting to "four or five regalia" and "two or three chalices."[80] Should anything escape this initial round of liquidation, it was to be kept in the chest and managed by secular magistrates as a kind of reserve fund.[81]

Other Saxon parishes made similar recommendations in the 1530s.[82] They became especially prevalent in regions concerned with the confiscation of monastic property specifically, as was the case in Württemberg in 1534.[83] Three years later, Ulrich, duke of Württemberg, issued an ordinance for his entire realm with similar provisions for the property of parish churches. Unnecessary liturgical furniture was to be sold off, and any wealth generated would be redistributed to the poor. The ordinance reasoned that this action had the twofold benefit of aiding the poor and stemming any potential idolatrous or superstitious beliefs that might arise from sensuous attachment to such things. The duke reissued the ordinance on multiple occasions in the late 1530s and early 1540s.[84] Similar patterns prevailed elsewhere in these years. When Pomeranian officials began visitations of parish churches in 1535, they adopted and promulgated this policy for the entire region under their jurisdiction.[85] In 1539, Albertine Saxony (the portion of the territory not ruled by the elector) instituted the policy in its own instructions to visitors to the parish churches.[86] Authorities in Quedlinburg, a Saxon district associated in the Middle Ages with its powerful abbey, applied it to all "parishes, convents and churches" in 1540, and in extensive visitations undertaken in the lower Saxon duchies of Wolfenbüttel, Lüneburg, and Göttingen-Calenberg two years later, confiscation and liquidation of superfluous liturgical furniture was the normal policy recommendation.[87]

Other policies advocated confiscation without specifically addressing the sale of superfluous liturgical furniture. In Braunschweig, Hamburg, and Lübeck, for example, all silver items were to be inventoried and then stored in the communal chest located in the municipal mint, to be managed by city officials.[88] This was also the policy for many of the territories of the elector of Brandenburg after 1540.[89] Although the influential Nuremberg-Brandenburg church ordinance of 1533 contained no explicit discussion of the communal chest, it seems likely that it was adopted as policy in practice. Given the influence of the Nuremberg church authorities in the drafting of the document, it may simply have been viewed as not meriting explicit discussion. As we saw in chapter 1, for Nuremberg and other large urban centers, civic control over liturgical furniture was already a fact of daily life well before the Reformation. In neighboring Brandenburg-Ansbach, evangelical confiscations of parish church property, including liturgical furniture, became standard practice already in 1526, and later visitation protocols formally mandated inspections of communal chests for the rural territories.[90]

From the perspective of religious reformers, the policy of confiscating liturgical furniture had the additional benefit of functioning as an oblique kind of iconoclasm. Authorities in Wittenberg had recognized this in the wake of the events of 1521–22, and it remained at least latent in the disciplinary efforts of reformers elsewhere. It became an explicit objective of confiscations of liturgical furniture in certain rural parishes of Brandenburg-Ansbach in the early 1530s.[91] By the middle of the century, it was more regularly articulated in the visitation protocols and ordinances. In visitation reports for the parish churches in the regions around Braunschweig, Wolfenbüttel, Hannover, and Lüneburg, for example, authorities regularly tasked local secular officials with extirpating idolatry by means of confiscating liturgical furniture. Idolatrous cults, as instructions indicated, "shall be done away with and whatever silver, treasures, or things of iron, wax, or whatever is on hand, shall be inventoried and carefully withheld until further notice. Such should happen in all places where such running about, idolatry and jugglery has been practiced."[92] Confiscation therefore became not only an important political-economic consideration of the early Lutheran churches but also a means of preserving the ideological identity embedded in the story of sensory reformation: should relatively modest liturgical changes and purified preaching of the Word prove ineffective, the removal of the offending objects of perception was an option available to reformers as a kind of last line of defense. Lutheran religion appeared to drift in a vague direction away from medieval sensuality.

The ordinances and visitation protocols of the early Lutheran churches in Germany therefore often pulled in a variety of directions. As a result, Lutherans were burdened with the task of constantly having to interpret what they should do about external forms of worship. Because large swaths of church practice were formally regarded as indifferent to the core questions of internal faith and salvation, and because Scripture neither commanded nor forbade them, many of the traditional ceremonies could be retained or abandoned, so long as they caused no harm. Often, this particular aspect of Lutheran liturgical policy has been cited as the reason for significant continuities with the medieval past.[93] However, exactly how indifferent such objects and practices could be in their sixteenth-century context is subject to question.[94] Judgments about the nature of these ceremonies and objects were still very often filtered through the narrative of sensory reformation. Evaluated in this light, the sensuality of ritual could pose a significant threat. Regardless of what was actually in the churches, or whether it corresponded to the overwhelming hyperaesthesia often represented in the cultural narrative, the sensuous residue of traditional Christianity still had the potential to inspire superstition and idolatry in the hearts of parishioners. Moreover, even if authorities determined that sensuous worship wasn't necessarily harmful, they still had to contend with the issue of the utility of liturgical furniture. The material culture of traditional Christianity was a necessary precondition for cultic practice, as well as a form of wealth, and Lutheran policy made it fairly clear that nonessential items ought to be liquidated or deposited in a communal fund. But what was essential and nonessential in the early Lutheran context? There was no standard of uniformity in practice, and so policy dictated that locals make this determination.

A variety of factors therefore shaped the implementation of sensory reformation in practice. Not surprisingly, the results of the project in Lutheran Germany were, from a sensorial perspective, deeply ambivalent and often seemingly incoherent. What worship looked, smelled, sounded, tasted, or felt like exhibited significant continuity with the medieval past in certain domains and important ruptures in others. We turn to these problems below as they manifested in the central rite of the Christian tradition, the Mass, or Lord's Supper.

The Lutheran tradition as it emerged in the sixteenth century shared much in common with late medieval visual piety. The material cultural record in the Lutheran heartland, encompassing Saxony, Thuringia, Brandenburg, as well as other northern German territories, such as Mecklenburg and Pomerania, and more centrally located cities like Nuremberg, attests to this fact. Some of the best-preserved examples of fifteenth-century religious art are found in these territories rather than in historically Catholic regions. In Saxony alone, approximately 270 altarpieces and 875 devotional images survived the sixteenth century.[95] Further to the north, in Mecklenburg, some 165 images survived along with 170 chalices, all of which were crafted in the fourteenth or fifteenth centuries, and approximately one-third of the parish churches in the territory still had late medieval altarpieces in situ by the end of the sixteenth century.[96] More than a thousand medieval chalices survived in Brandenburg, Saxony, and Schleswig-Holstein.[97] Candelabra, crucifixes, banners, altar linens, vestments, and other textiles remained important components of the visual appeal of the Lutheran Mass as well. In some cases, these items were still in use as late as the early nineteenth century.[98] Additionally, many of the permanent art fixtures and large sculpture work that had made them so rich as visual environments in the late Middle Ages remained in situ through the sixteenth century.[99] Many churches also retained the gestures that had traditionally framed the Eucharist, above all the ritual elevation of the bread and wine.[100] In most people's daily lives, it would seem that the Lutheran Lord's Supper looked more or less the same as it had under the old ritual regime of the Church of Rome.

There are several points, however, that qualify the story. Lutheran liturgical policy wrought some appreciable changes to the sightlines of sacred space over the course of the sixteenth century, particularly in wealthier urban locales, albeit in an oblique, circuitous manner that often unfolded over the course of decades. In the church of St. Lorenz in Nuremberg, for example, the city council mandated in 1529 that a large limewood sculpture of the Virgin Mary and Christ child encompassed by a rosary be permanently veiled in a purpose-made shroud. Completed in 1518 by the artist Veit Stoss, it had been installed over the great altar and prominently featured on a variety of feast days throughout the liturgical calendar, but especially those dedicated to the Virgin. It is likely that the church's evangelical preacher, Andreas Osiander, who was typically a sharp critic of traditional Marian devotions, spurred the city council to this decision. Henceforth, the covered image framed the celebration of the Eucharist as a conspicuous evangelical rejection of this particular aspect of traditional visual piety.[101] Often, authorities determined to remove installations only after prodding from local pastors about the idolatry and superstitions these objects elicited. This was the case in Nuremberg's *Frauenkirche,* situated between the city's two parish churches. There, in 1529, the city council removed another image of Mary that had become notorious for inspiring all manner of idolatry.[102]

Occasionally, this pattern impacted whole regions. The earliest example was the county of Hesse, where in 1526 images of all kinds came under intense scrutiny. On the recommendation of theologians, and with the authority of the recently converted landgrave Philip I, secular magistrates were instructed to look to Hezekiah's destruction of the bronze serpent, undertake the removal of all images, and strip the altars so that they were reduced to humble tables. The program was ambitious but never fully executed.[103] In the middle decades of the sixteenth century, Mecklenburg reformers pushed through a similar agenda, with similarly limited successes. A number of large altarpieces deemed "idolatrous" because of their connections to the late medieval cult of the saints were removed from parish churches in the territory.[104]

In most cases, the removal of traditional visual culture hinged on sentiments mobilized by the story of sensory reformation: in their sensuous appeal, the objects of the ritual environment were incongruous with Holy Scripture and utterly un-Christian: not only were they popish, they were evidence of pagan practice in the midst of the true Christian church. Moreover, idolatrous worship was gendered a feminine behavior, characteristic of silly old women.[105] The ire with which reformers approached traditional use of the rosary, in particular, illustrates this point. In addition to veiling or removing images of rosaries, official statements of doctrine such as the Augsburg Confession defined the use of the rosary and related devotions as "childish" and "needless."[106] As we saw in chapter 4, the pairing of femininity with childishness or foolishness was a common rhetorical tactic in the story of sensory reformation. Similarly, in several recommendations to the Nuremberg city council in the late 1520s, Andreas Osiander regularly derided rosaries as "fool's tricks" that distracted people from the Word.[107] In the 1533 ordinance for Nuremberg and Brandenburg-Ansbach, he succeeded in formally proscribing the use of rosaries in churches, condemning it as "unchristian babbling" characteristic of "old hags" and "fools."[108]

Other, more pragmatic rationales aligned with the narrative of sensory reformation to justify significant transformations of the sightlines in the churches. The sheer number of altars, for example, presented a major obstacle to the Reformation fetish of the Word. Occasionally, it was acceptable simply to defund them, effectively allowing them to die of benign neglect, as Luther had recommended in the mid-1520s.[109] However, the concern that the Word be accessible to congregations often motivated more immediate solutions. Pastors needed to be seen and heard, and when the presence of one or more altars interfered with this, removal was justified, and indeed necessary. This is precisely what happened in Nuremberg's parish churches in the early 1540s. In 1542 the city council ordered the removal of three altars in the church of St. Sebald because they "get in the way of people hearing the Word of God and in front of them the preacher cannot be seen or heard well."[110] Although no contemporary evidence confirms it, later reports suggest that it is likely that many of the altars in both of the city's parish churches were removed or destroyed in the year following this decree of the city council.[111] Additionally, liturgical reforms had simply made the altars unnecessary. The preponderance of altars populating late medieval churches had been essential to the processions and ceremonial blessings that often attached themselves to Masses on special feast days throughout the year. These, however, were no longer permissible, and the number of feast days was, in most Lutheran communities, drastically reduced. This indirectly removed the need for so many altars.[112]

Once altars were gone or reduced in number, the rationale for much of the liturgical furniture in the sacristies of the churches disappeared as well. In chapter 1 we saw how abundant reliquaries, icons, candelabra, and ornamental textiles were used in a dizzying array of combinations on various feast days, making the celebration of the Mass a visually protean thing throughout the liturgical year. Particularly in wealthy urban parishes, the Lutheran reformation wrought significant, if inconsistent, changes to this paradigm in the sixteenth century, on the whole reducing the diversity of mobile liturgical furniture in churches and thereby circumscribing to some extent the visible variability of the Mass. Reliquaries, the most striking visible manifestation of the late medieval cult of saints, and frequent ornaments on altars, were excluded from worship of any kind. Monstrances, too, so often used in the processions of traditional Christianity, no longer had a purpose. Items less specifically connected with particular feast days or processions, such as candelabra, vestments, and altar textiles, might remain, but local authorities were encouraged to reduce their collections to the minimal number of pieces necessary for worship. In Nuremberg, these principles appear to have been put into practice after 1530, when the city council locked away the majority of the liturgical furniture of its two parish churches, described above in chapter 1, leaving only liturgical vessels essential to the celebration of the Eucharist at the disposal of the pastors.[113] In September 1552 the city council took the decision to liquidate the property held in storage, sending almost all of it to the smelters to be melted down and converted into cash in order to finance an expensive war with the city's regional rival Albrecht Alcibiades of Brandenburg-Kulmbach.[114] The old textiles, however, appear to have escaped this fate, as evidence attests to their presence and use in the churches until the late eighteenth century.[115]

Similar patterns prevailed in other urban locations. In Lübeck in 1533, the 339 chalices of the city's parish churches, along with most of its other liturgical furniture, was melted down to finance a war with the king of Denmark.[116] Accounts of the parish church of Göttingen, which adopted Lutheranism in 1529, indicate significant amounts of continued spending on the maintenance of old Mass vestments and altar textiles, alongside the sale of various monstrances, chalices, patens, and other church silver deemed superfluous. Additionally, there was a significant decline in the purchase of candles for use in churches.[117] Perhaps even more than the liturgical forms outlined in the church ordinances, the management of moveable church property suggests that when Lutherans took action on the sightlines that defined sacred space, they tended to drift in the direction of simplification and elimination of certain elements of traditional visual culture, even when motivated by concerns not explicitly religious. In many of the wealthier Lutheran churches, there would be fewer altars and less ornamentation of church interiors than had been the case in the later Middle Ages.

The drift toward simplification, of course, should not be seen as universally representative of German Lutheranism in the sixteenth century or as an indication of a "less sensuous" form of Christianity. In electoral Brandenburg, for example, authorities took very little action to remove liturgical furniture and, indeed, were quite concerned with preserving what they had for most of the sixteenth century.[118] Further, while Lutheran churches generally abandoned the side altars that had crowded late medieval church interiors, they often enthusiastically replaced the great altars where the Eucharist was celebrated, as well as many of the objects that typically ornamented them, especially crucifixes. Usually, the act of replacing old altars and liturgical furniture constituted a self-conscious assertion of Lutheran identity against both Catholics and more "fanatical" sects of Protestantism: Lutherans, by retaining some elements of traditional Christianity but refusing a wholesale stripping of the altars, followed a "middle path" between what they perceived to be the religious extremes of the sixteenth century.[119] The nature of the images adorning Lutheran churches, of course, underwent important shifts: at least in theory, they became less emotive, contained more explanatory inscriptions, and were more self-consciously concerned with communicating theological doctrines in a simple and clear manner.[120]

These patterns, however, were most pronounced in the wealthier urban churches of Lutheran Germany. In rural locations, there was marked concern with ensuring that communities had the basic implements needed for Eucharistic practice. Above all, as visitation reports attest, this resulted in efforts to ensure that poor rural parishes had at least one chalice and one Mass vestment, the minimal furnishings deemed necessary for putting on a good Eucharistic show. Often, this was a constant struggle, as such items were stolen, or borrowed by a neighboring parish and never returned.[121] Providing these communities with chalices was especially important given the Lutheran emphasis on Communion in both kinds, which they considered an essential means of differentiation from their Catholic counterparts, who often withheld the wine from lay communicants. All of this complicates the general drift toward a more simplified visual staging of the Eucharist in early Lutheran practice.

Similarly, a rather circuitous and ambivalent story emerged with respect to the gestures that framed Eucharistic practice, especially the elevation of the elements. In Wittenberg, Luther technically maintained that the elevation was adiaphoron until his death, declaring that "Christ does not forbid the elevation, but leaves it to free choice."[122] His support for it was inconsistent at best, oscillating between lukewarm tolerance and outright condemnation. His 1523 *Formula missae* and 1526 German Mass ordinance prescribed its use.[123] In the 1530s, he supported removing it from services, and this seems to have happened briefly in Wittenberg, although only temporarily. Wolfgang Musculus, a reformed theologian in the mold of Zwingli, witnessed a Lutheran Mass in Eisenach in 1536, describing the practice of elevation in detail. After the consecration of the Eucharist, the officiant "admonished the small gathering on the institution of the meal, next he sang the words of the meal, first over the bread . . . [then] he elevated the bread before all in papistic fashion, then the chalice, and this he simultaneously elevated with the final words of Christ."[124] In the same year, Musculus observed the elevation at Wittenberg as well.[125] Formally, the elevation was discontinued in Wittenberg's castle church by 1539, but it seems to have continued for a couple more years in the city's parish church. In 1541–42, Johannes Bugenhagen, newly installed as pastor of Wittenberg's parish church, definitively eliminated the practice. Many other churches in Saxony followed suit shortly thereafter.[126]

In other localities, similar ambiguity and inconsistency prevailed, as authorities chose to remain silent about the elevation in official ordinances. The 1533 ordinance for Nuremberg and neighboring Brandenburg-Ansbach neither directly prohibited nor endorsed the practice.[127] This reflected the divergent practice in the two territories: in Brandenburg-Ansbach, the elevation had already been abandoned by 1530.[128] In Nuremberg, it was retained throughout the sixteenth century, though not without considerable controversy and resistance from the pastorate and educated elites of the city.[129] The central concern of these elites was precisely what ordinary people experienced when witnessing the elevation, and whether or not it was cultivating inappropriate attachments to the material elements of worship. As one pastor complained to the city council in the late 1530s, the elevation was inspiring idolatrous worship of the visible bread, rather than of Christ, because the uneducated laity were unable to distinguish between the sensible and spiritual worlds. Remarking that he commonly overheard his parishioners describe that they had "seen our Lord today" after witnessing the elevation, he added that they also continued to have "manifold false thoughts and idolatry, namely that the simple people believe that if they see this sacrament, they will have no tooth or eye pain on that day, more luck than usual, as well as others."[130]

Similar complaints proliferated many times over in Lutheran Germany.[131] This is not surprising, because silence on the elevation became the norm for most church ordinances after the mid-1520s: a recent comprehensive survey of the ordinances demonstrates that it was explicitly mandated in only 11.2 percent of German Lutheran churches in the sixteenth century.[132] All of these mandates appeared in the ordinances up to 1549, and never thereafter.[133] This required local authorities to determine whether or not they elevated the elements. In all likelihood, the popular piety surrounding the elevation, cultivated over generations and extremely difficult to eradicate, produced a more widespread reaction against it in the second half of the sixteenth century, when explicit prohibitions against the practice became more common in the ordinances. Of the fifteen ordinances that made such prohibitions for the entirety of the early modern period, thirteen were published between 1546 and 1576.[134]

Explicit prohibition was not universally the case, of course. In precious few locations, authorities ardently defended the elevation and even developed it into a more elaborate ritual. In electoral Brandenburg, for example, it was required in the territory's first church ordinance of 1540. By 1562, pastors were expected to perform what was called the *ostensio*. In addition to the traditional elevation, this involved turning to the congregation and addressing them with the words: "see, dear Christians, this is the true body of Christ given for us, and this is the true blood of Christ shed for us."[135] As with the elevation elsewhere, educated Lutherans regarded the Brandenburg ostensio with suspicion and even hostility. In the face of mounting pressure at the end of the century, the electors abolished it in 1598.

These complicating factors notwithstanding, the *longue durée* drift toward simplification of the sightlines within churches seems to have been the preferred Lutheran method of relating to the visual culture of late medieval Christendom. This is perhaps most apparent in the construction of the first purpose-built Lutheran churches. The Saxon elector Johann Friedrich initiated construction of the first such church, the Torgau castle church, in 1533. When completed in 1544, the underlying visual theme of the church was austerity, and at first glance there was little to distinguish it visually from the whitewashed churches of the Reformed tradition. Indeed, the plainness of the interior was striking and blended quite seamlessly with the castle residence to which it was attached.[136] During the dedication sermon he gave at the church, Martin Luther thus aptly described it as a humble "house" of God's Word, in contrast to pomposity of Catholic cathedrals.[137] A small sandstone table, unadorned by any special linen, silk, or velvet, and no longer ornamented by a retable, relics, or other vessels, replaced the imposing altars of traditional Christianity. The pulpit took a much more prominent position, located centrally on one side of the nave, and offering congregations a rich display of polychrome relief carvings. All of this was set within a space with a much lower ceiling, enclosed by walls with plain windows of modest size. The design self-consciously emulated ancient theaters, rather than late medieval cathedrals, and was intended to focus the gaze of churchgoers onto the humble altar during the Eucharist and on the pulpit during sermons.[138]

In the second half of the sixteenth century, church builders sought to emulate and improve on the visual paradigm set by the Torgau castle church. Chapels attached to the palaces and castles of secular princes, such as those at Hartenfels in Neuberg, built by Ottheinrich, Elector of the Palatinate, as well as the Moritzbau in Dresden, and other palatial chapels in Stettin (Pomerania), Stuttgart (Württemberg), Augustusburg (Saxony), Freudenstein (Freiberg, Saxony), and Schmalkalden (Thuringia).[139] The palatial chapel at Schmalkalden, completed in 1590, represented a major shift in its relocation of the pulpit to the choir. Positioned directly above the altar table, it further rationalized the sightlines of church space, directing eyes to a single location and effectively unifying reception of the Word and reception of the Eucharist. As Joseph Koerner suggests, this configuration constituted a model for Lutheran church building in the seventeenth century.[140]

In the late sixteenth century, preachers and theologians enthusiastically advertised the fact that only modest liturgical furnishings complemented the visual austerity of these model Lutheran spaces. The tradition began with Luther himself, in his dedication sermon at Torgau in 1544. The sermon echoed the narrative of sensory reformation as a self-conscious rejection of the hyperaesthesia of traditional church consecration ceremonies. Luther exhorted those gathered for the dedication simply to call upon God in prayer, honor his Word, give thanks, and be faithful. "Take hold of the censer with me," he exclaimed, "that is, seize hold upon prayer, and let us call upon God and pray . . . for this is what God would have from us all, and this is the true incense of Christians—the pray earnestly for all of these necessities."[141] Additionally, Luther rejected unequivocally the sanctifying power of Holy Water, chrism oil, special vessels, or precious textiles. The absence of such things helped define the Lutheran ritual environment and cleared space for hearing the Word of God, the only truly sanctifying force in the world.[142] The dedication inscription for the Torgau church, completed in 1545, conveyed a similar message, describing the space as one in which a "totally new" and "wholly pure" piety was practiced.[143] Similarly, Caspar Cruciger, a friend and colleague of Luther's, memorialized the Torgau dedication in verse form a few years later, writing "no chrism or holy water did he use, no flags or candles or incense; the divine word and his prayer, together with the faithful did this."[144] Following Cruciger, countless Lutheran pastors and preachers in the second half of the sixteenth century recited this moment in their own dedication sermons, and even added other objects associated with traditional Christianity into the mix, including crucifixes, monstrances, reliquaries, and other images.[145]

As Luther's comments at Torgau made clear, what was at stake was not simply the visual production of the Eucharist. Rather, ritual was manifestly an intersensorial problem, and for Lutherans, fully separating the visual from the rest of the senses was impossible. The history of the other four senses traditionally identified in the Western European sensorium reveals more significant transformations in Lutheran ritual life and further complicates the predominant thesis of continuity with traditional Christianity.

With respect to aurality, the Lutherans introduced several fundamental changes to the soundscape of the traditional Mass. In urban landscapes, the Reformation presented a significant challenge to the supermusicality that had defined much of the late medieval aural setting of the Mass.[146] Whereas late medieval worship had placed a relatively low priority on verbal clarity, and correspondingly high emphasis on aural excess and magnificence, reformers inverted this paradigm. Verbal clarity, focused aural attention, and the management of competing sounds, all in the service of administering the "pure" and unadulterated Word of God, characterized sixteenth century Lutheran practice. This is evident in virtually every aspect of the reformers' aural engineering of the Lord's Supper.

The most obvious transformation of the soundscape of the Mass was the introduction of a sermon into services.[147] In the late Middle Ages, the sermon was only inconsistently part of Mass, if at all. Occasionally, Latin homilies were inserted after the Gospel reading, during the Offertory, or even following the elevation. More typically, however, sermon and Mass were separate services, and the main contexts for preaching in the fifteenth century were monasteries, public spaces like market squares, or within the church, during special "pulpit services," often endowed by wealthy patrons.[148] Luther had frequently criticized the omission of sermons from the Mass, and in his first orders he made it a required part of the rite.[149] He inserted the sermon at the end of the first portion of the Mass and required it be conducted in the vernacular. Immediately following the reading of the Gospel text, the pastor was to give the sermon, ideally related in some way to the text of the Scripture. Lutheran communities of the sixteenth century (and indeed, beyond) universally emulated this model in their own ordinances.[150] Situated at the end of the liturgy of the Word, the Lutheran sermon served as a transition into the second half of the Mass, or liturgy of the Eucharist. Indeed, viewing Lutheran orders of the Mass alongside their late medieval counterparts, it is clear that the sermon effectively replaced the Offertory portion of the Roman rite. This was significant because it eliminated the sacrificial theology of the rite, so offensive to all Protestants, but also because it eliminated the context for a wide range of the gestures, manipulations of the Eucharistic elements and liturgical vessels, and the burning of incense. In this respect, the move was a near perfect crystallization of the narrative of sensory reformation in miniature: clearing the Mass of the sensory pandemonium of the Offertory made room for the Word of God, communicated through the voice of the pastorate. All other Lutheran ordinances of the sixteenth century followed the paradigm established by Luther, and undoubtedly, the sermon represented the most consistent transformation of traditional soundscape of worship introduced by the new confession in the sixteenth century.[151]

There is no question that Lutheran authorities considered the sermon the most important component of the Mass. It preceded and was superior to the sacrament of the Eucharist, which itself was simply a different manifestation of the Word according to Lutheran theology.[152] Beyond this, the importance Lutherans attached to the sermon manifested in concern with the preacher's ability to captivate the aural attention of his parishioners. Again and again, church visitors throughout the sixteenth century confronted the shortcomings of both laity and clergy. Often, the superstitious or idolatrous behaviors of laypersons were attributed to inattentiveness during the sermon or the lack of skill of the preacher. The remedy for most of these problems was to reiterate the need for pastors to preach "clearly," "purely," and in a loud voice.[153] Simply hearing the sermon should have been enough, and, despite the fact that movement leaders like Philip Melanchthon wrote several treatises on rhetoric for the specific purpose of improving preaching, this was usually the extent of the advice given in these situations.[154] Given the Lutheran emphasis on verbal clarity, one might expect to find attempts to manage the specific content of *what* exactly preachers were saying in their sermons, but this was largely irrelevant because, much like their late medieval predecessors, sixteenth-century Lutheran preachers were in the main expected to preach from model sermons, written and assembled by leading theologians into purpose-made collections known as *postils*. Again, Luther had established this paradigm in the early 1520s, and later intellectuals followed his example, compiling numerous postils in the mid- to late sixteenth century.[155] Thus, the pastoral emphasis in the visitation reports tended to rest on the concrete, hierarchical aural exchange between preacher and listener. This relationship defined the essence of the sermon, and all other aspects of the soundscape of worship were subordinate to it in a manner never articulated in the late Middle Ages.

New Lutheran aural sensibilities were also apparent in a secondary form of preaching Lutherans introduced into the Mass, immediately at the beginning of the liturgy of the Eucharist. This took the form of a vernacular exhortation to communicants, spoken by the pastor to the congregation. The exhortation explained the theological significance of the sacrament, forced communicants to reflect on their own sinfulness, and encouraged those who felt prepared to approach to receive the bread and wine. Luther had failed to include this component in his 1523 Mass order, but other early orders, from Coburg, Nuremberg, and Strasbourg, pioneered it. He adapted it into his 1526 German Mass ordinance, following these earlier examples. Thereafter, 78 percent of the ordinances published in the sixteenth century included the exhortation as part of the Lutheran Mass.[156] This exhortation removed the necessity of the Eucharist prayers so popular in fifteenth century personal prayer books and, paired with a systematic campaign against these items, represented another fundamental shift in the soundscape: no longer would the variegated, murmured prayers of individuals form a sonic backdrop to the liturgy of the Eucharist. Rather, the rational declamation of the meaning of the sacrament by the pastor, and the passive reception of these words by the congregation, became the focused aural center of the liturgy.

Following this logic, Lutheranism introduced several significant changes to the musical setting of the Mass as well.[157] Almost every portion of the rite could be sung, though the ordinances made clear that all church music was technically a matter of indifference, so long as it did not interfere with people's understandings of the words of the songs, which, like sermons, were primarily intended to serve a didactic purpose. Thus, beginning with Luther, the precise mode of vocal music was usually determined by local authorities, according to local custom, tradition, and, perhaps most important, the material resources of the community. This could and did result in wide variations, but there were nonetheless some widespread patterns that broke with the late medieval soundscape in significant ways. Perhaps the most dramatic transformation was the progressive transition toward a vernacular Mass. In his 1523 *Formula missae*, it is probable that Luther intended every sung portion to remain in Latin, except perhaps the collects, epistle, Gospel, and final benediction.[158] In 1525, Nuremberg issued its first ordinance for a nearly completely vernacular German Mass, leaving only the performance of the Gradual unspecified, and of course, a year later, Luther published his ordinance for the German Mass, which completed the process.[159] Other fully vernacular Masses proliferated throughout the sixteenth century in the Lutheran territories, beginning in the 1530s.[160] The overarching tendency, however, was to allow some parts of the Mass to be sung in Latin, while mandating progressively more vernacular performance of the rite. In his ordinances for northern German towns like Hamburg, Braunschweig, and Lübeck, Johannes Bugenhagen consistently prescribed Latin singing only for the Sanctus, recommending German for other portions of the Mass or stipulating that Latin could be used in those communities with the resources to do so.[161] The 1528 ordinance for Nuremberg and Brandenburg-Ansbach mandated that most of the Mass be sung in Latin, but the 1533 ordinance revised this, making all Latin singing, with the exception of the Kyrie and Gradual, optional.[162]

Descriptive evidence attests to a mixture of German and Latin sung during Lutheran Masses, at least in the cities. In 1536, when Wolfgang Musculus recorded his careful observations of the performance of the rite in Wittenberg, he left behind one of the most detailed descriptive accounts of musical practice for the entire period. He explicitly noted that the Introit, Collect, and even the Epistle and Gospel readings were all sung in Latin, as was the *Pax domini*, and *Agnus Dei* during the Communion.[163] He also identified various parts of the Mass sung in the vernacular, including the Lord's Prayer, a hymn following the *Agnus Dei*, and the concluding hymn of thanksgiving. The priest also sang the words of consecration in German while elevating the elements.[164] Thomas Eliot, an English visitor who witnessed a Mass performed in the church of St. Lorenz in Nuremberg in 1532, noted a slightly different pattern, blending Latin and the vernacular, as well as sung and spoken portions of the Mass. For the first part of the Mass up to the Epistle, he declared the priest sung "everi thing in Latine."[165] The pastor then read the Epistle in Latin, and the assisting deacon read the same passage to the congregation in German. The pair of ministers followed this pattern for the Gospel as well, the priest this time reading in Latin "softly," and the deacon reading "aloude" in German. Thereafter, the priest sung the Credo. When the priest spoke the words of consecration, Eliot reported that he "singith with a high voyce" and elevated the elements. Finally, the deacon delivered the exhortation to communicants in German, much later in the services than any of the contemporary ordinances suggested as a norm.[166] During a 1586 colloquium, Jakob Andreae, one of the most prominent second-generation Lutheran theologians, noted that a mix of Latin and German during the Mass was common practice.[167]

Both Eliot and Musculus also referenced the use of choirs, another fundamental aspect of the soundscape of worship. Eliot only mentioned it in passing, noting that the choir accompanied the priest while he sang the Credo.[168] Musculus provided more detail, indicating that the choir aided in the performance of the Introit, the Kyrie, the Gloria, *Pax domini*, a variety of hymns before and after the Gospel reading, and the hymns preceding and following the sermon.[169] Whether these performances injected polyphony into the soundscape, however, is by no means certain. On balance, polyphony was probably heard less in Lutheran churches for much of the sixteenth century than it had been in the fifteenth. A large part of this was due to the fact that most communities simply continued to lack the means to support polyphonic choirs. In many medium-sized German towns, churches only began to build polyphonic choirs in the later decades of the sixteenth century.[170] Additionally, though, the early years of the Reformation produced a generally negative attitude toward polyphony that had some appreciable influences on the practice. Even in places like Nuremberg, with a rich tradition extending back into the fifteenth century, polyphonic music occupied an ambiguous position in the early decades of the Reformation. There, in 1524, the city's leading reformer, Andreas Osiander, convinced the city council to abolish it altogether in the city's parish churches.[171] This was a temporary ban, but the process of reinstating polyphony into the liturgy was long and arduous. More than ten years later, in 1536, it still remained absent from the Nuremberg churches.[172] It gradually reappeared in lesser religious services (in other words, Vespers, Matins, and the like) in the late 1530s, but Masses celebrated in the city's parish churches lacked polyphony until late 1545. Throughout the entire interlude, the city maintained choirs in the schools as well as choir directors and composers, but performance was largely secularized.[173] The reintroduction of polyphony into the Mass was achieved in spite of considerable resistance from the city's ruling elite. In the mining town Joachimsthal, a similar temporary elimination of polyphony occurred, lasting for about a decade after the city adopted the Reformation.[174] Elsewhere, in larger communities with similar traditions of liturgical polyphony prior to the Reformation, resistance to its reinstatement came from the laity. In Ulm at the turn of the seventeenth century, for example, Lutherans were resentful of polyphony's encroachment upon monophonic congregational singing, which by then was regarded as an important form of lay participation in the Mass.[175]

Similarly, accompanying instrumental music could be regarded with suspicion and occasionally prohibited. Instrumental music almost always meant organ music, but, as with polyphony, organs were simply not present in most German Lutheran churches during the sixteenth century.[176] The controversies over this particular element of worship were therefore restricted to a tiny minority of communities. Also like polyphony, organ music became more common only in the late sixteenth century. Very little evidence of organ music exists before about 1590, and what is there provides little insight into actual practice.[177] We know from Wolfgang Musculus that organ music punctuated the performance of Masses in Wittenberg and nearby Eisenach at various points: it accompanied the choir during the Introit, alternated with the choir during the Kyrie and Gloria, and preceded hymns before the Gospel reading and sermon.[178] Beyond this, the main role for many of the organs in the sixteenth century was probably simply setting the pitch for the choir.[179] However, in general, sixteenth-century Lutherans were never fully comfortable with their use in religious services. As with many aspects of the soundscape, the affective potential of the sound always threatened to divert aural attention away from the Word. This was the reasoning behind the elimination of organ music from Nuremberg's parish churches, which occurred in tandem with the elimination of polyphony in 1524. Whereas the city maintained the necessary resources for polyphony practice throughout its multi-decade hiatus from the liturgy, the elimination of organ music was much more thoroughgoing: organists were removed from the payrolls of the parish churches, and organ music, like polyphony, was only restored to the Mass in the mid-1540s.[180] However, on several occasions in the late sixteenth century, pastors complained that the organs were distracting people during the Mass, and they petitioned the city council for their removal, or for rules stipulating a reduction in use.[181] This was a constant concern in sixteenth-century Lutheran culture. Thus, at the end of the century, Jakob Andreae attempted to defend both polyphony and organs from Calvinists critics yet conceded that there was always the potential that "listeners pay attention only to the sound and not to what is sung."[182]

Like church music, the religious use of bells in sixteenth-century Lutheranism exhibits continuities with late medieval practice—but again, the imperative to guard against supermusicality was apparent in reforms introduced. Lutherans gradually developed a rich bell-ringing culture over the course of the sixteenth century but consistently took aim at reducing this element of the soundscape specifically as it related to the rite of the Mass. The official policy toward religious bell ringing developed early: as the 1525 ordinance for the castle church in Wittenberg indicated, bells "ought to be used only to call people to sing and listen to the Word of God, but not for pomp on holidays."[183] In the first generation of the movement, communities tended to favor the ringing of a single, large bell for this purpose, and viewed overzealous ringing of multiple bells as characteristic of "papist" practice. This was a much simpler vision of bell ringing than the complex and highly variegated practices that had inflected the late medieval Mass. Occasionally, ordinances made space for some variations: in Frankfurt am Main in 1529, for example, churches were allowed to ring one of their great bells at the beginning of Communion.[184] The types of ringing mentioned in these ordinances concerned the large bells, mounted in belfries. Later in the sixteenth century, as Lutherans developed a more distinctive bell-ringing culture, these bells also became the object of laudatory sermons and were put to a range of new, carefully prescribed religious uses, although rarely during the Mass specifically.[185] By contrast, the smaller, handheld bells—known variously as transubstantiation bells or elevation bells—remained in use, at least in some liturgies that retained the elevation. In Wittenberg, Musculus indicated that the elevation of both bread and chalice took place "to the sounding of bells."[186] None of the Wittenberg ordinances specifically prescribed ringing during the elevation at the time, and a few years after Musculus's visit, when the elevation was officially eliminated, the rationale for these bells vanished. In other cases like Nuremberg, where the elevation was tacitly permitted, it seems that elevation bells were not used. Like much of the liturgical furniture in the city's parish churches, they were put into storage after 1530 and then melted down in 1552.[187] In any event, the general Lutheran orientation toward bell ringing during the Mass favored simplification of late medieval urban practice.

Preaching, the performance of music, and the ringing of bells during the Mass all took place in the confines of church space, which Lutheranism endeavored to transform in various ways. In addition to having an effect on the sightlines, such transformations affected soundscapes as well. As in contemporary England, German Lutherans confronted the traditional church spaces they inherited as an acoustic problem.[188] As we observed in chapter 1, the cavernous expanses of the cathedrals and large urban parish churches were echo chambers, which complemented the late medieval emphasis on supermusicality. The various sounds produced during the performance of the Mass bounced off walls, blending with one another and in general obscuring the verbal content of the service. The corollary of this soundscape, at least in theory, was greater affective impact on churchgoers. From the perspective of the first generation of Protestant preachers and theologians, and arguably the better-educated sorts of sermon-listeners, these same spaces presented an "acoustic nightmare," as Philip Hahn has recently suggested.[189] The removal of the various side altars, as well as significant portions of traditional liturgical furnishings, may well have compounded the issue further. With fewer objects to dampen the acoustic environment, the problem of reverberation would have been amplified. The common exhortation that preachers ought to improve the clarity and loudness of their voices may therefore have reflected this reality. Not surprisingly, as Hahn has shown for the case of Ulm, the acoustics of large urban churches elicited no shortage of complaints from the evangelical pastorate.[190]

Elsewhere, Lutherans of the sixteenth century appear to have been of the same mind about the acoustics of church space. Luther himself expressed on more than one occasion his preference for medium-sized churches because they were better suited for preaching. In the interests of achieving verbal clarity, Lutherans instituted particular changes to their structured ritual environments. One major trend was to install sounding boards above the pulpits, which enhanced the projection of the preacher's voice. More broadly, however, the model churches built at places like Torgau and Schmalkalden introduced a number of acoustic features differentiating them from the older, larger urban churches of the late Middle Ages. The major changes were their reduced size and their lowered ceilings, which tended to be flat and lacked the vaults that produced so much resonation in the later Middle Ages.[191] Additionally, as ordinances from the late sixteenth century make clear, it became more common for churches to install permanent, assigned seating, further disciplining people's aural and visual attention toward the altar and pulpit.[192] Interestingly, in many respects, the smaller, rural parish churches of the late Middle Ages were already better suited to the worship needs of the Lutheran reformers: their smaller spaces and less acoustically reflective services were already ideal environments for cultivating focused attention on the verbal content of worship.

Turning to the olfactory landscape of the Mass, Lutheranism brought with it important transformations. Luther's first Mass ordinance was the only legislation of the sixteenth century to address incense explicitly, and he defined it as adiaphora if burned during the reading of the Gospel. As we saw in chapter 1, however, the Offertory was the major context for late medieval incense use during the Mass. The universal elimination of this portion of the ritual in the Lutheran churches therefore represented a major, albeit somewhat indirect, transformation of the religious olfactory culture of the later Middle Ages. The removal of incense from the Mass was never the stated intention of this move: rather, the sacrificial theology it embodied was the primary target. The cultural context, however, leaves open the possibility that it was an implicit item on the agenda of reformers. For all Protestants, whether Lutheran, Calvinist, or otherwise, the smell of incense in the sixteenth century conjured up thoughts of sacrifice, which was theologically anathema. Further, the contrariety between incense and the Word, so clearly established in the public discourse of the early 1520s, and then again in the consecration sermons of later decades, was a constant theme among Lutherans in the sixteenth century. In addition to the Offertory, other major contexts for incense use that might be connected with the Mass—namely, seasonal blessings and processions—were abolished in official liturgies.[193]

Like so much of the visual culture connected with these ceremonies, this undermined traditional incense use and forced authorities to scrutinize it in a new context. Not only was it an unnecessary expense, but it also had clear connections with the idolatry and superstition of the past. In most places, of course, incense had never been used in the first place and so was never a problem. In wealthier locations with the means to provide for it, however, purchases of incense quietly disappeared from the accounts of church masters and sacristans.[194] The censers, too, migrated out of church space. In Nuremberg, for example, the censers of the city's two parish churches were confiscated and stored away after 1530, until they were melted down in 1552.[195] The inventories of other parish churches where censers were documented disclose a similar fate: in Stettin, for example, they disappear after the mid-1530s.[196] Without the censers, it seems fairly uncontroversial to conclude that incense ceased to be an element of worship in such locations. An oblique reformation of olfaction in sixteenth-century Lutheran culture therefore appears to have been the rule, at least as it related to the performance of the Mass.

Oblique reformation, however, did not necessarily translate into permanent results. Inventories for Nuremberg's city churches for the remainder of the century attest to the absence of incense until at least 1584, when the superintendent noted that each parish church had acquired a small brass censer.[197] It is difficult to know what precisely the need for this purchase was, but it seems unlikely that they were used during the Mass or in any official religious capacity. In the fifteenth century, censing had occasionally occurred in other parts of the Mass beyond the Offertory, including during the Introit and Gospel reading. In theory, Lutheran liturgical policy had no objection to these uses, if they served a purpose explaining theological doctrine. However, given its widespread cultural associations with sacrifice, it seems unlikely that church officials in Nuremberg would have regarded incense in this light. Further, if the history of the management of liturgical furniture in the city is any indication, incense use had been absent from the Nuremberg liturgy definitively since 1552 and, in all likelihood, probably at least since 1530. Church leadership in Nuremberg generally adhered to Melanchthon's policy on ceremonies that had been eliminated from the liturgy: "What has already been stopped, one should not restore."[198] Thus, any feel for incense use derived from traditional practice would have dissipated by the late sixteenth century, and the new church orders provided no guidance on the matter. The only practical model available was the Church of Rome, but papal incense continued to animate anxieties about idolatry, superstition, paganism, and even witchcraft in the second half of the sixteenth century, as the Nuremberg theologian Hieronymus Rauscher made perfectly clear in his 1562 *One Hundred Papal Lies*. "Censing," he declared, was a preserve of the monks, who offered it up to the devil, and as such, was just another form of "pagan babbling."[199]

It may have been that that the presence of the censers was part of a more widespread embrace of religious sensuality among Lutherans at the end of the sixteenth century and the beginning of the seventeenth. It is true that Lutherans in this era abandoned some of their negative associations with traditional uses of images, more elaborate forms of church music, and bell ringing, and began to promote such things as a means of distinguishing themselves from the growing presence of Calvinism, which they came to consider more of a threat than Catholicism. As a result, we can speak of a coherent "Lutheran Baroque" in visual and aural culture at this time.[200] The same, however, cannot be said of incense. Lutherans continued to reject and condemn its use even as they promoted image devotion. Unlike their regard for images, Lutheran attitudes toward incense shared common ground with neighboring Calvinist aesthetics. For example, in a 1597 anti-Calvinist polemic, the pastor Abraham Taurer argued for the use of images but claimed that ritual incense transformed images into idols. He thus explained, "That is why the holy King Hezekiah rightly and justly crushed the brass serpent that Moses had made, because the children of Israel had offered incense, and thereby committed idolatry. Outside this abuse, the brass serpent was not broken or done away with by David or the other holy Kings."[201]

In light of these factors, the more likely explanation for the purchase of the censers in Nuremberg was that they were put to secular use as a form of preventative medicine or apotropaic magic against the plague. Aerial theories of contagion had been central to medical knowledge about how the plague spread since the fourteenth century and so gave rise to a rich olfactory culture. If disease spread on foul-smelling airs, the best preventative medicine was good fragrance. Incense was a critical part of this medical culture and was commonly recommended as a public-health measure in the prescriptive literature.[202] A sermon by the Bavarian Lutheran theologian Andreas Pankratius (d. 1576) disclosed that the Reformation did little to change this aspect of people's daily lives, which could nonetheless bleed over into church space.[203] Pankratius observed that some congregations had, in recent times of plague, gathered in their churches for a communal censing to ward off the disease.[204] Beyond this utterance, there are no descriptions of incense use in Lutheran churches for this period. Hypothetically, this could explain the presence of censers in the Nuremberg churches. In the late decades of the sixteenth century, several outbreaks of plague elevated concerns over the quality of air in the city and gave rise to a series of ordinances that attempted to manage this problem.[205] This quotidian concern was at the forefront of people's minds, and incense may well have been used in the churches without playing any role in official religious ritual. It was, put another way, desacralized.[206]

In its appeals to touch, the Lord's Supper in the Lutheran churches broke with late medieval tradition in several dimensions. First, by doing away with the Offertory, Lutherans eliminated a variety of kisses and ritual bows traditionally performed by the priest and deacon at the altar during this portion of the rite. As we observed in chapter 1, the performance of these gestures varied significantly from one context to the next, and so elimination of the Offertory aligned with the general orientation of Lutheran liturgical policy, which favored simplification of the late medieval paradigm. Also along these lines, the repeated emphasis in church orders and in visitation protocols that pastors always face their congregations when administering the sacrament was not only for the benefit of the parishioners, so that they may better hear the words of the ceremony, but also so that the pastor might not become distracted by the handling and management of liturgical vessels assembled at the altar. As Volker Leppin has shown, this complemented the Lutheran imperative to reduce the ornamentation at the altar, especially in the churches in Saxony and Thuringia in the 1530s and 1540s.[207] As noted earlier, the other conspicuous appeals to touch performed during the Mass—namely, the kiss of peace (Pax) and the fraction of the Host—were both displaced at a very early stage, already in the early 1520s. As Koslofsky points out, Lutherans managed the elimination of the kiss of peace both by removing it from the prescriptive ordinances and by confiscating the pax boards specially designated for the performance of rite at the end of the Middle Ages.[208] Similarly, the absence of the fraction of the Eucharist Host became a hallmark of Lutheran practice already in the 1520s. Of the various liturgical changes introduced by Lutherans, the elimination of these two elements from the Mass appear to have been among the most consistently maintained, and uncontroversial, at least until the end of the sixteenth century.[209]

Finally, on balance, how the new Lutheran Eucharist appealed to taste probably remained much the same as it had in the fifteenth century. Lutherans continued to use the traditional wafers employed by the Church of Rome, and there is no evidence to suggest that they effected any change in the ingredients used to prepare them. As with other Protestant denominations, the Lutheran churches emphasized Communion in both kinds for the laity more than the late medieval church had, and so in theory more people should have enjoyed a taste of the Eucharistic wine. The actual impact of this policy on practice, however, was at best ambiguous, and in many places, especially in the countryside, Communion remained as infrequent and irregular as it had prior to the Reformation.[210] The impact may have been more appreciable in the urban scene. In the Rhineland town of Wesel, for example, which became a multiconfessional town in the late sixteenth century, people were intensely concerned with the outward form of the bread and wine, suggesting regular reception in both kinds.[211] However, this might not have been a profound break with the late medieval past: as we saw in chapter 1, the quantities of wine procured for churches in larger urban centers indicate that regular reception of the wine by the laity was not necessarily unusual. To the extent that it might be discerned, the range of tastes available to communicants when they received the wine was probably much the same as it was prior to the Reformation. The regions where wine was produced, and the methods for procuring it in the churches, remained more or less the same as they had been in the fifteenth century, and, setting aside normal year-to-year and generation variations in wine-grape crops, we can assume that the qualitative taste changed little. In any event, Lutheran liturgical policy had even less to say about the nature or quality of the wine that was to be used than the late medieval prescriptions.

Although it proved a powerful and persistent force in Lutheran culture, attempts to realize the reformation of the senses in practice were fraught by a variety of complicating and countervailing factors in the sixteenth century. Lutherans preserved much of the institutional structure of parish governance that had given rise to the diversity of sensuous worship in the fifteenth century, enshrining the right of local communities to determine, to a large extent, the form and content of their worship. Theologically, too, they deemed most of the ritual edifice of the church a matter of indifference: as it had no bearing on the fate of the souls in their care, Lutheran pastors should not be overly concerned with the merely external elements of worship. Instead, their chief concern lay in clearly communicating church doctrine and ensuring that people understood the rudiments of Christian theology. Often, these features of Lutheran liturgical policy secured a good deal of continuity with the late medieval past. However, it is mistaken to consider only the continuities. Evaluated from a more comprehensive, intersensorial perspective, Lutheran liturgical policy was schizophrenic, giving rise to significant continuities in some areas but profound ruptures in others. Often, ruptures occurred in an oblique fashion, when reformers determined to eliminate a particular portion of the Mass because of the theological connotations it represented, or when they made judgments about the utility of a particular piece of liturgical furniture. Whatever the intentions behind a particular ritual reform, the major consequence was a liturgical policy that generally favored a simplification of the worship patterns of traditional Christianity and, correspondingly, changes to the sensory production of ritual life, at least in wealthier, mostly urban churches.

Sensory transformation, however, should not be confused with desensualization. Lutheran practice reflected a shift in the sensorium, emphasizing and elaborating on some sense modalities more than others, but in the course of designing a new ritual scheme, reformers collided with the reality that sensory transcendence was not achievable or even desirable. In this respect, the relationship between Lutheran ritual practice and the cultural narrative of sensory reformation was fundamentally paradoxical. The story, repeated again and again, stated an obvious fact: evangelical Christianity was less sensual than its traditional counterpart. This was the primary cultural context in which ritual changes often unfolded, but it was not the only one. As the sixteenth century progressed, Lutherans contradicted this narrative with increasing frequency. Particularly by the late sixteenth and early seventeenth centuries, when Lutherans engaged more often with neighboring Calvinist interlocutors, they enthusiastically embraced the role of the sensuous in worship, particularly when they thought about their engagement with the Eucharist. Even as they continued to tell the traditional story of sensory reformation in certain domains, they saw and promoted the affective potential embedded in the sensuality of their own practices. It is perhaps more surprising that the Calvinists with whom they often argued shared many of the same assumptions, thinking with and embracing the senses in the second generation of the Protestant Reformation. In the next chapter, we turn to this phenomenon.

6 Thinking with the Senses in the Second Reformation

When Johann Sigismund, margrave and lector of Brandenburg, received Communion on Christmas Day 1613, things were noticeably different. Gone was the traditional Eucharist wafer, elevated and on display for the adoration of devoted communicants. Gone, too, was the ornamentation at the altar, sensuous vestiges of traditional Christianity lingering in many of the churches across Lutheran Germany. The Berlin Cathedral had been stripped bare of virtually all of the distinctive visual appeal of Lutheran worship. The elector and his ministers had even gone so far as to do away with beloved Lutheran hymns, reported Simon Gedicke, a Lutheran chaplain and eyewitness to Johann Sigismund's Communion. What was left was a bare table, covered in white velvet, upon which had been laid a plain loaf of bread. The bread was torn into pieces. Johann Sigismund approached the table, took a small piece of bread in his hand, ate it, sipped from a cup of wine, and returned to his seat. Along with him, Gedicke reported, "about fifty people communed."[1]

The elector of Brandenburg had used the Christmas Communion services in 1613 to mark his public conversion to reformed, or Calvinist, Christianity, but he had likely already converted privately as early as 1606. In the first years of the seventeenth century, he had spent considerable time at the court of the Counts of the Palatinate, in the city of Heidelberg. By then, Heidelberg was recognized as the epicenter of German Calvinism in the Holy Roman Empire. Since the conversion of Frederick III (1515–1576, r. 1559–1576), the Counts Palatine, along with leading intellectuals in the University of Heidelberg, had vigorously supported the spread of a decidedly Calvinist variety of reformed Christianity, particularly in those areas that had converted to Lutheranism earlier in the sixteenth century. From Heidelberg's situation in the southwestern corner of the Empire, the new religion radiated north and east, taking hold mainly among nobility and intellectuals but generating controversy and conflict within the Protestant community more broadly. This was a distinct, new era in the history of the German Reformation. As those reformed Christians who led the charge saw it, they were enacting a reformation of the Reformation, or a "Second Reformation."[2] Both sides, Lutheran and Calvinist alike, saw ritual as the frontline of this new battle. In many respects Johann Sigismund's Communion in 1613 marked the culmination of the Second Reformation: German Calvinism would spread no further beyond the ruling class of Brandenburg, which sprawled across the northeastern plains of the empire. Unlike other princes who converted, Johann Sigismund never attempted to impose the new faith on the populace; he hoped, rather, to persuade them, employing professors and theologians from across the empire to spearhead a propaganda campaign on behalf of the new religion. He failed in this respect, and henceforth the Calvinist margraves of Brandenburg would rule over Lutheran subjects.

We often think about the ritual controversies that erupted during the Second Reformation as struggles over markers of confessional identities and, as such, central to the exercise of power by Lutheran and Calvinist authorities. Ritual was the primary means by which authorities sought to communicate abstract theological doctrines to a subject population that, while largely alphabetically illiterate, was nonetheless well schooled in the language of ritual.[3] Ritual assent signified submission to the combined authority of secular and clerical magistrates, to the doctrines they promoted, and thus as belonging to a particular community. Debates over what people did during the Eucharist were therefore really theological questions over whether Christ's body and blood were present during Communion, and where precisely that presence manifested itself. For Lutherans, it resided in the elements of bread and wine. For Calvinists, the question was more complicated. Christ's presence could be in the souls of communicants, but the doctrine of the Real Presence as a whole might just be a lingering vestige of "papal filth," to be rejected out of hand.[4] Although often framed in comparative language, the contours of ritual life and practical devotion among Lutherans in this period are much clearer than that their Calvinist counterparts. Indeed, focus on the vestiges of traditional practices in many of the Lutheran churches of the late sixteenth century has often overlooked Calvinism or treated it in strictly negative terms.[5] The continued use of traditional religious images and consecration rites, for example, makes clear the distinctive visual identity of Lutheranism in this period.[6] Werner Freitag has shown how the use of images was not strictly visual but had a certain haptic appeal as well, and Susan Karant-Nunn has discussed the matter more generally in terms of the lingering "sensuous residues" of traditional Christianity.[7] Regardless of the sense invoked, it was clear that, for Lutherans, it was better to appear "papist than Calvinist."[8] Calvinist identity, presumably, constituted itself negatively, in opposition to the Lutheran embrace of sensuous worship.[9] This is a common pattern: in the sensory history of early modern Europe, Calvinism resides in what Mia Mochizuki has called a kind of "mythic vacuum."[10]

In this final chapter, I want to begin the work of inscribing Calvinism into the narrative of sensory history. By focusing on the ritual controversies of the Second Reformation, this chapter shows how both Lutherans and Calvinists actively and positively thought *with* the senses in fundamentally the same way. Using a mix of polemical sermons, pamphlets, learned theological and natural philosophical treatises, as well as autobiographical writings, this chapter traces the origins, extent, and significance of this pattern. Although each side differed on precisely what it thought church ritual should look, taste, feel, and sound like, everyone understood the efficacy of worship—how it affected churchgoers—in the same way. To be sure, there were important theological differences, but both Lutherans and Calvinists shared the same anthropological assumptions about the human soul as a unity of bodily and intellectual faculties, and about the fundamental malleability of those faculties when confronted with objects in the environment. In this regard, Johann Sigismund's Communion in 1613 was not simply about symbolically marking his conversion to Calvinism: the ritual tearing and chewing of the loaf of common bread was an embrace of the haptic and the imprint it might leave on the soul. As in the later Middle Ages, the senses mediated engagement between internal soul and external environment. Also like their late medieval predecessors, second-generation reformers talked about this engagement in terms of an affective and affecting relationship. Ritual's sensuous appeal *moved* people. Under this view, the sensuous objects held out for consumption did more than simply demarcate confessional identity or symbolize theological doctrine. Rather, they always already held the potential to transform the soul, its internal dispositions, and moral habits. Sensuous worship was a tool for making and unmaking Christians in the Second Reformation, and so getting it right was of profound importance.

Within this framework, there were other commonalities in how Lutherans and Calvinists thought with the senses. Both camps dedicated most of their time to the Eucharist ritual specifically. Part of what motivated them to do so was theological controversy over the doctrine of the Real Presence, but as we will see here, there was something more primary at stake in these disputes. Lutherans and Calvinists alike were concerned with how the sensuous elements of worship made people feel, how these aspects influenced their faith. This is apparent in arguments over how people handled the Eucharist Host, as well as the composition of the Eucharist: should it be a wafer, or ordinary bread? These controversies foregrounded the importance of sight but also of touch, and to a somewhat lesser extent taste, in Second Reformation thought.

How people thought with the senses in the Second Reformation had its origins in the late medieval past. The basic framework for understanding sensation—and, accordingly, sensuous worship—remained largely Aristotelian, notwithstanding an attempted reformation of the system in its own right. Amid the radical, totalizing visions of reform that had characterized evangelical discussions of church ritual in the early 1520s, the natural philosophy of Aristotle in general, and the late medieval science of the soul specifically, had often been objects of scorn and derision, and calls for wholesale abandonment were not uncommon. As we saw in chapter 4, evangelicals understood Aristotelian natural philosophy as foreign, and they opposed to the pure Word. They also understood it as a tool by which the Church of Rome defined and exercised ritual power. It was the intellectual framework justifying much of the hyperaesthesia of traditional Christianity.

As with the broader story of sensory reformation, there were elements of this myth that would have seemed uniquely convincing in the immediate context of the early 1520s. Although there was little in the way of centralized oversight from Rome on the teaching of Aristotelian natural philosophy to confirm the conspiracy-theory-like sentiments of early evangelicals, Aristotelianism *was* normative in fifteenth-century university curricula, and an important means by which learned elites established their authority as ritual experts. It was about power, and it did shape the baseline understanding of ritual's importance prior to the Reformation. The early evangelical calls to abandon Aristotle were therefore about breaking this power; by contrasting natural philosophy with the Word, they proposed an alternative to the system of knowledge that traditionally undergirded ritual expertise.

The major problem for the early evangelical community, however, was the lack of any viable alternative explanatory paradigm. After remaining mostly silent in the late 1520s, Melanchthon began to reconsider the issue. Returning to the texts in the 1530s, it seemed to him that "those theologians are robbed of a great instrument if they do not know of the most learned disputations on the soul, the senses, the causes of the appetites and feelings, cognition, and the will."[11] Over the course of the next two decades, he began more systematic study of the problem, lecturing on the "science of the soul" at Wittenberg. His lectures were published as a *Commentary on the Book of the Soul* beginning in the late 1540s and went through multiple editions in the last half of the century. In addition to the volume's clear utility for pastors and theologians, Melanchthon claimed to be motivated to improve and update the traditional Aristotelian understanding in light of some of the intellectual developments of the Reformation, recent studies of Galenic physiology, and the anatomical work of Andreas Vesalius.[12] Whatever the motivation, the outcome was the retrenchment of the traditional understanding of how the senses worked. Despite small refinements to the global picture of the human soul and its relationship to the physical body, the affective, passive sensory experience of objects remained intact. "Thus when we apprehend an object," Melanchthon explained, "and judge whether it is good or bad, then the affected spirits in cognition bring it to the heart, which, so to speak, is struck, beaten and agitated, and either aspires to the object or flees from it."[13] What had begun as a call for reformation, if not outright abandonment, had ended with a renaissance of the most central elements of the account of sensation around which so much of late medieval sacramental theory had cohered.

Philipp Melanchthon was primarily responsible for this renaissance, but his resuscitation of the science of the soul would prove profoundly influential among Protestants in the Second Reformation. Many of the leading voices who would define sensuous worship in the next generation studied directly under Melanchthon as he was lecturing and writing on the topic. This included well-known theologians, pastors, and polemicists like Matthias Flacius, Joachim Westphal, Nikolaus Gallus, Johann Wigand, Joachim Mörlin, Tilemann Heshusius, Martin Chemnitz, Nikolaus Selnecker, David Chytraeus, and Andreas Musculus, as well as many laymen who took up posts in civic governments across the Empire.[14] Beyond this direct influence, Melanchthon's commentary would become the essential textbook on the soul and its sensory powers at universities across the Holy Roman Empire, shaping Lutheran and Calvinist minds alike. Late-sixteenth-century statutes reforming the curriculum at the University of Heidelberg, for example, required that professors of physics lecture on Aristotle, or "those who have brought in [the form of] a compendium the nearest and best substitute for Aristotle," namely the "*De anima Melanchthoni*."[15] Victorinus Strigel (1524–1569), professor of ethics at Heidelberg, produced annotations on Melanchthon's commentary that were published posthumously in 1590.[16]

The influence of Melanchthon's commentary was apparent at other centers of Protestant learning in the second half of the sixteenth century. Sebastian Leonhart, a reformed theologian working in the service of Christian I of Saxony at the end of the sixteenth century, described his education in Leipzig as beginning with studies of Aristotle's works, as well as "Philipp's" books on physics and the soul.[17] At approximately the same time, Wolfgang Ammon was studying in Jena, where he received a thorough education in Aristotle's teachings on the soul from his teacher Zacharias Brendel. In his diary, he noted specifically that he had struggled with Brendel's "libellum de anima," likely referring to his 1598 *Annotations* to Melanchthon's commentary.[18]

The traditional, late medieval understanding of affective sensation remained essential to understandings of ritual practice well into the seventeenth century, even among Calvinists. The Heidelberg theologian Abraham Scultetus (1566–1624), arguably the most influential Calvinist intellectual of this period, was well trained in the science of the soul, having attended both the University of Wittenberg and the University of Heidelberg.[19] He even produced a brief tract on the five senses, which provided a wholly orthodox account of affective sensation.[20] More important, a massive treatise on ethics represented an important synthesis of the traditional Aristotelian teachings in physics, psychology, physiology, and ethics.[21] Because he built on essentially the same foundations as his late medieval predecessors, he ultimately arrived at very similar conclusions about the importance of human sensuality and emotion, especially in those more practical domains of religion, including administration of the sacraments, prayer, and catechetical instruction.

In this regard, Scultetus typified broader patterns in late-sixteenth- and early-seventeenth-century Calvinist intellectual culture.[22] He made the case that aesthetics and ethics were inseparable on the basis of the traditional observation that the human soul's encounter with external objects, mediated by the senses, was never neutral but rather always affected the soul, causing what he called "commotions" with the potential to shape moral and intellectual dispositions.[23] Although these commotions, or affections, were formally restricted to the lower faculties of the soul, Scultetus also allowed that they could impinge on the higher-order cognitive processes as well. Sensation was equally didactic and affective. On this point, Scultetus believed he was reconciling the positions of a number of the most prominent thinkers on emotions in the Western intellectual tradition, thus concluding: "The soul's affections are in the lower appetite, as the proper seat, although they also consider, and as we explained, affect, the higher. In this way Scotus can be united with Thomas; nor do I suppose Augustine and Galen to have thought differently."[24] The account of passive, affective sensory experience mediated largely by Melanchthon, but essentially no different than late medieval commentators, would form an important piece of the mental equipment of this new generation as it approached the problem of worship.

In tandem with the renaissance of Aristotle among Protestant intellectuals at midcentury, a number of other factors elevated the importance of thinking with the senses in the Second Reformation. Many of those who trained under Melanchthon in the 1530s and 1540s became the sharpest critics of the Interim, a liturgical ordinance mandated by the Holy Roman Emperor Charles V at Augsburg in 1548 that aimed at restoring the ceremonies of traditional Christianity in Lutheran churches. The Interim produced the first major, sustained conflict over the meaning of church ritual within the Lutheran community as a whole, pitting Melanchthon and his followers, who recommended accommodation to the ritual impositions of the ordinance, against more uncompromising factions, led in the main by a circle of pastors and theologians in the city of Magdeburg, among them Matthias Flacius, Nikolaus Gallus, and Nikolaus Amsdorf. This faction would come to call themselves Gnesio-Lutherans, or "authentic Lutherans," and would argue against the idea that church ritual could ever really be a matter of indifference, or adiaphora.[25] As Nischan has suggested, it was their position that would win the day among the majority of Lutherans in the second half of the sixteenth century, and so it is of essential importance to understand what this conflict was about.[26] Although the Gnesio-Lutheran view first emerged as it related the role of ritual in Lutheran-Catholic relations, it later defined how Lutherans approached their Protestant, mainly Calvinist, opponents later in the century. The *Adiaphorastreit*, or adiaphoristic controversies of the late 1540s and early 1550s, reinforced many of the underlying anthropological assumptions about church ritual held by Lutherans. It was in many respects a somewhat ironic harvest of Melanchthon's own teaching about the senses and soul that grounded the Gnesio-Lutheran understanding of church ritual. The sensuous appeal of church ritual made it a powerful tool in the confessional struggles of the Second Reformation.

After its promulgation in 1548, Melanchthon encouraged Lutherans to accept the liturgical ordinance of the Interim on the grounds that external ceremonies were adiaphora, or matters of indifference to the essential elements of true Christian religion. True religion had to do with internal or spiritual goods only accessible through prayer, faith, and pious devotion to the Word. At the same time, Melanchthon carefully preserved the Lord's Supper and baptism as "external and visible ceremonies commanded and instituted by God," who attached to them the "promise of grace and forgiveness of sins." He even maintained a fairly conventional, affective theory of sacramental efficacy, allowing that, through participation, the benefits of Christ's sacrificial death were actively "applied" to the hearts of the faithful in a manner analogous to the saving and faith-enhancing work performed by the Holy Spirit when one heard the Word of Scripture.[27]

In many respects, Melanchthon was simply applying what had become one of the fundamental premises of Lutheran liturgical policy. However, in the new, post-Interim context, the internal contradictions of his simultaneous rejection and assertion of the importance of the external in Christian worship was less tolerable to a new generation of Lutherans. Melanchthon now seemed either a spiritualist, or a papist, but certainly not a Lutheran. He did very little to help his cause in this regard, even adding that, since the late 1520s, the evangelical church had changed very little of the traditional worship practices of Christianity, and that the new evangelical liturgical ordinances he and his colleagues had so painstakingly crafted could be reconciled, quite comfortably, to late medieval liturgical texts like William Durandus's *Rationale divinorum*.[28] Instead of concerning themselves with such external trivialities, people should withdraw within themselves and focus on the truly essential aspects of Christian religion.

Milner has suggested that this way of thinking was a major blow to the dominant, Aristotelian approach to the sensuous in religion in Elizabethan England.[29] In the contemporaneous German-speaking world, however, quite the opposite was the case. To many, Melanchton's position seemed an obvious betrayal of the story of sensory reformation so central to evangelical identity for the previous three decades despite the fact that the principle of adiaphora had been a critical component of Lutheran liturgical policy. Charges of spiritualist hypocrisy, as well as papist sympathizing, were forthcoming. The city of Magdeburg was the epicenter of this criticism, but tremors were felt further afield in the Lutheran community.[30] Joachim von Westphal, for example, was apt to level the criticism while preaching in Hamburg, intuiting the "fanatical" spirit of Andreas von Karlstadt was behind Melanchthonian adiaphorism.[31] Often, the claim went hand in hand with the charge that Melanchthon had abandoned Luther's ideas and legacy. In Nuremberg, when in 1563 the city's astronomer Joachim Heller was banished for holding Gnesio-Lutheran beliefs critical of the city council's staunchly Melanchthonian stance, he did so with resolve in his belief that he remained true to Luther's heroic vision for the church, in contrast to civic and clerical authorities' weak, sophist, spiritualizing rationalizations. Such rationalizations had let papal idolatry back into the church and threatened to "open a window to the devil," by which he might slip into people's souls.[32] As Lyndal Roper has shown, Melanchthon had always been seen as both physically and morally weak when compared with Luther, and so in the eyes of many evangelicals, this narrative of his betrayal of Luther's legacy was likely an easy pill to swallow.[33] Even if Melanchthon's comments about the relatively modest ritual changes introduced by the Reformation were objectively true (and they were in a certain sense, as we saw in chapter 5), a negative reaction against them made sense within the ideological structure of feeling the community had erected around itself.

Even more disconcerting, however, was the fact that Melanchthon's view and corresponding recommendations seemed completely disconnected from historical reality. Gnesio-Lutherans like Matthias Flacius observed that some things had been explicitly commanded or forbidden by Scripture, and that such things were not adiaphora. On these grounds, they could agree with Melanchthon that the Lord's Supper and baptism were sensuous ceremonies instituted by God. The bigger problem they observed, however, was that Scripture remained totally silent about a vast amount regarding worship, even with respect to the gestures, objects, and words embellishing sacramental performance. These things were historically left to the discretion of authorities, ecclesiastical and secular alike. In a world of confessional unity, this might not have been a problem, but this in no way corresponded to the real conditions on the ground in the Holy Roman Empire. The fractured and divergent religious perspectives riven by the Reformation only intensified in the second half of the sixteenth century and meant that the imposition of ritual practices by authorities always risked violating one's conscience, thereby obliterating the possibility of adiaphora. As Flacius famously put it, "When confession and offense are involved, nothing is adiaphoron."[34]

For many, this was a persuasive argument, not simply because it followed a fairly convincing logic but also because it corresponded to many evangelicals' experiences in the mid-sixteenth century. Catholic authorities, including Charles V, had been quite clear that ritual was an essential component of a campaign to win back hearts and minds, despite their many rhetorical appeals to freedom of internal belief and conscience. Similarly, it was an explicit component of the program of intellectuals like Georg Witzel, who saw sensuous worship as a tool for inspiring feelings of devotion among people and winning their souls back to the Catholic Church.[35] For those who lived through these years, the memory of the ritual impositions of the Interim thus became an extension of the military violence visited upon the evangelical community. For example, when Jacob Andreae, one of the intellectual architects of the Formula of Concord (1577), composed his autobiography near the end of his life, all of his memories of the Schmalkaldic War (1546–47) revolved around disputes over church practice he had with occupying Catholic forces in his hometown of Stuttgart. In one such instance, an imperial legate told him that the emperor was convinced "that you [the Lutherans] had thrown away all faith and religion, and that there were no sacraments among you."[36] Elsewhere he recalled silencing the captain of an occupying force of Spanish soldiers about the use of chrism oil, patens, and images in the churches by challenging him to demonstrate where Scripture mandated such things.[37] After the war, Andreae also noted that the reintroduction of the Catholic Mass under the auspices of the Interim had caused "the greatest vexation" in the evangelical community.[38] For Andreae, such anecdotes crystallized the essence of Catholic-Protestant conflict in the 1540s. Writing some forty years later, Andreae noted the two sides would never be reconciled, primarily "because of the errors and idolatrous worship" of the Church of Rome.[39]

Other evangelicals reflected similarly on the ritual violence of the late 1540s and early 1550s. Sebastian Fischer, a shoemaker in Ulm, described the Interim as a liturgical ordinance designed to transform the Lutheran churches into "popedom," rehashing the litanies of abuses found in 1520s rhetoric. The Interim was restoring everything the Reformation had cleared away, from the sacrificial theology of the Mass to the "use of images, fasts, confession, purgatory, feasts, as well as all ceremonies, organs, banners, [and] altar lights."[40] The first Mass celebrated to mark Charles V's victory after the war thus utilized heaps of red silks, "golden pieces, there all ceremonies were used, such as organs, singing, lights, and whatever else appertained thereto."[41] The impression was overwhelming, and Fischer endeavored to communicate this. The Interim had thus restored "almost everything that I have seen in pope-dom," Fischer reported, and the Masses were "heavy with all ceremonies." As he explained: "Now candles burnt on the altar, two young servants in choir gowns processed to the altar, each holding a transubstantiation candle, standing behind the doctor; there the doctor lifted the Host on high, and did the same with the chalice, and one rang a little bell."[42] The churches hadn't seen such provision for sensuality in twenty years, he claimed, and as he understood it, this was the main reason why many evangelical congregations resisted, often refusing to receive the sacrament, despite sharp admonitions from priests.[43]

In light of these memories, it is not surprising to find that Melanchthon's narrative about liturgical continuity with late medieval Christendom had little purchase among many second-generation Lutherans. It is also not surprising to find that Gnesio-Lutherans enthusiastically appealed to a counternarrative in their polemics. Although they generally avoided talking about specific objects and practices, they understood the Catholic Church as attempting to enact a reversal of sensory reformation, or a kind of reimposition of the hyperaesthia of late medieval Christianity. Joachim Westphal, preaching in Hamburg, claimed that "the majority of the customs and ceremonies were done away with and thrown out in the [evangelical] church ordinances."[44] Nikolaus Gallus in Magdeburg registered a similar unraveling of sensory reformation, describing the Interim as a reversal of the example of the Israelite king Hezekiah, with whom the evangelical community had identified since the early 1520s. "It is not possible," he claimed, "that the establishment of papist ceremonies will not at the same time bring with it papist delusion and other abhorrence now or hereafter . . . as they were in earlier times the principal tool of introducing idolatry into the church."[45] The external, sensible presence of these ceremonies in Lutheran churches therefore posed the constant threat of transforming the souls of true Christians. In response, supporters of Melanchthon, such as Johannes Pfeffinger (1493–1573), offered up a metaphorical repackaging of the traditional story of sensory reformation in support, declaring that the preaching of the pure Gospel had overcome the idolatrous and abusive practices of "popedom" but strictly referred to an internal, subjective overcoming or detachment from these practices on the part of individual Christian subjects. Those who remained concerned about the sensuous were not Christians but Epicureans.[46] Such arguments followed patterns of Lutheran liturgical policy as it had developed to that point. However, they found relatively few sympathetic ears amid the increasingly apocalyptic atmosphere of the late 1540s and early 1550s.

Beyond these arguments over the role of ritual in evangelical history, the Gnesio-Lutheran rejection of adiaphora rested on well-established facts about human nature. Religious worship could never be completely indifferent because it appealed to the senses, and through that external appeal it had the power to effect real internal transformations. For Joachim Westphal, the reintroduction of ceremonies promised to transform the Christian faith into a "child's game" because they dazzled the senses, appealed to people's desires, and distracted attention from the Word.[47] The invocation of children's games by no means diminished the threat of ceremonies to the evangelical community. Westphal saw them, rather, as part of a papal design to cultivate false belief: their very presence was a "spectacle" and "agitation" (*Reizung*) to the soul, inclining it toward idolatry and threatening to transform churchgoers into something un-Christian. Un-Christian rites produced un-Christian souls, and, as Westphal pointed out, "The majority of the papist ceremonies are pagan customs." As such, they could never serve the purposes of Christian edification.[48] They could, however, destroy the true church: Lutheran acceptance of the Interim, Westphal warned, would result in the "Judaizing" of true Christians: "The Christians, in the acceptance of papist ceremonies, must judaize . . . for the papists through their foolish emulation have in part restored Jewish ceremonies done away with by Christ."[49] Westphal considered this not a theological argument but an anthropological observation. In 1550, while addressing a colleague in Lübeck on why it was so important to resist the liturgical impositions of the Interim, he explained that it was "inborn in us by nature, that we (as Isocrates says) prefer foods more lovely, dear, and sweeter than healthier food, and, to wit in all things, that external form and appearances goes and moves us more than the internal good."[50]

The inborn proclivity to be drawn to external objects of the senses and for those interactions to shape the internal state of one's soul were ideas as old as Aristotle, but they had been given fresh urgency in the mid-sixteenth century, and many others concurred with Westphal. Vaguely referencing Platonic commentary on human nature, Matthias Flacius observed of ritual that "objects move the senses, [and] what one sees, to that he is disposed."[51] Nikolaus Ambsdorff, a stalwart defender of Martin Luther who had moved to Magdeburg in the late 1540s and become a Gnesio-Lutheran, argued that the reintroduction of ceremonies into Lutheran services was contrary to the Word and would eventually result in the transformation of souls and, ultimately, the destruction of the church, because they "have a great appearance and prestige, filling the ears and eyes, so that the heart is drawn to them, and catch the eye of the crowd, forgetting the sound of the Word, and paying it absolutely no heed."[52] Like Westphal, Ambsdorff believed that ceremonies would result in judaizing, taking people back to the idolatries of ancient Israel via the abominations of Rome.[53] Joachim Heller, the astronomer of Nuremberg, similarly considered ceremonies dangerous on the grounds that they would lead true Christians into popery and idolatry. In this regard, he was especially concerned about the "spectacle of the mass" and in particular the acts of Eucharistic adoration that took place during the ceremony, comparing it with the biblical story of David gazing at the body of the bathing Bathsheba. The story, he claimed, was a good example of the universal human "bodily weakness" (*leibs schwachait*) for outward things. Investing oneself in such things could produce "impudence beating in the heart," which had been so powerful that it even dominated the affections of King David.[54] In a private letter to his friend Bartholomäus Schöber, Heller warned that, in the face of such things, true Christians "must look to the light and truth alone, otherwise they themselves will be infiltrated by idols."[55] Heller, like most of the leading Gnesio-Lutheran polemicists, had studied with Melanchthon in the late 1530s and early 1540s, and even owned copies of Melanchthon's *Commentary on the Book of the Soul* and the original treatise on the soul by Aristotle.[56] By its very nature, the problem of church ritual could not be separated from this intellectual context.

Such warnings notwithstanding, the ineluctably sensuous nature of humanity was not an entirely bad thing. Gnesio-Lutherans, like their late medieval predecessors, considered sensuality a two-sided coin. Human nature could not be overcome, and adiaphorists seemed to ignore this fact. The point was not to permit all ceremonies, but neither was it to throw out everything, as Nikolaus Gallus explained. Both eventualities seemed like practical impossibilities, rhetorically inspired by spiritualist thinking.[57] The Gnesio-Lutherans sought a church liturgy that was not only grounded in Scripture but also recognized and met the needs of human nature. Westphal wanted only to "see and hear" that which might please God and "also bring us spiritual and heavenly joy."[58] As was the case in many of the controversies that rocked midcentury Lutheranism, it was Matthias Flacius who developed the positive arguments for thinking with the senses most fully, and to their most radical conclusions. Since the adiaphora controversy, Flacius had constantly reiterated the necessity of things "external, visible, and comprehensible through the senses of the body" in religious practice.[59] As the 1550s gave way to the 1560s and 1570s, he engaged not only with his "adiaphorist" enemies but also "sacramentarians," "spiritualist fanatics," tridentine Catholics, and, perhaps most critically, "Calvinists" and "Zwinglians," by which he meant reformed Christians generally. Each of these groups diverged from the true form of Christianity upheld by orthodox Lutheranism, both on intellectual, doctrinal grounds and in terms of practical, sensuous worship.[60]

Flacius developed this argument most thoroughly in one of his final writings, a massive treatise: *On the True, Essential, and External Presence and Oral Enjoyment of the Body and Blood of Christ* (1575). He argued theologically for the doctrine of the Real Presence but, alongside that, made a strong anthropological argument for the importance of the sensate in religious practice. "Enjoying" the Eucharist meant not simply spiritual, internal enjoyment but an embrace of "natural and fleshly" enjoyment as well.[61] Christ's words, "Take and eat," made it abundantly clear that the physical touching and tasting of the elements were of central import.[62] "Oral enjoyment" also encompassed the visible side of worship: Flacius thus excoriated the "sacramentarian" and "spiritualist" teachings of Caspar von Schwenckfeld (1489–1561) that Christians were obliged to "remove from their eyes" the entire practice of the Lord's Supper as it had been relayed in Scripture. Quite to the contrary, Flacius found in Scripture a very precise practical outline that required people to engage with their senses of taste, touch, and vision. They were to eat the bread and drink the wine and observe the "entire business" of sacramental practice.[63] Getting the senses right in worship wasn't just a theoretical issue—it was a practical imperative.

Flacius considered the provision for sensible worship to have specific grounding in Scripture and natural philosophy. With respect to the former, he commonly equated enjoying the Eucharist with the stories of Christ "inspirating" or breathing the Holy Spirit into the souls of the Apostles, found in John 20. Orally enjoying the sacrament was "like the Holy Spirit in the dove and tangible wind, or the tangible breath of Christ, and visible flames over the Apostles seen and felt with bodily senses, and comprehended in accordance with his unspeakable wisdom."[64] Interestingly, John 20 also contained the famous story of the disciple Thomas, whose need to touch the wound in Christ's side proved rather important to contemporaneous English Reformation discussions of what constituted good and bad sensuality.[65] Flacius, however, like most of his contemporaries in the German-speaking world, chose to ignore it. Here, in the specific context of ritual controversies, it was more important to set aside the more abstruse theological issues surrounding the story of a doubting Thomas and think pragmatically with the senses. The entirety of Scripture had, after all, shown that

> Christ cannot be comprehended by our souls through faith alone, but rather also by our bodies, through our senses, and otherwise in other manners . . . [it is] the nature or characteristic of man, who has not only a soul, but also a body, and must govern and regulate himself according to the body or flesh and his senses, especially since the fall from grace, yea also the spiritual death of the soul that had befallen him in paradise through the deception and murder of Satan.[66]

In addition to its scriptural basis, thinking with the senses in church practice was justified on natural philosophical grounds. The physical, oral enjoyment of the Eucharist was a central concern because, as Flacius was apt to point out, "Man first must learn almost everything through the body and external senses that he wants to know in his soul. From here comes the famous expression: *Nothing is in the mind that is not first in the senses* [*Nihil est in mente, quod non sit prius in sensu*]." He was of course referencing Aquinas's summation of late medieval epistemology.[67] Here, Flacius applied it to the specific ritual context of the Eucharist: all human knowledge was embodied knowledge, or knowledge of something sensible, and there was no point in trying to work around this fact. The senses, in conjunction with habitual engagement with their objects, were essential to the process of knowledge-making. "Through daily use of things," Flacius explained, "the more alien, obscure, hidden things are best taught and shown to be more useful and familiar to us."[68] Attending to the senses in ritual practice was therefore justified on complementary scriptural and natural philosophical grounds.

For Flacius, getting the sensible aspects of sacramental practice right was important not only for its didactic function but also because it affected how people felt and, in the process, had the potential to strengthen faith. Flacius described this as taking pleasure in or enjoying the sacrament and as the principal "fruit or effect" of the sacrament.[69] He didn't deny that there was an inscrutable intellectual mystery involved in the sacrament and that taking spiritual pleasure in this mystery might be the highest form of engagement with the Eucharist, but he also rejected any strict separation between the categories of "spirit" and "flesh." Before such mysteries could be internalized or "spiritualized," one first had to "pore over" them "with our fleshly heads and senses."[70] Ultimately, however, Flacius was somewhat agnostic about the human capacity to access the spiritual realm, leading him to reiterate the importance of sensible worship. The inscrutable mystery was just that: inscrutable and inaccessible to human perception, ultimately an article that had to be taken on faith. Sensible worship, however, could be controlled and manipulated to affect a positive internal disposition toward faith and to make the soul more receptive to the spiritual goods of Christianity. Moreover, Christ himself, the prescient liturgist that he was, had provided future generations with a very precise model of what worship should look, sound, taste, and feel like to achieve these ends.[71] Scripture had carefully delineated the entire business of how one orally, externally, and truly enjoyed the Eucharist.[72]

Although they disputed many of his other, more radical theological positions, the most important representatives of Lutheran orthodoxy in the Second Reformation agreed with Flacius on the significance of the senses in Christian worship. Indeed, many of the framers of the Formula of Concord (1577), which took its place alongside the Augsburg Confession of 1530 as one of the authoritative statements on Lutheran belief and practice, spoke often and enthusiastically about "orally" and "physically enjoying" the Eucharist. As the Formula itself dictated, because Christ's body and blood were truly present in the elements of bread and wine, Communion was always a matter of both spiritual and sensual, or oral, reception.[73] Martin Chemnitz, who, along with Jacob Andreae, was one of the lead authors of the Formula, reiterated in a variety of treatises that Luther himself had clearly emphasized eating the Eucharist as an oral experience. The fullest sense of Communion encompassed the "food, that one can see, grasp, and feel, and is thus enjoyed in a natural manner, that they bite with teeth, or otherwise chew in the mouth" in conjunction with "spiritual eating," which Chemnitz described as an affective transformation "when the heart or soul, through faith, takes on and dedicates itself to also spiritual reception of the benefactions of Christ."[74] Through the physical act of eating the bread, the communicant also sacramentally ate the body of Christ, although the precise nature of union of profane elements and sacred substance remained mysterious.[75] The whole experience of Communion, Chemnitz deemed, could nonetheless be therapeutic to the troubled Christian conscience.[76]

None of this is to dismiss the importance of theology as an essential context for understanding the ritual conflicts of the Second Reformation. However, separating theological doctrine from sensuous practice flew in the face of common sense, historical experience, and the latest scientific understandings of humanity. All the framers of the Formula of Concord had lived through the 1530s and 1540s and, with the exception of Jacob Andreae, had studied with Melanchthon during these turbulent decades. It was apparent that ritual could never be a matter of indifference, and so attending to and thinking with the senses was essential in the confessional landscape of the late sixteenth and early seventeenth centuries. External worship conveyed doctrinal information, but perhaps more important, it had the power to shape how people felt and to transform them internally in a prelinguistic, prerational sense. Nikolaus Selnecker, who contributed to the Formula of Concord, understood true sacramental efficacy as the "good motion of the heart" stirred up by the external action, in conjunction with faith in the testimony of Scripture. Each element influenced and reinforced the other. It was both spiritual and bodily; accordingly, Selnecker called it a "seal pressed into the body."[77] Even the mundane act of chewing the Eucharist, Selnecker claimed, could not be disaggregated from the spiritual effects it had on the soul.[78] This was a theological argument on the one hand, but it could never be completed unmoored from its anthropological foundations in the late Middle Ages. Mediated by Philipp Melanchthon, the renaissance of Aristotelian science of the soul at midcentury had led Protestants back to more systematic elaborations of the importance of sensing and feeling in religion. As the confessional landscape shifted, and as Calvinists displaced "adiaphorists" later in the century, this remained the essential cultural and intellectual context.

Both Calvinists and Lutherans approached religious worship from the same anthropological perspective in the late sixteenth and early seventeenth centuries, actively and positively thinking with the senses in the ritual controversies that preoccupied them. More traditional histories that emphasize the utter depravity of the human body as the cornerstone of Protestant thought in this period tend to obscure this fact.[79] However, neither side could ever fully deny the fact that, as the Heidelberg theologian Abraham Scultetus observed, "We poor humans live in the five senses."[80] Scultetus was a Calvinist, and he made this observation at the end of the Second Reformation while trying to convince Johann Sigismund's subjects in Brandenburg of the truth of the Calvinist view of the Eucharist in 1614. Thinking with the senses and getting the sensuous appeal of worship right, however, had been of central concern in a variety of ritual controversies between Lutherans and Calvinists that emerged after 1560, the most important of which revolved around the celebration of the Lord's Supper. Eucharistic conflicts were widespread but most intensely concentrated in Heidelberg and the Palatinate, in Saxony and Anhalt, and finally in Brandenburg. Closer scrutiny reveals that Lutherans and Calvinists alike were deeply concerned not only with the visual appeal of the rite but also with its gustatory and tactile elements. Scultetus's comments about a five-sense sensorium notwithstanding, both sides demonstrated little concern over the audible dimensions of the rite, and both sides agreed that incense, and by extension olfaction, had no positive role to play.

The first major ritual conflict to foreground these problems emerged in the Palatinate, in southwestern Germany, and centered primarily in the city of Heidelberg, home to the Counts Palatine and the university they patronized. The Palatinate had come relatively late to the Reformation but rapidly changed once it broke with Rome: it had only become Lutheran in 1546, before the Count Palatine Frederick III (1515–1576, r. 1559–1576) officially adopted reformed Christianity early in the 1560s.[81] The abrupt changes paralleled disputes over the Eucharist that set the stage for many later controversies. Controversies originated in theological concerns but opened themselves up to approaching ritual as an anthropological problem more broadly. Namely, the doctrine of the Real Presence raised the question of what rituals were actually doing to the bodies of churchgoers. From a sensory standpoint, these conflicts foregrounded the importance of seeing, touching, and, to a somewhat lesser extent, tasting. For both Lutherans and Calvinists in Heidelberg, the sensible edifice of worship continued to have the power to shape how people thought and felt and, in so doing, could enhance people's faith. In this regard, Lutherans and Calvinists in the Palatinate could agree that the sensible elements of worship were "external instruments and media of the Holy Spirit." As the Heidelberg professor of theology Caspar Olevianus explained, these instruments included the sermon, which presented the sacrifice of Christ "through the ears to our hearts," as well as the sacraments, instituted "in order better to inform and impress this same sacrifice in the eyes and other senses, and thus affirm the faith."[82]

At the beginning of the controversies in 1559, Tilemann Heshusius, who had studied with Melanchthon in the 1540s, was the Lutheran superintendent of the churches in Heidelberg. Heshusius, who is often recognized as a rather pugnacious figure, is credited with beginning the arguments over the Lord's

Supper, which would in the short term lead to the Second Reformation of the Palatinate.[83] His advocacy of the doctrine of the Real Presence led him to assert the importance of the visual, gustatory, but especially tactile experience of ritual participants in a variety of ways. Like Flacius and others, Heshusius saw participation in the Eucharist as a matter of "enjoyment," arguing for an embrace of "bodily and oral reception."[84] This meant the use of traditional Eucharist Hosts, which had been retained in many Lutheran churches, and the continued practice of ministers placing Hosts directly onto the tongues of communicants. In addition, Heshusius argued against the breaking of the Eucharist (fraction) prior to its distribution, a practice that would quickly come to occupy the center of controversies between Lutherans and Calvinists. He reasoned that the original words spoken by Christ during the Last Supper referred not only to the breaking and tearing of the bread but also to the distribution and feeding of the hungry.[85] The emphasis on distribution over fraction also doubled as an implicit argument for the continued use of Hosts, to which he yoked a more explicit, practical point: bread, which he deemed necessary for the fraction to occur, was impractical because it would not meet the needs of a large congregation wishing to commune. If four hundred people communed in Heidelberg on a Sunday, he pointed out, "that would require quite a great cake indeed, so that each could receive a piece."[86]

For all his emphasis on the importance of the sensible, especially haptic, dimensions of ritual practice, Heshusius was careful to qualify that, despite the doctrine of the Real Presence, people did not sensibly experience Christ in the act of Communion.[87] This, however, did nothing to diminish the importance of the sensible from an anthropological perspective. Heshusius, rather, operated within the common learned paradigm, especially emphasizing the affective impact of sensuous worship on the souls of communicants. The sensible elements of the Eucharist were powerful instruments of the Holy Spirit because they could change the way people felt, instilling feelings of reconciliation to Christ, neighbors, friends, and enemies, and providing comfort in trying times.[88] The Holy Spirit could not be efficacious without the sensible elements of worship.

There was, to be sure, more than a little circularity to Heshusius's account: while regarding faith as a necessary precondition for receiving all the benefits associated with the physical enjoyment of the Lord's Supper, he simultaneously promoted the affective power of the practice to "arouse and strengthen" faith in people's hearts.[89] The logical consistency of the argument, however, was subsumed to what appears to have been a more pressing concern with how people should deal with sadness, pain, and fear. As Susan Karant-Nunn has recently shown, this concern pervaded Heshusius's sermons, along with many of his contemporaries.[90] It lay at the heart of his sacramental thinking as well. Perhaps even more than hearing the Word preached from the pulpit, Heshusius saw participation in the Lord's Supper as the most effective means of dealing with pain and suffering. "It is necessary," he wrote in his 1562 preface to his *Little Book of Comfort* (*Trostbüchlein*),

> . . . that Christians who, in temptation, go often to the table of the Lord. For such food the son of God has ordained for the purpose that, with it, we might refresh and enliven our flagging and nearly spent conscience, and through diligent observance of our received baptism, as well as constant enjoyment of the body and blood of Christ powerfully in us, God wills to seal our consciences, strengthen faith, control temptation, grant the spirit, and increase his gifts in us.[91]

Lest anyone misconstrue his comments as in some way metaphorical or as referring to an interior, subjective, and asensual experience, Heshusius carefully and repeatedly emphasized the sacraments as external instruments of the Holy Spirit. He thus contrasted Lutheran sacramentality with what he saw as extreme poles toward which the practical life of the church could drift: Catholicism and Calvinism. This allowed him to play with the old narrative of sensory reformation. Lutheranism struck a middle path between the overwhelming spectacle of Catholicism, and the cold, empty "seals and signs" of Calvinist sacramental practice.[92] Scholars have observed the theme of a "right middle path" or *via media* recurrent in late-sixteenth-century Lutheran constructions of identity, particularly as they related to the continued use of devotional images.[93] Here, however, Heshusius made clear that he was not talking strictly about visual culture, and that he did not have a static notion of confessional identity in mind. Rather, in the context of Eucharistic practice, he favored a dynamic understanding of orally and physically enjoying the sacrament that embraced other sense modalities beyond the narrowly defined, overly visualist notion of sacramentality first defined by St. Augustine.[94] He saw sensible engagement, broadly defined, not as a means of confessional identification with a limited and defined set of doctrines but rather as a means of influencing how people felt, kindling faith, and shaping Christian souls. It was a much more dynamic vision, and one that had a good deal more in common with traditional, late medieval understandings of sacramentality than we are often given to believe.

Heshusius's assertion that Lutheranism was "less sensual" than Catholicism was, of course, common wisdom among his cohorts. What of his claim that Calvinists denied the sensate entirely? Among Lutherans, this was a common assertion. For Matthias Flacius, the oral enjoyment of the Eucharist distinguished Lutheran practice from the "cold," "empty" spiritualism of Calvinist sacramentality.[95] The latter he saw as a corruption of Calvin's original embrace of the senses and flesh in sacramental practice. The "fanatics" who dominated German reformed Christianity had forgotten that Calvin had denied a purely memorialist understanding of the sacrament, or the idea that "the external should only be a sign," and instead insisted "on the true presence of the spiritual thing . . . so that the sacred elements gave the spiritual, according to its measure, to the external senses to grasp and seize, similar to a medium, tool, or instrument."[96] He elaborated still further, claiming that both Calvin and his successor, Theodore Beza (1519–1605), believed, first, that "the bodily and external truly contains within itself, or brings with it, the spiritual," and second, that just as "the external represents the spiritual and renders it to the human senses to be seized and examined," so too "the bread brings with it the body of Christ, and thereby hands over and renders to our bodies and senses to be seized and embraced."[97] Flacius and his contemporaries therefore thought that their German Calvinist opponents were ignorant of the positive role Calvin himself had accorded the senses in sacramental practice.

Despite their longstanding reputation as anti-sensual, the Calvinists to whom Lutherans like Flacius and Heshusius addressed themselves quite plainly asserted the importance of the sensuous in worship. Johannes Willing, court preacher to Frederick III in Heidelberg, took it upon himself to challenge John Chrysostom's dictum that Christ "gives nothing sensible" to those who wish to worship him. In sermons on the Eucharist given in the 1560s, he declared that, in Eucharistic practice, "external things are indeed sensible," explicitly and carefully mandated by Christ in the scriptural account of the Last Supper. "There," Willing explained, "he calls sensible that which is conceived through sight, hearing, taste, and touch."[98] Willing categorized the bread, wine, vessels, along with the actions of handling and receiving the sacrament, as part of the sensible domain.[99] More than his Lutheran interlocutors, Willing wanted to maintain a stricter, formal separation between the sensible and what he called "intelligible" goods of sacramental practice—those spiritual things comprehended by the faithful "with conscience, reason, and observance and reckoning of the heart." At the same time, however, he also recognized the practical difficulties of such a separation and even allowed that the sensible reception of the sacrament did something useful internally for people's souls.[100] He referred to this as enjoyment of the sacrament, much as his Lutheran contemporaries did. Indeed, it is difficult to distinguish in any significant way his understanding of the senses' role in sacramental efficacy from people like Heshusius, Flacius, and other second-generation Lutherans. Willing saw the sensible and spiritual as sacramentally united in the act of receiving Communion, so that the physical act was always already bound up with feelings of joy and love for Christ. The sensible act was emotionally and spiritually transformational: "There the mouth externally receives the bread and drink of the Lord, as the soul, however, inwardly enjoys the Lord Christ, and delights in him."[101] It was in these particular moments of sacramental practice that Calvinists seemed able to set aside views about the predestined nature of the human soul, seeing instead a potential for the positive affection of the soul and the strengthening of its internal dispositions toward faith in God.

Willing reflected broader currents among Calvinists in the Second Reformation. In his immediate surroundings in the Palatinate, the most outstanding examples came from Thomas Erastus, Zacharias Ursinus, and Caspar Olevianus. Ursinus and Olevianus were both credited as principal drafters of the Heidelberg Catechism, the first authoritative statement of the reformed faith published in German.[102] For all their importance, Ursinus and Olevianus were certainly influenced by Erastus, arguably the most important intellectual force behind the adoption of reformed Christianity in the Palatinate in the early 1560s. Erastus had been appointed to one of the chairs of medicine at the University of Heidelberg in 1558, and while a physician by training, he exercised tremendous influence over church policy among the pastorate and at the court of Frederick III.[103] Taken together, Ursinus, Olevianus, and Erastus represented not a rejection of the sensuous but rather a full-bodied embrace of it, particularly the visual and tactile dimensions of worship. Their embrace rested on three underlying principles.

The first of these principles was the human need for divine accommodation. Ursinus was especially clear on this point. In defining the sacraments, he acknowledged the need for sensible ceremonies on the grounds of the "great weakness and forgetfulness" of humanity before God.[104] Humans required "visible and sensible tokens and signs . . . in which our eyes and senses could not be allowed to doubt," and it was because of this that God had instituted sacraments, declaring, "My covenant shall be in your flesh as an eternal covenant."[105] The Heidelberg Catechism, as well, echoed this point: sacraments complemented the Word of Scripture as "visible holy tokens and seals" instituted by God "because of our weakness."[106] The catechism's treatment of the Eucharist dwelt more broadly on the necessity of "bodily enjoyment" of the bread and chalice.[107]

At first glance, the principle of divine accommodation may seem like something of a truism, requiring little further justification or elaboration. In the sixteenth century, however, this was by no means the case. As Ursinus and others recognized, sensuous practice was always a two-sided coin, with the potential to elevate human consciousness or to lead the body into sin. There were many examples of the latter in the biblical and historical record.[108] The Eucharist, as an object of both taste and touch, mobilized traditional anxieties about the bodily sins of lust and gluttony.[109] However, without some divine allowance for the sensible, humans could have no knowledge of God or form a community of worship. Calvin addressed the problem first and most famously, lending some credence to Flacius's claims that his theology represented a thoroughgoing embrace of the sensuous. His comments in this regard became foundational to reformed ritual theory in the late sixteenth century. Much of it built on precepts familiar to the late medieval science of the soul. To be sure, human nature, with its inclinations toward sin, meant the specter of idolatry always potentially lurked in any kind of provision for the senses in religious practice. Nonetheless, it was equally unquestionable that God made some kind of accommodation to the limits of human perception in order to make religion possible. Calvin saw Scripture in this light, as well as the book of nature, which could be read for the design of the creator.[110] He put the matter clearly enough, noting, "God, in speaking to man, accommodates himself to human sense."[111] Significantly, Calvin made this point in his *Psychopannychia*, his earliest systematic work on the human soul, and it later became central to his sacramental theology. God accommodated human sensuality in the form of sacraments for pedagogical purposes, as Calvin explained, "to instruct us according to our dull capacity, and to lead us by the hand as tutors lead children."[112] The provision for the senses in Calvinist worship, justified by the principle of divine accommodation, was primarily intended for didactic purposes.

Divine accommodation acknowledged an anthropological fact: humanity required sensuous worship to access knowledge of a transcendent, super-sensible God. The particular forms ritual ought to take were very precisely defined in Scripture, making the Eucharist's appeals to the sensible, especially sight and touch, not just a means of accommodating human nature but also a practical imperative. Indeed, the account of the Last Supper provided a perfect, comprehensive model of sacramental practice, and Christ had explicitly mandated that it be emulated as closely as possible.[113] In the Heidelberg Eucharist controversy, Thomas Erastus took the opportunity to outline positive prescriptions for how practice ought to look, feel, and, somewhat implicitly, taste. His prescription was, in effect, the mirror opposite of Tilemann Heshusius's: Scripture clearly demonstrated that ordinary loaves of bread, not Hosts, were to be used during the celebration, and that any kind of special vessels for carrying and containing the elements beyond the humble devices depicted in Scripture were forbidden. Most important, Erastus emphasized the fraction. Ritually tearing apart the bread before distributing it to communicants was absolutely essential.[114] This again was usually intended for didactic purposes. Christ had been described breaking the bread, and so people should see the pastor breaking the bread in order to gain a better understand the Scripture. Ursinus concurred, reminding ordinary churchgoers that Christ exhorted them to approach the Word both through a "memorial before your eyes" and a "sign in your hand."[115] He further pointed out that the account of Scripture clearly excluded the use of ornate vessels for carrying the Eucharist, like monstrances, as well as the use of Hosts, and instead required the simple, bodily enjoyment of bread and wine.[116]

Equally as important as the didactic role played by the sensuous worship was its traditional, affective potency. Engagement with the ritual edifice of the church was not just about teaching people doctrine; it also made a prelinguistic, prerational appeal to the soul, shaping how people felt. Christ was both model teacher and prescient liturgist who, in his infinite wisdom, had established the practices he knew would most powerfully affect people's souls. In contrast to his Lutheran opponents, Erastus rejected the doctrine of the Real Presence and tended to avoid describing the sacrament as a medium or instrument of the Holy Spirit, instead favoring the more typical reformed usage of sacraments as "signs," "seals," or "tokens."[117] These differences, however, obscure a good deal of common ground the reformed Heidelberg intellectuals shared with their Lutheran counterparts. Theologically, the denial of the Real Presence was rather ambiguous. Erastus was committed to the idea that a real bond that could be achieved between human soul and divine in the act of Communion. It was a slightly "higher" view of sacramental efficacy than that of many of his contemporaries who took their cues from the strictly memorialist, symbolic interpretations of Swiss reformers like Huldrych Zwingli.[118]

Even if Erastus's theological view drained the Eucharist of the Real Presence, anthropologically speaking, the function of the sensible dimensions of the rite remained more or less the same as they did in other traditions. It was both a "visible and tangible" thing, "given to us by God for the purpose that communion with the body of Christ . . . is accepted in our hearts through the Holy Spirit, externally and visibly assured, strengthened, and sealed."[119] Erastus hastened to add that the comforting feelings of communion with Christ were completely disembodied, "invisible and intangible."[120] This, however, did little to lessen the power of the external, visible, and tangible elements to affect real, internal transformations in the human soul. The bread "that we break," he emphasized, was a sign or token by which the heart, not the mind, was convinced of and comforted by the soul's communion with Christ.[121] The reception of the bread, similarly, moved the human soul to feelings of sadness, joy, and ultimately comfort.[122] In the tactile experience of both tearing the bread during the fraction and chewing it after reception, Erastus saw a kind of sympathetic parallel with the rending of Christ's body during the crucifixion. Through ritual engagement, people would be "even more and better reminded of his suffering and death," kindling feelings of identification with that suffering, and inspiring charity and empathy toward the suffering of one's neighbors.[123] In was on these grounds that Erastus repeatedly emphasized the sacrament as "no mere, empty sign." Rather, it communicated the effect of the Holy Spirit in the hearts of those who received the external elements of bread and wine.[124]

There was a similarly clear emphasis on the affective potential of sensuous worship in the thought of Ursinus and Olevianus. Ursinus seems to have found little meaning in the strict definition of sacraments as signs, seals, or tokens, using such terminology interchangeably with the Lutheran vocabulary of media, instruments, and tools of the Holy Spirit.[125] If used properly according to scriptural examples and received in faith, the Eucharist, Ursinus believed, had a profound power to comfort people. As with Heshusius's positions, there was a circularity to Ursinus's understanding of sacramental efficacy with respect to faith: faith was a precondition for receiving the full benefit of the sacrament, but physical engagement with the sacrament simultaneously had the power to shape people's interior dispositions and "effect faith" in their souls.[126] This view of sacramental efficacy prevented Ursinus from seeing the Eucharist as purely a memorial of the Last Supper.[127] It was not simply relating a story and teaching people the content of Scripture: in its external appeal, it was instead doing something to people's interior souls, changing the way they felt and believed. Olevianus concurred, emphasizing that the sacraments were instituted precisely to go beyond the rational, didactic dimensions of preaching and reading the gospel and, by "impressing" themselves "on the eyes and other senses," to create pathways by which the Holy Spirit could reach into the soul and lodge itself in the heart.[128] Far from representing any kind of "desensualized" form of Christianity, the reformed tradition in Heidelberg embraced the sensuous in the Eucharist in its own distinctive ways, intensifying focus in particular on the visual, tactile, and gustatory dimensions of the rite. In doing so, it established a reformed paradigm of thinking with the senses that would be reflected in learned discourse until the eve of the Thirty Years' War.

After the 1560s, Calvinist treatments of the sensuous dimensions of Christianity tended to take one of two directions: considerations of the Eucharist in the context of ceremonial practice more broadly; and more specific, intensely focused meditations on the peculiar materiality of the Eucharist and its affective potentials. These were interrelated tendencies that built on the basic foundations laid in the Palatinate, demonstrating continued concern with the sensuous appeal of church practice. In the courts of Saxony, Anhalt, and other parts of the northern and northwestern German-speaking world where they were able to spread their influence, Calvinists tended to reject in more specific terms an increasingly wide array of traditional vessels, altar decorations, and vestments associated with traditional Eucharistic practice. At the same time, they consistently asserted the importance of the fraction and the use of ordinary bread, arguing on the same grounds as their Heidelberg predecessors: divine accommodation required some kind of provision for the senses, Scripture mandated a very specific form by which practice should appeal to sensuality, and by appealing to the senses, worship not only performed a didactic role, it also had a more primary, affective power to shape people's souls. Taken together, these elements of Calvinist culture in the Second Reformation elevated still further the importance of the senses, particularly vision and touch, in religion.

We see these patterns most clearly in work of many of the leading theologians at the turn of the seventeenth century. Among these were Christoph Pezel in Bremen, Wolfgang Amling in Zerbst, David Pareus in Heidelberg, and Abraham Scultetus in a variety of locations throughout the Holy Roman Empire. Pezel, who had been educated at Wittenberg, was expelled from the university in the early 1570s after coming out as a Calvinist. He eventually landed in the Hanseatic city of Bremen, in the northwestern corner of the Empire, where he set about the work of completing the Reformation. The city had drifted in a Lutheran direction in the 1530s and had even begun to toy with reformed Christianity in the late 1540s, appointing the Dutch theologian Albert Hardenberg as pastor of the city cathedral. It was under Pezel's guidance that the city council adopted a more explicitly Calvinist variety of Protestantism in the 1590s.[129] Through sermons and published treatises, Pezel constructed a vision of worship that expanded on the foundations laid by the Second Reformation in the Palatinate. He encouraged secular and clerical magistrates to identify with the "praiseworthy examples" of iconoclast kings of the Old Testament, especially Hezekiah and Josiah, and to root out the superstitious and idolatrous Catholic ceremonies that lingered in the churches.[130]

Pezel's view of what remained to be extirpated was much more comprehensive and specific than that of his predecessors. He understood ceremonies, broadly speaking, to encompass a variety of external things, and was particularly concerned with those relating to the practice of the Eucharist. Pezel's account had some symmetry with the old narrative of sensory reformation: Christ and the Apostles had established a pure and simple set of rituals that had been corrupted and transformed into a spectacle through centuries of "innovations," instigated primarily by the medieval papacy.[131] These included: candles, lights, vestments, albs, choir gowns, the use of an altar instead of a simple table during the Lord's Supper, little clothes and towels to wipe fingers while handling the sacrament, the practice of receiving the sacrament on the tongue rather than in the hands, the use of Hosts instead of ordinary bread, the absence of the fraction, the singing of Latin songs, overly long songs, or songs accompanied by organ music, kneeling while praying, bowing, and the use of devotional images.[132]

Reformers in other principalities across the Empire soon picked up Pezel's arguments in their own ritual disputes. Wolfgang Amling, working in the city of Zerbst (Anhalt), developed the same arguments in a treatise on ceremonies in 1596. Exhorting pastors to become new Hezekiahs and Josiahs, Amling replicated Pezel's list and added to it fasting and the ritual elevation of the bread and wine.[133] David Pareus in Heidelberg and Johann von Münster in Westphalia concurred with these lists as well. Both devoted much of their lives to combatting the reinvigorated advance of Catholicism under the leadership of the Jesuit order, in addition to criticizing Lutheranism as outlined in the Formula of Concord.[134]

The temptation here is to view such calls through the lens of the "mythic vacuum" in which Calvinism often resides and to see them as still more evidence of the desensualization of Christianity. In many respects, they looked like the litanies of abuses heaped upon traditional Christianity in the polemical literature of the 1520s, albeit presented more programmatically. Certainly, Lutherans often perceived the Calvinist critiques in such a light. Johannes Olearius (1546–1623), a defender of Lutheran orthodoxy in Anhalt, equated them with the utter ruin of the churches envisioned by the Ottoman Turks, already achieved in some cases where "Karlstadtish iconoclasm" had broken through.[135] Calvinists, to Olearius's mind, condemned "not only the abuse, but rather also the proper use of ceremony . . . for it should be called Judaizing, paganizing, [or] papitisizing when one has and keeps altars, crucifixes, or images, vestments, excorcisms, lights, songs and the like."[136] Polycarp Leyser (1552–1610), the court preacher at Dresden at the turn of the seventeenth century, regularly made such absolute claims, openly accusing Calvinists of being Muslims on the matter of external worship in general.[137]

Such contemporary perceptions notwithstanding, there was a key difference between the story told by the early evangelicals of the 1520s and the Calvinist intellectuals working toward a Second Reformation nearly a century later. The traditional story of sensory reformation had offered only vague suggestions about what was to replace traditional worship, leaving the door open to a more totalizing vision of ritual destruction; the Calvinists of the Second Reformation carefully and systematically argued not for destruction but for the "transformation and improvement of ceremonial life," as Pezel put it.[138] The basis of this transformation was provided in Scripture, which Pezel and his reformed colleagues considered to be much more comprehensive and sufficient a model for church practice than many Lutheran thinkers had.[139] Abraham Scultetus, writing a couple of decades later, agreed, applying this prescription to the problem of images. The model Christ provided in the Scriptures was all that was necessary for evaluating what should be removed from churches and what should remain, and the unhelpful notion of ritual adiaphora that had vexed Lutherans for so long could be set aside. Under this view, Scultetus's understanding of iconoclasm under was a targeted, fairly precise process. He preferred to describe it as a cleansing analogous to the purification of the Jewish temple by Judas Maccabee in the second century BCE. As he explained, the priests "did not tear apart the Temple, in which shameful idolatry had been performed, but rather purified the sanctuary, and carried away the defilement and impure stones to an impure place."[140] Scultetus could still argue positively for the church, cleansed of its impurities, as a structured environment of images by which God's grace "was painted before the eyes."[141]

The point of all this was to purify the sensory landscapes of church interiors—not for the purposes of transcending the senses, but rather in order to facilitate more intense engagement with what was left behind. To be sure, there were numerous examples of ceremonies corrupting people, but this was just a fact of nature: humans were sensuous creatures, and sensuality was always a two-sided coin. There was bad sensuality in practice, but there was also the good, which, if properly instrumentalized, became an efficacious means by which the Holy Spirit could shape people's souls. Most centrally, it was important to instrumentalize sensuous devotion to the Eucharist. Here, as Pezel and Amling saw it, it was foolish to withdraw from the senses because church ceremony not only provided access to knowledge about God, but it also helped to strengthen faith and led people to rejoice in the comforting feelings that came along with faith.[142] In any event, Scripture clearly mandated a provision for the senses in its account of the Last Supper. Like Erastus, Ursinus, and Olevianus before them, Calvinists in the later decades of the Second Reformation tended to emphasize the Eucharist as an intersensorial object of devotion. As Pezel explained, its visual and tactile qualities were of primary significance: "The visible bread and wine is received with the bodily hands and mouth, eaten and drunk in bodily manner, and bitten and chewed with the teeth.[143] Pezel was not asserting that the sensuous was more important than the spiritual here; he was instead acknowledging that, in practice, the two simply could not be neatly separated.[144] Amling agreed, adding that physically handling the torn bread before placing it in one's mouth must be important because Christ had modeled it for future generations. He thus cautioned against adding or omitting anything from this practice, warning that in producing the worship experience, "we must not be cleverer than Christ, nor seek more holiness than he demands of us."[145]

At the turn of the seventeenth century, this intensified emphasis on the Eucharist as sensuous object of devotion was especially apparent in the thought of David Pareus and Abraham Scultetus. Both men had resided in Heidelberg, and both aggressively sought to expand Calvinism throughout the Lutheran churches of the Holy Roman Empire. Pareus likely had a hand in Johann Sigismund's early conversion, and Scultetus would later provide intellectual support to the margrave's attempted reforms in the form of a series of vernacular pamphlets.[146]

Pareus's extensive consideration of the material composition of the Eucharist foregrounded the importance of religious sensing.[147] He was clear, along with all of his Calvinist colleagues, that traditional Eucharist Hosts were inadmissible in true Christian practice. Above all, he emphasized that the Eucharist must be made from the flour used in bread. Wheat or any other ground grain was acceptable, so long as the Eucharist embodied three essential qualities. It had to be "natural, customary, and nourishing."[148] These qualities, he claimed, were apparent in the scriptural account of the Last Supper: Christ had clearly used natural bread, customary to the foodways of his local culture. As natural, customary bread, it was by definition nourishing to the body: it had to be, after all, because people depended on it for survival.

On these three criteria, Pareus also asserted that the Eucharist should be locally produced. This meant that people would use wheat in some places, spelt in others, and rye in still others.[149] Local production, however, in the later years of the Second Reformation was increasingly seen in a broader, global context. Pareus thus referenced inquiries made to Calvin and Theodore Beza from missionaries in Brazil about what people ought to use for the Eucharist. In these new places, missionaries reported, nothing like the breads or wines of Europe were produced or consumed. They wondered, therefore, whether it might be possible to substitute local "root-breads" and beverages (unspecified) in place of the bread and wine. Pareus explained that, according to Calvinist doctrine, these substitutes were permissible so long as they embodied the essential qualities of the Eucharist: they had to be naturally produced from the local environment; their customary, quotidian use must parallel the use of bread and wine in European culture; and they had to be nourishing to the body so that they might have a kind of symbolic sympathy with the spiritually nourishing effects that Communion had on the soul.[150]

Embedded in Pareus's discussion of Eucharist substitutes was an abiding concern with the sensible dimensions of the practice. He was primarily concerned with its visual and haptic appeal. He thought it appropriate to allow Eucharist substitutes so long as they looked similar enough to European breads and wines. More important, any substitute utilized must be something that could be torn apart by Eucharistic ministers during the fraction rite, and chewed by communicants.[151] Pareus also seems to have been concerned with the gustatory dimension of the practice, and he devoted more specific discussion to it than many of his reformed colleagues. For example, he rejected anything resembling traditional "Jewish sweet bread," which he described as being used during Passover, on the grounds that such bread hadn't used leaven, unlike most breads commonly found in Europe.[152] He claimed that the Eucharist Hosts utilized by Jesuits sought to emulate this bread, and thereby threatened to "Judaize" Christian communicants.[153] As this last comment suggests, Pareus's discussion of the sensible dimensions of Eucharistic practice were informed by concerns first articulated in the early 1520s when evangelicals sought to distinguish themselves from traditional Christianity. His specific targeting of the Jesuits resonated with this narrative, but in the context of the Second Reformation it was also an oblique attack on Lutherans, who continued to use the traditional wafers in their own worship practices. The intellectual context reinforced the dangers, as well as potential benefits, of sensuous worship: external, material objects always had the potential to affect and shape the interior soul.

When Abraham Scultetus was called to assist in convincing the Lutheran subjects of Brandenburg of the truth of the margrave's new religion, he mobilized virtually all of the arguments Calvinists had developed over the previous generation about the sensuous appeal of the Eucharist. Christians were bound to abandon the use of traditional Hosts, ostentatious decoration of the altar, the use of elaborate vessels, and the practice of receiving the sacrament on the tongue because Scripture mandated an alternative form of practice. This form, however, didn't represent a rejection of sensuous worship but rather its embrace: as Johann Sigismund had done in 1613 in his Berlin cathedral, Christians were to "enjoy" the body and blood of Christ by tearing apart the bread, receiving it in their hands, and chewing it with their teeth.[154] Following Pareus, he argued that the bread had to be ordinary, local bread, "from the baker," with the power to nourish the body.[155] All of this, he maintained, was made clear by the scriptural injunction found in the account of the Last Supper: *hoc facite* (this do). The Lutheran subjects of Brandenburg were bound to emulate what had been carefully instituted by Christ: "Nothing," he explained, "can be a sacrament, or be called a sacrament, outside the custom established by Christ."[156] Others in Brandenburg, such as the prominent court preachers Salomon Finck (1566–1629), concurred with Scultetus on these points.[157]

Where Scultetus went beyond some of his contemporaries, however, was the extent to which he emphasized the positive affective potency of the specifically haptic dimensions of the ritual. This was most apparent in the care he devoted to describing the mundane act of chewing during Communion. If Christ had used ordinary bread, that clearly meant people were supposed to chew their Eucharist.[158] By contrast, the foam of Communion wafers simply dissolved on the tongue or could easily be swallowed in a single gulp, circumventing the physical, and indeed emotional, struggle that Christ had intended people to endure when receiving the sacrament. The chewing, tearing, and mashing of bread with the tongue and teeth were supposed to stir up feelings of devotion and identification with the "unspeakable agony and martyrdom of his [Christ's] body; the flagellation, crowning, and the nailing of his hands and feet, all of which so miserably tore his holy body."[159] He eschewed distinctions between "fleshly" and "spiritual" experience in this moment, instead insisting that "whoever mashes the bread with teeth and tongues also mashes the body of Christ with teeth and tongues."[160] The intertwining of senses, emotions, faith, and salvation were of essential importance, and Scultetus took a hard line on the matter, inflected with more than a little predestinarian cruelty. Responding to the Lutheran argument that the easier-to-swallow wafer facilitated greater participation in the Eucharist by the elderly, infirm, and those whose teeth had worn down or fallen out, he declared that Christ had foreseen and ordained that some might be excluded. He knew, after all, "what people can and cannot bite."[161]

While such positive evocations of the sensual among Calvinists are typically overlooked, it should not be entirely surprising to encounter them here. Scultetus, for his own part, thought with and about the senses intensively throughout his life and keenly appreciated the affective, nonverbal dimensions of religion. Some of his earliest childhood memories revolved around his own deeply felt connection with Eucharistic devotion. In his autobiography, he recalled sectarian divisions that erupted in his hometown of Grünberg after the promulgation of the Formula of Concord, describing himself initially as strongly disposed to "enjoying the flesh of Christ" in the Eucharist.[162] This was his way of talking about belief in the doctrine of the Real Presence, but as we've seen here, this kind of language was always bound up with questions of what sensuous worship was doing to people's minds, bodies, and souls. He reflected further on the matter when remembering what he considered to be the most essential lessons he had learned from his first teacher, Abraham Buchholzer (1529–1584). Buchholzer had impressed upon him that all life was a struggle with external threats and enemies, and even when not face-to-face, the struggle continued internally as an emotional one: as he put it, "We carry it about in our breasts day and night."[163] Buchholzer, however, also taught Scultetus that the church offered a joyful refuge where one observed and experienced the divine in the contrast to the "desire, lust, and joy of the flesh" of daily life.[164] Along with late medieval predecessors like Gabriel Biel, Scultetus had learned from an early age that sensuality was a two-sided coin in people's lives and required the church to intervene. These lessons resonated with Scultetus and informed how he imagined the divine. He thus described life after death as one in which the soul experienced God in full, "tasting how friendly the Lord is, and touching my Lord and my God with the hands."[165] After his death in 1625, a colleague commemorated his skill as a preacher, dwelling in particular on his power to move his congregations "with such charming and at the same time penetrating words. And he sometimes pressed bright tears from his listeners, which afterward many a pious Christian, when he recalled it, felt his heart to be pierced."[166] Here was a Calvinist who clearly embraced the sensuous in religion.

Abraham Scultetus was somewhat unusual among his peers in that he left behind such a critical mass of written material documenting not only his theological and natural philosophical views but also his personal biography. His enthusiastic embrace of the senses in religion, however, seems to have fit into the broader cultural paradigm among intellectuals in Second Reformation Germany. In the second half of the sixteenth century, Lutherans and Calvinists alike reasserted the importance of religious sensuality in strikingly similar ways. This reflected the fact that both confessions retained the same basic understanding of the senses that had framed late medieval discussions of church ritual. Despite calls to abandon it in the early 1520s, Aristotelian natural philosophy offered the only explanation of how ritual engaged the senses and, through that engagement, shaped people's souls. At midcentury, as this science of the soul enjoyed something of a renaissance in the newly Protestant universities, and as new ritual controversies erupted across the German-speaking world, it became ever more important for Protestant intellectuals to think through the fundamentals of this account of the human body, soul, senses, and what it all meant for questions about sacramental efficacy.

For Lutherans, this new context undermined the notion that anything practiced in the church could be adiaphoron, or indifferent. Although it remained in the formal lexicon of Lutheran theology, second-generation Lutheran theologians were deeply suspicious of the concept of ritual indifference, and they renewed their efforts to think about the affective impact of sensuous worship, especially when it came to the Eucharist. More focused discussions of this rite cast new light on its visual, gustatory, and especially tactile aspects. The Eucharist was not simply about the theological doctrines it was supposed to symbolize and communicate; it was about "enjoying" the sacrament. At its core, this meant a dynamic process between churchgoers and the ritual edifice of the church. Sensuous engagement was not only a pragmatic necessity; it was an opportunity for affective, internal transformation.

Calvinists also thought with the senses in Second Reformation Germany in much the same way as their Lutheran counterparts had. Although ingrained tendencies to view Calvinist religion in a kind of "mythic vacuum" have often obscured this point, it should by now not be entirely surprising. Calvinist intellectuals in the second half of the sixteenth century often attended the same schools as their Lutheran interlocutors, or, if they matriculated in a place like Heidelberg, they worked with the same Aristotelian natural philosophical corpus. In this context, their most basic assumptions about the human body, soul, and senses were shaped. As the new religion spread and began to compete with Lutheranism for the souls of early modern Germans, it made sense to utilize this knowledge. Much as it had in the late Middle Ages, the science of the soul became a useful tool for explaining how their external ceremonies not only commemorated or symbolized an essential theological truth but also *did something* to people. They identified with Christ as a liturgical theorist. In the Scriptures, they saw him modeling what people should be doing in church, because he knew best how to affect people's souls. It was therefore essentially important to calibrate the sensuous appeal of worship precisely according to his example. The whole physical experience of the rite, even the most seemingly mundane acts of tearing the bread, receiving it in the hands, and chewing it, exerted a profound power to change people. In spite of its reputation today, the emergence of the reformed tradition in the sixteenth century represented a distinctive embrace of the senses in religion.

Conclusion

It's now time to bring together the threads of the story of the senses in Reformation Germany and draw some conclusions. If we consider religious experience in this period in terms of the convergence of sensory discourses and sensory practices, the only major narrative of the Reformation that coheres is a highly ambiguous one, characterized by partial continuity with late medieval religion but also by important ruptures.

First, we should observe that the production of religion as a sensuous edifice unfolded rather haphazardly and was typically determined by a variety of factors converging in a local context. This was true of traditional Christianity in the fifteenth century and of Protestant Christianity in the sixteenth. How people assembled their worship practices reflected what was materially possible within their local communities: the types of liturgical vessels, textiles, and books on hand, the architecture of their sacred space, and the personnel and organizational capacities they had for putting on a good ritual show, among other things, all figured into the equation. In the fifteenth century, it may have been that sensory production aimed at some ideal of affective piety determined by learned discourse, as appears to have been the case in contemporaneous England, but evidence for this on the German scene is rather slim.[1] This is not to say that producing religion as a sensuous experience was unimportant: clearly, the outlay of time, money, and effort in many communities conveys that it was, and even in poorer, rural places, where worship was perhaps less "spectacular," the religious appeal to the senses was no less important. It is to say, however, that the divergent, quotidian concerns of political economy, not Aristotelian science, were of primary importance. As a result, variation prevailed in how religion appealed to smell, taste, touch, sight, and hearing. Among Lutheran communities of the sixteenth century, the political economic aspect of producing sensuous worship remained of primary importance. People mostly made do with what they had, even as they were told that external forms of worship were essentially indifferent and meaningless and as they constantly confronted the cultural narrative that Reformation religion was less sensual than the religion of their late medieval ancestors. At the same time, reformers built on the models for managing church property bequeathed to them by these same ancestors. Local communities were empowered to manage the material culture of their church but directed to confiscate and liquidate things that either caused idolatrous abuse or no longer had utility to meet the worship needs of the community.

The specific impact of Lutheran liturgical policy on what was on offer to the senses in the churches was, not surprisingly, erratic. It did, however, drift in the direction of simplified, perhaps more uniform practice than had prevailed in the late Middle Ages. With respect to the traditional objects of sight, the use of images, traditional Eucharistic vessels, vestments, and other liturgical textiles persisted in many cases. Also, many late medieval altarpieces remained intact and in situ. However, there were ambiguities and even ruptures in the fabric of devotional life. Sometimes the material culture of traditional Christianity was replaced with new objects that accorded more with Lutheran doctrine. The traditional elevation of the bread and wine of the Eucharist, so central to fifteenth-century piety, was variously tolerated and condemned from place to place, but increasingly abandoned. By the end of the sixteenth century, it appears to have been an outlier in most Lutheran churches. The objects and practices of Lutheran liturgy were, in some respects, visibly different. So too with the sightlines that helped define the space of the Lutheran churches. Most of the time, Lutherans inherited older churches and made do with the architectural features of these spaces. In some cases, however, they had the opportunity to make concrete their ideal of what a church should look like. When they did, Lutherans favored spaces that looked rather similar to their supposedly more austere reformed or Calvinist counterparts.

Even though much of the visual culture, and indeed sensory culture generally, of traditional Christianity was formally permissible, it was not completely desirable, and sixteenth-century Lutherans were constantly engaged in the business of making determinations about whether this sensuous residue either caused idolatrous or superstitious abuses among the laity or had any utility for the religious community. The former required making judgments on a case-by-case basis. Sometimes images manifestly incited idolatrous worship and belief. Sometimes they didn't. The latter, by contrast, could potentially always elicit a negative answer. Technically, almost everything associated with traditional worship had no real religious utility in Lutheranism. It did, however, always have very real economic utility, to which church and civic officials were very sensitive. These factors, in conjunction with widespread cultural bias against what they imagined to be traditional, sensuous worship, inclined such people negatively toward the wealth in their midst and often resulted in its removal from churches—at least the wealthier sorts of churches, mostly in urban spaces. It was a kind of oblique form of iconoclasm that impacted not only the traditional objects of vision but also the olfactory and tactile dimensions of worship. Censers were often liquidated, as were pax boards and other devices designed to make ostentatious appeals to touch in the ritual environment. In some instances, however, many of these eliminations were not permanent, and there is some evidence from the waning years of the sixteenth century that some Lutheran churches acquired new objects that had long since gone out of use in local practice. How they put them to use, however, is unclear. Again, this was primarily an urban phenomenon, as many churches simply didn't have that much to dispose of in the first place, and rarely acquired new stuff: the humble furnishings of rural church inventories stand testament to this fact.

The story of the aural dimensions of worship in the Reformation was similarly circuitous but also evinces some ruptures that tended to simplify late medieval practice. In the few churches that had enjoyed polyphonic and organ music prior to the Reformation, there appears to have been a temporary hiatus of these practices until the late decades of the sixteenth century. The acoustics of church space for the most part remained the same, but again, in cases where Lutherans had the opportunity to build new churches, their design reflected a concern with eliminating some of the distortive reverberations of the larger late medieval urban churches. Bell ringing, which became a hallmark of certain aspects of Lutheran liturgical and paraliturgical practice, especially in the late sixteenth century, nonetheless played a reduced role in the confines of the mass. The small, handheld bells rung during the elevation ritual were retained in some cases, but the larger bells mounted in the belfries of churches were generally not used during the mass. When they were deployed, the complex interplay of multiple bells was supplanted by a singular tolling, usually functioning to call people into church. All of these simplifying tendencies seem to have followed a logic of reducing the competing auralities that had defined late medieval church space in order to facilitate a clearer hearing of the words spoken and sung during services. The strongest evidence of this is perhaps the Lutheran insertion of a sermon into the liturgy of the mass, which became the defining feature of the new soundscape.

Of all the senses in the five-sense sensorium, the production of the gustatory elements of religious worship exhibits the strongest continuities between late medieval and Reformation eras. The ideal of Lutheran worship was communion in both kinds: reception of both the host and wine. The actual effect of this ideal on differentiating Lutheran practice from its late medieval forebear, however, is often difficult to assess. Further, there was no attempt among Lutheran reformers to alter the material composition of the Eucharist Host or wine, and so chemically at least, these things would seem to have tasted more or less the same as they had in the fifteenth century. Attempts to reform prayer books, however, did have some impact on how people imagined the gustatory experience of the Eucharist. By eliminating the sensory language characteristic of late medieval prayer books, which frequently dwelt on the gustatory experience of the bread and wine as one of intense sweetness, reformers moved to change the context in which people tasted the elements.

On balance, then, when we evaluate the impact of Lutheran reform on late medieval practice from an intersensorial perspective, we can't really conclude, with Ernst Walter Zeeden and others, that Lutheranism ultimately amounted to a veneer of new doctrinal ideas laid over the same old material substrate of worship.[2] There were important continuities, especially in the domains of visual and gustatory experience, but there were also important ruptures. To be sure, the Lutheran churches were not "less sensual" than their late medieval counterparts. We know as sensory historians that this is, strictly speaking, an objective impossibility and, moreover, a narrative loaded with often pernicious ideological baggage. They were, however, sensibly different places, even if this differentiation had been achieved in somewhat haphazard, inconsistent fashion.

Turning away from the sensory production of religion to consider how people consumed and understood it, we must also draw similarly ambivalent conclusions. Learned discourse in the fifteenth century consistently adhered to a mostly Aristotelian understanding of how sensation worked, and applied that understanding to the objects and practices of ritual life. Above all, the powerful affective bond between perceiving subject and perceived object underscored the significance of church practice and correspondingly reinforced the authority and status of those tasked with managing practice. As ritual experts specializing in the administration of sacraments, the clergy wielded an enormous power to reach out to the senses of parishioners and, in the process, shape their souls to the good. The dominance of this way of thinking with and about the senses outside the rarefied air of elite intellectual discourse, however, was by no means a foregone conclusion. The idea was a powerful one, but people exercised agency in how they used it. In the vernacular, people seem to have accepted the basic premise of learned sensory culture, but when they turned to narrate their own religious experience, they made more playful, creative use of the senses, often in ways that elicited anxieties from learned elites.

Similarly, the Reformation retained much of the intellectual framework that bound together the late medieval system, even as it partially undermined it. Theologians and pastors in the sixteenth century entered an educational system that cultivated an Aristotelian scientific worldview from an early age. The rhetoric of the early 1520s had called for abandoning this system, but reformers quickly realized they lacked any viable alternative and so returned to it in the 1530s and 1540s. In the newly Protestant schools and universities, students were immersed in the same ideas about the human soul and senses as their predecessors in the fifteenth century had been, and they were even encouraged to apply the lessons they learned there to the specific, concrete pastoral duties they confronted in their daily lives. The affective theory of sensation was therefore a widespread assumption in the mental equipment of sixteenth-century Protestants, Lutheran and Calvinist alike. When new ritual controversies erupted mid- to late century, it guided discussions of the meaning of the sensible in religious practice among Protestant intellectuals. In broad strokes, they asserted the same affective potential of sensuous worship that late medieval intellectuals had, although their discussions were more limited to a narrower vision of the sensual appeal of the Eucharist.

It should be noted, however, that these shades of continuity in intellectual culture did not play the determining role they seem to have performed in contemporaneous England.[3] For many, continuity with the late Middle Ages characterized how many understood the meaning of church practice throughout the sixteenth century, but it was not the only game in town. At the same time evangelicals were calling for the abandonment of the Aristotelian system, they were also beginning to weave together the mythology of the reformation of the senses. The contrariety between hyperaesthetic late medieval religion and a disembodied, intellectual form of evangelical Christianity held powerful sway in the imaginative landscape of the sixteenth century, shaping how people conceived of themselves and the sensory worlds they inhabited. It generated intellectual dissonance, as objective experience confirmed implicitly what Aristotelian science asserted explicitly: all life by definition was inescapably sensuous, from the bottom up. There was no transcending smell, taste, touch, sight, and hearing in this world, so how could religion be less sensual? The question was irrelevant when caught up in the narrative sweep of the reformation of the senses. To be sure, it was pure ideology, and as such it fractured and obscured historical reality even as it retained shards of its original truth. It was nonetheless an ideology with a profound power to affect reality. The story was repeated over and over again in the sixteenth century, and it motivated people to action. The radical iconoclasts of the early 1520s are testament to this, but so too are the more gradual, oblique reforms to sensuous worship instituted by cautious Lutherans over the course of the sixteenth century.

If the major empirical result of this study of the sensory history of fifteenth- and sixteenth-century Germany can be characterized in terms of ambivalence, paradox, and outright contradiction, what broader use could it possibly have? The notion that history was and is far less coherent than historians imagine and tell it to be is probably true, but that doesn't feel like a very edifying place to end. Allow me, then, to suggest one major point that, at the very least, is worth thinking about in the circumstances we confront today, five hundred years after Martin Luther published his *95 Theses*. The reformation of the senses is, if nothing else, an object lesson in the ideological power at stake in the manipulation and domination of media technologies across the centuries. Not in the simple sense that Marshall McLuhan or Walter Ong would once have had it: we can set aside the binary distinctions between a premodern, multisensory culture grounded in manuscripts and oral communication and a modern, visualist regime emerging from the typographic revolution of the mid-fifteenth century. We cannot, however, get around the fact that early German Protestant domination of the print medium changed the way some Christians thought and talked about the senses in religion in a fundamental way. The story of sensory reformation quickly established itself as a governing assumption in the cities of Germany among the first Protestants and gradually spread throughout sixteenth-century Europe. Even Catholics bought into the idea and used it to fashion a new identity premised on a more thoroughgoing embrace of sensuous religion, over and against their supposedly more intellectual Protestant neighbors. The story changed how people conceived of the history of religion, and it influenced the construction of religious, cultural, and even ethnic difference. Since then, its permutations have reverberated on the stage of the modern world, sometimes to extremely violent effect.

Although the reformation of the senses has been profoundly consequential in modern culture, particularly in Western Europe and North America, it initially took hold by relatively crude means. The success of the story depended in the first place on a highly motivated, powerful minority promoting and controlling it through the domination of media. The story was easily captured and reproducible—akin to what we might think of today as a sound byte or meme. Those who promoted it understood its power and effected a major cultural change simply by repeating it over and over again. Certainly, many people were aware of the manifest contradictions in the story of sensory reformation, but in their daily lives they were immersed in it, to the point that submission to its "truthiness" became a reflexive, thoughtless action. Obviously, Protestantism was less sensuous than what had come before, even though it was equally obvious that religion, and human life in general, was inescapably sensuous. The absurdity of such an utterance should serve as a mirror for reflection. Today, as we go about our daily lives, bombarded by endlessly repeating and repeatable narratives that betray contempt for independent critical thought, in a media landscape that seems ever more nakedly subservient to powerful interests, the reformation of the senses should serve as an example of what is at stake in learning how to engage with and respond to such stories.

Notes

Introduction

1. In this respect, the reformation of the senses seems to be an important component of what Edward Muir has identified as the emergence of ritual as an object of theoretical reflection in the sixteenth century. See Muir, *Ritual in Early Modern Europe*, 2nd ed. (Cambridge: Cambridge University Press, 2005).

2. See Weber, *The Protestant Ethic and the Spirit of Capitalism*, trans. Talcott Parsons (Minneola, N.Y.: Dover, 2003), 105. Translation originally published by Scribner (New York), 1958.

3. Ernst Troeltsch, *Die Bedeutung des Protestantismus für die Entstehung der modernen Welt* (Munich: Oldenbourg, 1911), 292–96.

4. MSNBC pundit Chris Matthews, for example, commonly uses this phrase to refer to his own Catholicism. He has noted Ronald Reagan's fondness for this phrase when describing his own complicated relationship to Catholicism. See Chris Matthews, *Tip and the Gipper: When Politics Worked* (New York: Simon & Schuster, 2013), 330.

5. For a sketch of the cultural history of the Reformation, see Bernhard Jussen and Craig Koslofsky, eds., *Kulturelle Reformation: Sinnformationen im Umbruch, 1400–1600* (Göttingen: Vandenhock and Ruprecht, 1999).

6. Susan Karant-Nunn has persistently defended the basic thrust of the narrative. See Karant-Nunn, *The Reformation of Ritual: An Interpretation of Early Modern Germany* (New York: Routledge, 1997), 107–37. Karant-Nunn, "'Gedanken, Herz und Sinn': Die Unterdrückung der religiösen Emotionen," in Jussen and Koslofsky, *Kulturelle Reformation*, 69–96. Karant-Nunn, "Ritual in Early Modern Christianity," in *The Cambridge History of Christianity: Reform and Expansion, 1500–1660*, ed. R. Po-Chia Hsia (Cambridge: Cambridge University Press, 2007), 371–85. Karant-Nunn, "Die Reformation des Rituals und ihre visuellen Effekte in Sakralraum," in *Topographien des Sakralen: Religion und Raumordnung in der Vormoderne*, ed. Susanne Rau and Gerd Schwerhoff (Munich: Dölling and Galitz, 2008), 90–102. Karant-Nunn, *Reformation of Feeling: Shaping the*

Religious Emotions in Early Modern Germany (Oxford: Oxford University Press, 2009), 101–7.

7. Karant-Nunn, "Gedanken," 69–96. See also Karant-Nunn, *Reformation of Feeling*.

8. Scribner set many of the parameters for the recent discussion of vision in late medieval piety in a series of articles in the 1990s, before his premature death. See Scribner, "Popular Piety and Modes of Visual Perception in Late-Medieval and Reformation Germany," *Journal of Religious History* 15, no. 4 (1989): 448–69. Several variations on the theme of visual culture appeared in various articles in English and German, most of which are now gathered in English in the posthumously published *Religion and Culture in Germany (1400–1800)*, ed. Lyndal Roper (Leiden: Brill, 2001), 85–145.

9. Thomas Kaufmann, "Die Sinn- und Leiblichkeit der Heilsaneignung im späten Mittelalter und in der Reformation," in *Medialität, Unmittelbarkeit, Präsenz: Die Nähe des Heils im Verständnis der Reformation*, ed. Johanna Haberer and Berndt Hamm (Tübingen: Mohr Siebeck, 2012), 11–43.

10. Ibid. This is, however, a claim based on circumstance. Kaufmann observes that these rites objectively appealed to touch, and he infers the value accorded to the sense by reformers. He presents somewhat limited evidence of reformers explicitly discussing the tactile appeal.

11. John Bossy, *Christianity in the West 1400–1700* (Oxford: Oxford University Press, 1985), 97–104. Ulinka Rublack, *Reformation Europe* (Cambridge: Cambridge University Press, 2005), 10–11, 46, 151, 193. Ulinka Rublack, "Grapho-Relics: Lutheranism and the Materialization of the Word," *Past and Present* 206, supp. 5 (2010): 144–66. Joseph Koerner, *The Reformation of the Image* (Chicago: University of Chicago Press, 2004). Lee Palmer Wandel, *The Reformation: Towards a New History* (Cambridge: Cambridge University Press, 2011), 63–88. Andrew Pettegree, *Reformation and the Culture of Persuasion* (Cambridge: Cambridge University Press, 2005).

12. Peter Blickle, "Die Reformation vor dem Hintergrund von Kommunalisierung und Christianisierung: Eine Skizze," in *Kommunalisierung und Christianisierung: Voraussetzungen und Folgen der Reformation 1400–1600*, ed. Peter Blickle and Johannes Kunisch (Berlin: Duncker, 1989), 9–28. At 24.

13. Many of these interpretations speak to themes established by media theorists Marshall McLuhan and Walter Ong. See McLuhan, *The Gutenberg Galaxy* (Toronto: University of Toronto Press, 1962); Ong, *The Presence of the Word* (New Haven, Conn.: Yale University Press, 1967); Ong, *Orality and Literacy: Technologizing the Word* (New York: Routledge, 1982). For critical evaluations of the notion that hearing and seeing are more intellectual senses in western European culture, and the tendency to associate sight in particular with modernity, see Mark M. Smith, *Sensing the Past: Seeing, Hearing, Smelling, Tasting, and Touching in History* (Berkeley: University of California Press, 2007), 19–58. David Howes, ed., *The Varieties of Sensory Experience: A Sourcebook in the Anthropology of the Senses* (Toronto: University of Toronto Press, 1991). David Howes, ed., *Empire of the Senses: The Sensual Culture Reader* (New York: Berg, 2005). Constance Classen, *Worlds of Sense: Exploring the Senses in History and Culture* (New York: Routledge, 1993). Constance Classen, "Foundations for an Anthropology of the Senses," *International Journal of Social Science* 153 (1997): 401–12. Constance Classen,

The Color of Angels: Cosmology, Gender, and the Aesthetic Imagination (New York: Routledge, 1998). Jonathan Crary, *Techniques of the Observer: On Vision and Modernity in the Nineteenth Century* (Cambridge, Mass.: MIT Press, 1992). Martin Jay, *Downcast Eyes: The Denigration of Vision in Twentieth-Century French Thought* (Berkeley: University of California Press, 1993).

14. Scott Hendrix builds on this theme in "Rerooting the Faith: The Reformation as Re-Christianization," *Church History* 69, no. 3 (2000): 558–77. Hendrix offers a different interpretation of vineyard imagery in early Reformation rhetoric, similar to Schön's woodcut.

15. Thomas Lentes, "Die Deutung des Scheins: Das symbolische Verhalten im Spätmittelalterbild (1830–1945)," in *Spätmittelalterliche Frömmigkeit zwischen Ideal und Praxis*, ed. Berndt Hamm and Thomas Lentes (Tübingen: Mohr Siebeck, 2001), 1–23 (quoting Ranke at 1). Lentes's narrative focuses on the visual has been by far the most studied of sensory modalities, but it is relevant to the larger problem at hand.

16. Smith, *Sensing the Past*, 16–17. Mark M. Smith, "Making Sense of Social History," *Journal of Social History* 37, no. 1 (2003): 165–86. David Howes, *Sensual Relations: Engaging the Senses in Culture and Social Theory* (Ann Arbor: University of Michigan Press, 2003), 3–28.

17. Smith, "Making Sense," 166. Mark M. Smith, "Producing Sense, Consuming Sense, Making Sense: Perils and Prospects for Sensory History," *Journal of Social History* 40, no. 4 (2007): 841–58.

18. Compare with "the forming of the five senses is a labor of the entire history of the world down to the present." In Marx, *Economic and Philosophic Manuscripts of 1844*, in Robert Tucker, ed., *The Marx-Engels Reader*, 2nd ed. (New York: Norton, 1978), 66–125 (quote at 89). The quotation appears frequently in the scholarship on the senses, often as an epigram. See, for example, Smith, "Making Sense," 165.

19. Philip Hahn, "Sensing Sacred Space: Ulm Minster, the Reformation, and Parishioners' Sensory Perception, c. 1470–1640," *Archiv für Reformationsgechichte* 105 (2014): 55–91. Philip Hahn, "The Reformation of the Soundscape: Bell-Ringing in Early Modern Lutheran Germany," *German History* 33, no. 4 (2015): 525–45.

20. Jacob M. Baum, "From Incense to Idolatry: The Reformation of Olfaction in Late Medieval German Ritual," *Sixteenth Century Journal* 44, no. 2 (2013): 323–44.

21. Compare with George Roeder Jr., "Coming to Our Senses," *Journal of American History* 81, no. 3 (December 1994): 1112–22.

22. Compare with Susan Karant-Nunn, "Changing One's Mind: Transformations in Reformation History from a Germanist's Perspective," *Renaissance Quarterly* 58, no. 4 (2005): 1101–27.

23. For an up-to-date online research directory and fairly comprehensive bibliographic reference on sensory studies, see www.sensorystudies.org.

24. Compare with Lucien Febvre, *The Problem of Unbelief in the Sixteenth Century: The Religion of Rabelais*, trans. Beatrice Gottlieb (Cambridge, Mass.: Harvard University Press, 1982), 421–37.

25. Alain Corbin, *The Foul and the Fragrant: Odor and the French Social Imagination*, trans. Miriam Kochan, Roy Porter, Christopher Prendergast (Cambridge, Mass.:

Harvard University Press, 1986). Alain Corbin, *Village Bells: Sound and Meaning in the Nineteenth-Century French Countryside*, trans. Martin Thom (New York: Columbia University Press, 1998).

26. Jay, *Downcast Eyes.*

27. A small sample of exemplary works in this vein includes: Crary, *Techniques*; David Levin, ed., *Modernity and the Hegemony of Vision* (Berkeley: University of California Press, 1993); Mitchell Merback, *The Thief, the Cross, and the Wheel: Pain and the Spectacle of Punishment in Medieval and Renaissance Europe* (Chicago: University of Chicago Press, 1999); Kate Flint, *The Victorians and the Visual Imagination* (Cambridge: Cambridge University Press, 2000); Robert S. Nelson, ed., *Visuality before and beyond the Renaissance* (Cambridge: Cambridge University Press, 2000); Suzannah Biernoff, *Sight and Embodiment in the Middle Ages* (New York: Macmillan, 2002); Stuart Clark, *Vanities of the Eye: Vision in Early Modern European Culture* (Oxford: Oxford University Press, 2007); Lee Palmer Wandel and Walter S. Melion, eds., *Early Modern Eyes* (Leiden: Brill, 2009).

28. Compare with W. F. Bynum and Roy Porter, eds., *Medicine and the Five Senses* (Cambridge: Cambridge University Press, 1993). The contributions in this volume still remain some of the most useful.

29. See the contributions in Charles Burnett, Michael Fend, and Penelope Gouk, eds., *The Second Sense: Studies in Hearing and Musical Judgment from Antiquity to the Seventeenth Century* (London: Warburg Institute, 1991); Veit Erlmann, ed., *Hearing Cultures: Essays on Sound, Listening, and Modernity* (New York: Berg, 2004); Mark M. Smith, ed., *Hearing History: A Reader* (Athens: University of Georgia Press, 2004).

30. McLuhan, *Gutenberg Galaxy*; Ong, *Presence*; Ong, *Orality and Literacy.*

31. See especially Howes, *Varieties*. Classen, *Worlds of Sense*; Classen, "Foundations."

32. This is demonstrated by several of the contributions and the bibliography in the recent volume edited by Herman Roodenburg, *A Cultural History of the Senses in the Renaissance* (New York: Bloomsbury, 2014). Some of the important works on England include: Emily Cockayne, *Hubbub: Filth, Noise, and Stench in England, 1600–1700* (New Haven, Conn.: Yale University Press, 2007); Katherine A. Craik, *Reading Sensations in Early Modern England* (New York: Palgrave Macmillan, 2007); Holly Dugan, *The Ephemeral History of Perfume: Scent and Sense in Early Modern England* (Baltmore, Md.: Johns Hopkins University Press, 2011); Lowell Gallagher and Shankar Raman, eds., *Knowing Shakespeare: Senses, Embodiment, Cognition* (New York: Palgrave Macmillan, 2010); Penelope Gouk, *Music, Science, and Natural Magic in Seventeenth-Century England* (New Haven, Conn.: Yale University Press, 1999); Laura Gowing, *Common Bodies: Gender, Touch, and Power in Seventeenth-Century England* (New Haven, Conn.: Yale University Press, 2003); Arnold Hunt, *The Art of Hearing: English Preachers and Their Audiences, 1590–1640* (Burlington, Vt.: Ashgate, 2010); Bruce R. Smith, *The Acoustic World of Early Modern England: Attending to the O-Factor* (Chicago: University of Chicago Press, 1999); Sarah Stanbury, *The Visual Object of Desire in Late Medieval England* (Philadelphia: University of Pennsylvania Press, 2008); Christopher M. Woolgar, *The Senses in Late Medieval England* (New Haven, Conn.: Yale University Press, 2007).

33. Matthew Milner, *The Senses and the English Reformation* (Burlington, Vt.: Ashgate, 2011). Matthew Milner, "To Captivate the Senses: Sensory Governance, Heresy, and

Idolatry in Mid-Tudor England," in *Religion and the Senses in Early Modern Europe*, ed. Wietse de Boer and Christine Göttler (Leiden: Brill, 2013), 307–30.

34. Milner, *Senses*, 9.

35. Milner, "The Senses in Religion: Towards the Reformation of the Senses," in Roodenburg, *Cultural History*, 87–106.

36. Quentin Skinner long ago observed this as a peril of intellectual history. See Skinner, "Meaning and Understanding in the History of Ideas," *History and Theory* 8, no. 1 (1969): 3–53.

37. A growing literature has demonstrated the vitality of sensory culture in post-Reformation Catholicism. See especially the contributions in de Boer and Göttler, *Religion and the Senses*, and the volume of essays edited by Marcia B. Hall and Tracy E. Cooper, *The Sensuous in the Counter-Reformation Church* (Cambridge: Cambridge University Press, 2013). See also Jeffrey Chipps Smith, *Sensuous Worship: Jesuits and the Art of the Early Catholic Reformation in Germany* (Princeton, N.J.: Princeton University Press, 2002).

38. Wietse de Boer and Christine Göttler, "Introduction: The Sacred and the Senses in an Age of Reform," in de Boer and Göttler, eds., *Religion and the Senses*, 1–15 (quote at 2).

39. Smith, "Producing Sense, Consuming Sense." Smith, *Sensing the Past*, 4–5, 118–25.

Chapter 1. Late Medieval Worship: A Sensory Production

1. For recent overviews of the senses in medieval Christendom that foreground the importance of ritual practice yet nonetheless overlook the German context, see Beatrice Caseau, "The Senses in Religion: Liturgy, Devotion, and Deprivation," in *A Cultural History of the Senses in the Middle Ages*, edited by Charles Newhauser (London: Bloomsbury, 2014): 89–110; Éric Palazzo, *L'invention chretienne des cinq sens: L'art, la liturgie et les cinq sens au Moyen Age* (Paris: Cerf, 2014); Matthew Milner, *The Senses and the English Reformation* (Burlington, Vt.: Ashgate, 2011), 53–161.

2. Susan Karant-Nunn, *Reformation of Ritual: An Interpretation of Early Modern Germany* (New York: Routledge, 1997), 107–8. See also Susan Karant-Nunn, *Reformation of Feeling: Shaping the Religious Emotions in Early Modern Germany* (Oxford: Oxford University Press, 2009), 68–69.

3. Early focus on the production of the Eucharist as a "salvific spectacle" was developed in the work of early-twentieth-century German scholars Peter Browe and Anton Meyer. See Browe, "Die Elevation in der Messe," *Jahrbuch für Liturgiewissenschaft* 9 (1929): 20–67; Browe, "Die Eucharistie als Zaubermittel im Mittelalter," *Archiv für Kulturgeschichte* 20 (1930): 134–54; Browe, *Die häufige Kommunion im Mittelalter* (Münster: Regensberg, 1934); Anton Mayer, "Die heilbringende Schau in Sitte und Kult," in *Heilige Überlieferung: Ausschnitte aus der Geschichte des Mönchtums und des heiligen Kultes: Festschrift für Ildefons Herwegen*; ed. Odo Casel (Münster: Aschendorf, 1938), 234–62. More recently, see Thomas Lentes, "So weit das Auge reicht: Sehrituale im Spätmittelalter," in *Das "Goldene Wunder" in der Dortmunder Petrikirche: Bildgebrauch und Bildproduktion im Mittelalter*, ed. Thomas Lentes (Bielefeld: Verlag für Regionalgeschichte, 2003), 241–58; Robert Scribner, "Popular Piety and Modes of Visual Perception in Late-Medieval and Reformation Germany," *Journal of Religious History* 15, no. 4 (1989): 448–69; Robert

Scribner, *Religion and Culture in Germany, 1400–1800* (Leiden: Brill, 2000); Michael Camille, “Before the Gaze: The Internal Senses and Late Medieval Practices of Seeing,” in *Visuality before and beyond the Renaissance: Seeing as Others Saw*, ed. Robert Nelson (Cambridge: Cambridge University Press, 2000), 197–223; Hans Belting, *Das Bild und sein Publikum im Mittelalter: Form und Funktion früher Bildtafeln der Passion* (Berlin: Gebrüder Mann, 1981); Suzannah Biernoff, *Sight and Embodiment in the Middle Ages* (New York: Palgrave, 2002), 133–64.

4. On the iconography of the Mass of St. Gregory generally, see Esther Meier, *Die Gregorsmesse: Funktionen eines spätmittelalterlichen Bildtypus* (Cologne: Böhlau, 2006); Thomas Lentes and Andreas Gormas, eds., *Das Bild der Erscheinung: Die Gregorsmesse im Mittelalter* (Berlin: Reimer, 2003). Lentes has also been instrumental in developing the online database of *Gregorsmesse* images at the University of Münster. The database is still being developed but provides a wealth of multimedia images of the Mass of St. Gregory iconography: http://gregorsmesse.uni-muenster.de.

5. For a useful summary of historians' efforts to “de-colonize” the Middle Ages from these old tropes, see Carol Symes, “When We Talk about Modernity,” *American Historical Review* 116, no. 3 (2011): 715–26.

6. Éric Palazzo, “Art, Liturgy, and the Five Senses in the Early Middle Ages,” *Viator* 41 (2010): 25–56.

7. Karant-Nunn, *Ritual*, 108; Robert Scribner, *Popular Culture and Popular Movements in Reformation Germany* (London: Hambledon, 1987), 21–22.

8. *Ordinarius magdeburgensis* (Leipzig: Brandis, 1485), fol. 2v.

9. For back-streaming as a method in the history of early modern popular culture, see Peter Burke, *Popular Culture in Early Modern Europe*, 3rd ed. (Burlington, Vt.: Ashgate, 2009), 122–29.

10. StAN, Rep. 44e, SIL 130, Nrs. 6, 7. StAN, Rep. 44e, SIL 131, Nrs. 2, 7, 7a, 10, 13. StAN, Rep. 44e, SIL 133, nr. 9. The first inventory was taken in St. Lorenz in 1421. Thereafter, inventories document a rapid accumulation over the course of the fifteenth century in both parish churches, as well as the Church of Our Lady and the chapel of the Holy Ghost Hospital. Additional inventories appear in StAN Rep. 59, Nürnberger Salbücher, Nr. 3, fols. 89v–93r, StAN Rep. 59, Nürnberger Salbücher, Nr. 1, fols 100r–138v. See also Karl Schlemmer, *Gottesdienst und Frömmigkeit in der Reichsstadt Nürnberg am Vorabend der Reformation* (Würzburg: Echter, 1980), 150–63.

11. They are especially well documented for St. Sebald in the late fifteenth century, in the accounts of Sebald Schreyer, master of the church from 1482 to 1503. See Theodor Hampe, “Sebald Schreyer vornehmlich als Kirchenmeister von St. Sebald,” *Mitteilungen des Vereins für Geschichte der Stadt Nürnberg* (hereafter *MVGN*) 28 (1928): 155–207. Elisabeth Caesar, “Sebald Schreyer, ein Lebensbild aus dem vorreformatorischen Nürnberg,” *MVGN* 56 (1969): 1–213.

12. Hektor Amman, *Die wirtschaftliche Stellung der Reichsstadt Nürnberg im Spätmittelalter* (Nuremberg: Selbstverlag des Vereins für Geschichte der Stadt Nürnberg, 1970), 11, 117, 120–22, 169, 189. Johannes Müller, “Der Umfang und die Hauptrouten des Nürnberger Handelsgebietes im Mittelalter,” *Vierteljahrschrift für Sozial- und Wirtschaftsgeschite* 6 (1908): 1–38.

13. Richard Klier, "Zur Genealogie der Bergunternehmerfamilie Schütz in Nürnberg und Mitteldeutschland im 15. und 16. Jahrhundert," *MVGN* 55 (1967–68): 185–213. Theodor Gustav Werner, "Die große Fusion der Zechen um den Rappolt in Schneeberg unter Führung der Nürnberger von 1514," (3 parts) *MVGN* 56–58 (1969–1971): 214–50 (part 1), 150–75 (part 2), 102–15 (part 3). Theodor Gustav Werner, "Regesten und Urkunden über Beteiligungen von Nürnbergern an der Zeche Rappolt und an anderen Schneeberger Bergwerks- und Metallhandelsunternehmungen," (two parts) *MVGN* 59–60 (1972–1973): 40–84, 153–94.

14. Heinrich Kohlhaussen, *Nürnberger Goldschmiedekunst des Mittelalters und der Dürerzeit, 1240 bis 1540* (Berlin: Verlag für Kunstwissenschaft, 1968); Gerald Strauss, *Nuremberg in the Sixteenth Century: City Politics and Life between Middle Ages and Modern Times* (Bloomington: Indiana University Press, 1976), 123–45.

15. Adolf Engelhardt, "Der Kirchenpatronat zu Nürnberg," *Zeitschrift für bayerische Kirchengeschichte* 7 (1932): 1–16, 65–80.

16. Schlemmer, *Gottesdienst*, 110–11. Hampe, "Schreyer," 174–90. Caesar, "Schreyer," 82–84.

17. For the sacristans' books, see Albrecht Gümbel, ed., *Das Mesnerpflichtbuch von St. Lorenz in Nürnberg vom Jahre 1493* (Munich: Kaiser, 1928). Albrecht Gümbel, ed., *Das Mesnerpflichtbuch von St. Sebald in Nürnberg vom Jahre 1482* (Munich: Kaiser, 1929), hereafter referred to as *MPBL* (for St. Lorenz), and *MPBS* (for St. Sebald).

18. Arnd Reitemeier, *Pfarrkirchen in der Stadt des späten Mittelalters: Politik, Wirtschaft und Verwaltung* (Stuttgart: Franz Steiner, 2005), 12, 89–157.

19. Charlotte Stanford, *Commemorating the Dead in Late Medieval Strasbourg: The Cathedral's Book of Donors and Its Use (1320–1521)* (Burlington, Vt.: Ashgate, 2011), 19–20, 48–50.

20. Scribner, "Popular Piety," 458.

21. For more on this, see chapter 3.

22. Franz Rudolf Reichert, ed., *Die älteste deutsche Gesamtauslegung der Messe (Erstausgabe ca. 1480)* (Münster: Aschendorff, 1967), 99.

23. Werner Rösener, "The Agrarian Economy, 1300–1600," in *Germany: A New Social and Economic History*, vol. 1: 1450–1630, ed. Robert Scribner (London: Arnold, 1996), 63–85.

24. Heinz Hürten, ed., *Cusanus-Texte V: Brixener Dokumente; Akten zur Reform des Bistums Brixen* (Heidelberg: Universitätsverlag, 1960), 38.

25. Host irons commonly appear in the sources as "oblateisen." See Janny de Moor, "The Wafer and Its Roots," in *Look and Feel: Studies in Texture, Appearance and Incidental Characteristics of Food: Proceedings of the Oxford Symposium on Food and Cookery 1993*, ed. Harlan Walker (London: Prospect, 1994), 119–27. Hanna Kronberger-Frentzen, *Die alte Kunst der süssen Sachen: Backformen und Waffeleisen vergangener Jahrhunderte* (Hamburg: Broschek, 1959).

26. See chapter 2.

27. Hampe, "Schreyer," 201, 203, 205, 207.

28. Reitemeier, *Pfarrkirchen*, 327.

29. Hampe, "Schreyer," 203, 205.

30. *Deutsche Gesamtauslegung*, 100.

31. Reitemeier, *Pfarrkirchen*, 331.

32. Joseph Greving, ed., *Johann Ecks Pfarrbuch für U.L. Frau in Ingolstadt: Ein Beitrag zur Kenntnis der pfarrkirchlichen Verhältnisse im sechzehnten Jahrhundert* (Münster: Aschendorff, 1908), 134, 220–21.

33. Malte Prietzel, "Alterleute und Kastenherren: Die Rechnungen der Kirche St. Jacobi in Göttingen von 1523/24 und 1534," *Göttinger Jahrbuch* 41 (1993): 61–95, at 30.

34. Quoted in Schlemmer, *Gottesdienst*, 168.

35. Caesar, "Schreyer," 90.

36. Cited in Schlemmer, *Gottesdienst*, 242.

37. *MPBL*, 41, 51–52; *MPBS*, 14, 16–17, 22, 38.

38. Ibid. In St. Lorenz, the sacristan provided twenty-nine "maß" (measures) of wine on Palm Sunday, twenty-two on Maundy Thursday, fifty-eight on Good Friday, fifty-two on Easter Sunday, and nine on Easter Monday. In St. Sebald, he provided twelve to fourteen maß of wine one Palm Sunday, thirty-seven on Maundy Thursday, fifty-five on Good Friday, and thirty-three on Easter Sunday. The conversion into liters is based on the ratio provided in Fritz Verdenhalven, *Alte Maße, Münzen und Gewichte aus dem deutschen Sprachgebiet* (Neustadt an der Aisch: Degner, 1968).

39. Schlemmer, *Gottesdienst*, 240–42, 261–68.

40. In Trier, for example, the parish of St. Gangolf in the 1492–1511 period averaged twelve hundred communicants on Easter (virtually 100 percent of the parish population, as best as can be determined), and between one hundred and four hundred communicants on Christmas (between 8.3 percent and 33 percent of the population). See Browe, *Häufige Kommunion*, 41. In Mainz, Florentius Diel, pastor of the parish of St. Christopher from 1491–1518, would typically expect no fewer than thirty communicants at the second and third Masses on Christmas, while on Palm Sunday in 1513, he reported that at least sixty people had received communion. The largest numbers of communicants came on Maundy Thursday and Easter Sunday. For both days, Diel noted that his preparations for Mass included consecrating two hundred "particles" of the Eucharist Host for distribution. See Franz Falk, ed., *Die pfarramtlichen Aufzeichnungen (Liber consuetudinum) des Florentius Diel zu St. Christoph in Mainz (1491–1518)* (Freiburg im Breisgau: Herder, 1904), 7, 18, 24, 29. Johann Eck, pastor in Ingolstadt from 1519 to 1540, observed the necessity of consecrating six hundred Eucharist Hosts for Palm Sunday services. See *Ecks Pfarrbuch*, 140. The parish church in Ulm documented eight thousand and eleven thousand Easter communicants in 1475 and 1523, respectively. See Philip Hahn, "Sensing Sacred Space: Ulm Minster, the Reformation, and Parishioners' Sensory Perception, c. 1470 to 1640," *Archiv für Reformationsgeschichte* 105 (2014): 55–91. For Göttingen's parish church of St. James, see Prietzel, "Altarleute," 75, 77, 80.

41. Qtd. in Browe, *Häufige Kommunion*, 73.

42. Ibid, 93–95.

43. Ibid., 96.

44. Ibid.

45. Brian Pavlac, "Reform," in *Introducing Nicholas of Cusa: A Guide to a Renaissance Man*, ed. Christopher Belitto (Mahwa, N.J.: Paulist, 2004), 59–118, at 90–91.

46. Scribner, *Religion and Culture*, 114.

47. Scribner, "Popular Piety," 458.

48. See bibliography for missals consulted.

49. Milner, *Senses*, 95.

50. Schlemmer, *Gottesdienst*, 121–22, 135–37.

51. *Missale numburgense* (Nuremberg: n.p., 1501); *Missale magdeburgense* (Nuremberg: Stuchs, 1503); *Missale hildensemense* (Nuremberg: Stuchs, 1511); *Missale brandenburgense* (Nuremberg: Stuchs, 1494); *Missale pataviense* (Nuremberg: Heller & Hermann, 1514); *Missale salisburgense* (Nuremberg: Stuchs, 1505); *Missale romanum* (Nuremberg: Stuchs, 1484).

52. Schlemmer, *Gottesdienst*, 104.

53. *Missale bambergense* (Bamberg: Sensenschmidt, 1490), fols. 163v–166v. *Missale bambergense* (Bamberg: Pfeyl, 1499), fols. 155v–160r.

54. *Missale romanum* (1484), fols. 178v–179v, 193v–196r, 199r–v, 201r–v.

55. Gerd Althoff, "The Variability of Rituals in the Middle Ages," in *Medieval Concepts of the Past: Ritual, Memory, Historiography*, ed. Gerd Althoff (Cambridge: Cambridge University Press, 2002), 71–87.

56. *Missale coloniense* (Cologne: Quentell, 1494), fols. 182r–184v; *Missale herbipolense* (Würzburg: Reyser, 1495), fols. 60r, 66r–70r.

57. *Missale wormatiense* (Basel: Wenssler, 1490), fols. 319r–323v; *Missale moguntinum* (Würzburg: Reyser, 1482), fols. 117r–119r. Priests were to elevate the Host, speak a portion of the consecration prayers, and then lift the Host still higher while speaking the final words of consecration. See fols. 320r–v.

58. *Missale brandenburgense*, fols. 161r–163r; *Missale brandenburgense*, (Leipzig: Lorr, 1516), fols. 150r–152r; *Missale magdeburgense*, not paginated; *Missale halberstatense* (Strasbourg: n.p., 1498), fols. 145r–146v. Similar provisions appear in missals not associated with a specific geographic location, such as the missal of the Augustinian hermits and more general "books of special masses." See *Missale ordinis fratrum eremitarum sancti Augustini* (Nuremberg: Order of the Augustinian Hermits, 1491), fols. 116r–117v; *Liber missarum specialis* (Strasbourg: Prüß, 1503), fols. 131v–132v.

59. Reitemeier, *Pfarrkirchen*, 242.

60. Edmund Ungerer, ed., *Elsässische Altertümer in Burg und Haus, in Kloster und Kirche: Inventare vom Ausgang des Mittelalters bis zum dreissigjährigen Kriege aus Stadt und Bistum Strassburg*, vol. 1 (Strasbourg: Trübner, 1913), 143–96, 240–47.

61. *Aufzeichnungen Florentius Diel*, 18. *Johan Ecks Pfarrbuch*, 140–41.

62. StAN, Rep. 44e, SIL 131, Nr. 2, fol. 6v. This set was estimated at almost twice the value as the next most valuable set.

63. GNM, HS Merkel 100, fol. 51r.

64. Reitemeier, *Pfarrkirchen*, 240–41.

65. These numbers are based on a survey of the reports collected in Karl Kayser, ed., *Die reformatorischen Visitationen in den welfischen Landen 1542–1544: Instruktionen, Protokolle, Abschiede und Berichte der Reformatoren* (Göttingen: Vandenhoeck & Ruprecht, 1897), 108–241.

66. Ibid. Although two parishes in Göttingen-Kalenberg—Hannover-Neustadt and Gehrden—documented seven and five chalices, respectively.

67. Numbers based on a survey of the reports collected in Victor Herold, ed., *Die brandenburgischen Kirchenvisitations-Abschiede und Register des XVI. und XVII Jahrhunderts*, vol. 1: *Die Prignitz* (Berlin: Kommisionsverlag von Gsellius, 1928); Gerhard Zimmermann and Gerd Heinrich, eds., *Die brandenburgischen Kirchenvisitations-Abschiede und—Register des XVI. und XVII. Jahrhunderts*, vol. 2: *Das Land Ruppin* (Berlin: de Gruyter, 1963).

68. This analysis is based on a survey of the sixty-five parish churches in the first three administrative units of the Lutheran church in Saxony, known as the *Ephorien* of Wittenberg, Kemberg, and Zahna, published in Karl Pallas, ed., *Die Registraturen der Kirchenvisitationen im ehemals sächsische Kurkreise*, vol. 1: *Kemberg, Wittenberg, Zahna* (Halle: Hendel, 1906–1918).

69. *MPBS*, 21, 52.

70. Ibid., 38–39.

71. *MPBL*. The notes of the sacristan of St. Lorenz provide no general description of a High Mass in the fashion of Schreyer's book for St. Sebald, and so we are left to make an educated guess. The range of two to four is based on the positive descriptions of illumination of the Lorenzaltar (high altar) on feast days throughout the year, which always included at least two candelabra, but never more than four.

72. *MPBS*.

73. *MPBL*, 14, 41–43, 49.

74. *MPBS*, 7–8, n4 (quoting from 1493 entry in the *Salbuch* of St. Sebald, kept by Schreyer).

75. *MPBL*, 21, 52; *MPBS*, 17–19.

76. *MPBS*, 18, 39.

77. *MPBL*; *MPBS*.

78. Ibid. The St. Lorenz sacristan's book provided considerably more detail on vestments than its counterpart in St. Sebald. In St. Lorenz, red vestments were documented for twenty-seven Masses, white for twenty-one. In St. Sebald, red vestments were documented in for eighteen Masses, white for six.

79. Ibid. Black vestments were documented for seven Masses in St. Lorenz, six in St. Sebald. In St. Lorenz, green and blue vestments appear in six and eight Masses, respectively. In St. Lorenz, green vestments were worn in four Masses, blue in three.

80. *MPBL*, 28, 32–33 (brown silk regalia with pearl tracery), 15, 27 (gray silk regalia).

81. In St. Lorenz, white was documented for all Marian feasts with the exception of the Annunciation (March 25). The most ornate of these vestments was a full set of silk regalia, embroidered with an image of the Virgin, framed by the sun. It was worn for Mass on the Purification (February 2). See *MPBL*, 16, 28, 34, 36, 43–45. On All Saints' in St. Lorenz, two different sets of black silk regalia were worn at the first and High Masses, one of which, donated by the family of the famous humanist Willibald Pirckheimer, was embroidered with gold. See *MPBL*, 42. In St. Sebald, vestments were documented for the Annunciation (white silk regalia), the Assumption (white damask with gold floral patterns and the arms of the donor family, Starck). See *MPBS*, 14, 30. For All Souls' in St. Sebald, the priest wore an especially fine set of regalia donated by the Kress family, of black silk with five pearl images. See *MPBS*, 36.

82. *MPBL*, 22. In St. Sebald, the documentation indicates white damask with golden floral patterns and the Starck arms (mentioned above) at the first Mass, red silk regalia with gold tracery and pearl images at the second, and green and gold for the High Mass. See *MPBS*, 18.

83. *MPBS*, 38.

84. For Easter and Christmas, see *MPBS*, 18, 38; *MPBL*, 22, 47. For the textiles deployed in St. Lorenz on the Marian feast days, see *MPBL*, 16, 28, 34, 36, 43–44, 45. For the church of Sebald, see *MPBS*, 11, 27, 30, 36, 37. The exceptions to this rule were the feasts of the Annunciation and the Birth of the Virgin in St. Sebald. For the Annunciation, the sacristan was to provide the best altar cloths on hand, including one with an image of the Virgin, and another with an image of the four doctors of the church, at the high altar. On the feast of the Birth of the Virgin, the sacristan was to avoid any kind of banners, tapestries, or altar cloth whatsoever. See *MPBS*, 14, 33.

85. *MPBS; MPBL*.

86. Xaver Haimerl, *Das Prozessionswesen des Bistums Bamberg im Mittelalter* (Munich: Kösel-Pustet, 1937). Andrea Löther, *Prozessionen im Spätmittelalterlichen Städten: Politische Partizipation, obrigkeitliche Inszenierung, städtische Einheit* (Cologne: Böhlau, 1999), esp. 55–138. Scribner, *Popular Culture*, 20–22.

87. This usage is indicated for 18 percent of the Masses documented in St. Sebald, and 30 percent of those documented in St. Lorenz. See *MPBS*, *MPBL*. Most of the time, the particular items used are not identified, instead referred to as “relics” or images placed on the altar.

88. StAN Rep. 44e, SIL 131, Nr. 2, fols. 1r–6r (Sebald). StAN Rep. 59, Nürnberger Salbücher, Nr. 2, fols. 89v–93r. Of the items documented in St. Sebald in this category, 52.5 percent contained a relic, whether it was a saint’s body part, piece of clothing, or a relic of a religious object, such as a fragment of the Holy Cross. In St. Lorenz, the number was lower (26.2 percent).

89. *MPBS*, 39.

90. Crucifixes are mentioned on Good Friday, the celebrations of the church’s relics, the Holy Cross, and the Ascension of the Lord. Monstrances are mentioned at the altar on the feast of John the Evangelist. See *MPBS*, 17, 20, 21, 38.

91. *MPBS*, 12, 26, 27, 29, 32. All three of these images also contained relics. See StAN Rep. 44e, SIL 131, Nr. 2, fol. 5v.

92. Specifically, on the feasts of Kunigund, Margaret, Anne, Martha, 11,000 Maidens, Barbara, and Lucia. See *MPBL*, 17, 29, 31, 32, 36, 40, 45. The one exception to this gendered rule appears to have been the Mass celebrated on August 3, commemorating the discovery of the relics of St. Stephen. See *MPBL*, 32.

93. *MPBL*, 29. This practice was evident on the feast of S. Kunigund (17).

94. Reitemeier, *Pfarrkirchen*, 261–63. As Reitemeier notes, these collections were comparable with other middle-sized towns such as Coburg, Wertheim, and Bamberg.

95. Anton Schilling, ed., “Die religiösen und kirchlichen Zustände der ehemaligen Reichsstadt Biberach unmittelbar vor Einführung der Reformation,” *Freiburger Diözesan Archiv* 19 (1887): 1–191, qtd. at 25.

96. Reitemeier, *Pfarrkirchen*, 179.

97. Ibid., 180.

98. Hahn, "Sensing Sacred Space," 61–62.

99. Ibid, 62.

100. Schlemmer, *Gottesdienst*, 63–64, 70–73.

101. Reitemeier, *Pfarrkirchen*, 224. Charlotte Stanford, *Commemorating the Dead*, 73–116.

102. Lucien Febvre was probably the first to make this observation. See Febvre, *The Problem of Unbelief in the Sixteenth Century: The Religion of Rabelais*, trans. Beatrice Gottlieb (Cambridge, Mass.: Harvard University Press, 1982). See also Holly Dugan, *The Ephemeral History of Perfume: Scent and Sense in Early Modern England* (Baltimore, Md.: Johns Hopkins University Press, 2011), 24–41; Constance Classen, David Howes, and Anthony Synnott, *Aroma: The Cultural History of Smell* (New York: Routledge, 1994), 51–93; Jonathan Reinarz, *Past Scents: Historical Perspectives on Smell* (Champaign: University of Illinois Press, 2014), 31–43, 50–51.

103. Charles Zika, "Hosts, Processions and Pilgrimages: Controlling the Sacred in Fifteenth-Century Germany," *Past and Present* 118 (1988): 25–64. Scribner, "Popular Piety," 458.

104. Josef Jungmann, *Missarum sollemnia: Eine genetische Erklärung der römischen Messe* (Vienna: Herder, 1949), 1:259–68, 1:393–97, 1:556–57, 2:171–254.

105. *Missale romanum* (1484), fols. 114r–117v.

106. *Missale ordinis fratrum eremitarum*, fols. 94r–v; *Missale augustense* (Augsburg: Ratdolt, 1502), fol. 107v; *Missale augustense* (1510), fols. 111r–v; *Missale constantiense* (Augsburg: Ratdolt, 1505).

107. *Missale numburgense*, fol. 403r; *Missale Brixiense* (Basel, 1511), fol. 139v.

108. *Missale basiliense* (Basel: Koch, 1479), fol. 136v; *Missale argentinense* (Basel: Wenssler, 1486), fol. 187r; *Missale misnense* (Mainz: Peter Schöffer, 1485), fol. 217r.

109. *Missale hildensemense*, fol. 27v.

110. This was recognized as the "common custom" in the 1482, 1493, and 1497 editions of the missal. See *Missale moguntinum* (1482), fols. 106r–v; *Missale moguntinum* (Mainz: Schöffer, 1493), fol. 132r; *Missale moguntinum* (Speyer: Drach, 1487), fol. 28r.

111. *Missale havelsburgense* (Leipzig: Brandis, 1489).

112. *Ordo missalis frisingensis* (Augsburg: Ratdolt, 1502), fol. 121r.

113. StAN, Rep. 44e, SIL 133, nr. 9, fol. 4r.

114. In St. Sebald, these included two Masses on the Octave of John the Evangelist, one on the Octave of the Epiphany, and two on the feast of St. Theodore. None of the sacristan's entries addressed the specific point in the liturgy when incense was deployed. See *MPBS*, 8, 9, 36. In St. Lorenz, incense was noted for the Introit of High Mass on All Saints' Day, the Introit of the morning Mass on Palm Sunday, the *Agnus Dei* (after elevation) on Maundy Thursday, Good Friday after the collect, and then on Easter. See *MPBL*, 19, 21, 42, 52. In addition to these dates, several other entries are somewhat ambiguous, and may indicate incense usage during High Masses on the feasts of the Discovery of Stephen's relics (33), Jerome (38), and Dionysius (38).

115. *MPBS*; *MPBL*.

116. Compare with Joseph Sauer, *Symbolik des Kirchengebäudes und seiner Ausstattung in der Auffassung des Mittelalters* (Freiburg: Herder, 1902), 204.

117. The daily canonical hours included the services of Lauds, Prime, Terce, Sext, and None.

118. *MPBS*, 15–19, 37–38; *MPBL*, 21, 44–46, 52.

119. *Ordinarius magdeburgensis*, fols. 10v–11r, 12r–14r, 16r–19v, 29r–31v.

120. *Obsequiale augustanum* (Augsburg: Erhard Ratdolt, 1487), fols. 3r–7v, 13r, 22r–23v, 40v, 52v–53r, 55r.

121. Adolph Franz, *Die kirchlichen Benediktionen des Mittelalters*, vol. 1 (Freiburg: Herder, 1909), 423–33.

122. *Agenda iuxta ritum gloriose et pretatissime ecclesie collegiate: sanctos mauricij et maria Magdalene hallis ad sudarium domini* (1536). The agenda is preserved in MWSB, Hs I, 434a. Prescriptions for the *Rauchnächte* appear on fols. 15r–17v.

123. Jacob M. Baum, "From Incense to Idolatry: The Reformation of Olfaction in Late Medieval German Ritual," *Sixteenth Century Journal* 44, no. 2 (2013): 323–44, at 333–34.

124. E. G. Cuthbert Atchley, *A History of the Use of Incense in Divine Worship* (London: Longmans, Green, 1909). Nigel Groom, *Frankincense and Myrrh: A Study of the Arabian Incense Trade* (New York: Longman's, 1981). Dugan, *Ephemeral History*, 31–32.

125. On this matter generally, see Paul Freedman, *Out of the East: Spices and the Medieval Imagination* (New Haven, Conn.: Yale University, 2008), 11.

126. Hampe, "Schreyer," 195.

127. Prietzel, "Altarleute," 75–79.

128. Reitemeier, *Pfarrkirchen*, 317–18.

129. Renate Smollich, *Der Bisamapfel in Kunst und Wissenschaft* (Stuttgart: Deutscher Apotheker Verlag, 1983), 69.

130. Reitemeier, *Pfarrkirchen*, 318.

131. Volker Schier, "Probing the Mystery of the Use of Saffron in Medieval Nunneries," *Senses and Society* 5, no. 1 (2010), 57–72.

132. Reitemeier, *Pfarrkirchen*, 318.

133. Joseph Braun, *Das christliche Altargerät in seinem Sein un Seiner Entwicklung* (Munich: Hueber, 1932), 600–604.

134. In St. Lorenz, the censers were purchased sometime between 1421 and 1466. See StAN Rep. 44e, SIL 130, nr. 6, fols. 1–5. StAN Rep. 44e, SIL 130, nr. 7, fols. 7v–8r.

135. StAN Rep 44e. SIL 131 Nr. 7, fol. 2v. The censer appears again in a later inventory from 1519. See StAN Rep. 44e, SIL 131, nr. 10, fol. 2r.

136. StAN Rep. 44e, SIL 133, Nr. 9, fols. 4r–v.

137. D. Pickel, "Ein Nürnberger Klosterinventar aus dem Mittelalter," *MVGN* 20 (1913): 234–41.

138. Ungerer, *Elsässische Altertümer*, vol. 1, 144, 185, 191–92, 244.

139. Reitemeier, *Pfarrkirchen*, 249.

140. Kayser, *Kirchenvisitationen*; Pallas, *Registraturen*. Herold, *Visitationsabschiede*; Zimmermann, *Visitationsabschiede*.

141. Anton Landersdorfer, ed., *Das Bistum Freising in der Bayerischen Visitation des Jahres 1560* (Ottilien: St. Ottilien Verlag, 1991). Reiner Braun, ed., *Die Bayerischen Teile des Erzbistums Salzburg und des Bistums Chiemsee in der Visitation des Jahres 1558* (Ottilien: St. Ottilien Verlag, 1991).

142. Reitemeier, *Pfarrkirchen*, 243.

143. Diocesan missals the provided for the use of corporals during the elevation included those for Würzburg, Cologne, Mainz, Constance, Strasbourg, and Brandenburg. See *Missale herbipolense*, fols. 66r–70r; *Missale coloniense*, fols. 182r–184v; *Missale moguntinum* (Speyer: Drach, 1487), fols. 224r–228r; *Missale constantiense* (Augsburg: Ratdolt, 1505), fols. 154v–156r. *Missale argentinensis* (Hagenau: n.p., 1520), fols. 175v–176r. *Missale brandenburgense*, fols. 161r–163r.

144. StAN, Rep. 59, Nürnberger Salbücher, nr. 2, fol. 91r.

145. *Missale romanum* (Basel: Wenssler, 1487), fol. 179v.

146. Ibid., fol. 196r.

147. Ibid., fols. 199v–200r.

148. Ibid., fol. 202r.

149. *Missale herbipolense*, fol. 72r; *Missale argentinensis*, fols. 423r–424v; *Missale magdeburgense*, fol. 373r; *Missale brandenburgense*, fol. 164v.

150. Jeffrey Hamburger, *Nuns as Artists: The Visual Culture of a Medieval Convent* (Berkeley: University of California Press, 1997), 3–4, 19–20.

151. *Missale brandenburgense*, fols. 165r–v.

152. Craig Koslofsky, "The Kiss of Peace in the German Reformation," in *The Kiss in History*, ed. Karen Harvey (Manchester, U.K.: Manchester University Press, 2005), 18–35, at 18–20.

153. *Deutsche Gesamtauslegung*, 184: "Der diacon oder altar diener der tregt den hin das selbe gekueste tefelein den andernn priesternn, die in dem kore sein, zekuessen. Und das kuest einer nach dem andernn mit andacht. Es ist auch an vil enden sith, das der altar diener umb tregt das selbe gekueste tefelein allen den, die hinder dem ambt oder messe stan oder knyen, einem yeden zekuessen. Und das heist osculum pacis—der kuß des frides."

154. The churches were in Rühstädt, Mansfeld, Söllentin, and Vehlgast. Compare with Herold, *Visitationsabschiede*, 69–104.

155. *MPBS*, 20.

156. Koslofsky, "Kiss of Peace," 19, 28–29.

157. This was the small village of Vienenburg, which owned three paxes. See Kayser, *Kirchenvisitationen*, 183.

158. Pallas, *Registraturen* vol. 1, 327–29.

159. On soundscapes in general, see R. Murray Schafer, *The Soundscape: Our Sonic Environment and the Tuning of the World* (1977, repr. Rochester, Vt.: Inner Traditions International, 1993); Barry Truax, *Acoustic Communication* (Norwood, N.J.: Ablex, 1984). For instructive historical treatments of premodern soundscapes, see Bruce R. Smith, *The Acoustic World of Early Modern England: Attending to the O-Factor* (Chicago: Chicago University Press, 1999); Emma Dillon, *The Sense of Sound: Musical Meaning in France, 1260–1330* (Oxford: Oxford University Press, 2012); Philip Hahn, "The Reformation of

the Soundscape: Bell-Ringing in Early Modern Lutheran Germany," *German History* 33, no. 4 (2015): 525–45.

160. Dillon, *Sense of Sound*. Dillon's brilliant musicological research focuses on an earlier period in France but is nonetheless a useful description of what happened in the German churches of the fifteenth and early sixteenth centuries.

161. Richard Cullen Rath, *How Early America Sounded* (Ithaca, N.Y.: Cornell University Press, 2003), 98–103.

162. Ibid., 100. Rath's reconstruction is based on acoustic analyses of mainly English churches.

163. Reitemeier, *Pfarrkirchen*, 165–69.

164. The contrast between rounded wooden and plaster structures and rectilinear stone structures parallels very closely the contrast drawn by Bruce Smith between the Globe and Blackfriars theaters in London. See Smith, *Acoustic World*, 208–17.

165. Milner, *Senses*, 115–16.

166. Schlemmer, *Gottesdienst*, 102.

167. Hahn, "Sensing Sacred Space," 59. Lübeck, too, probably the largest city in northern Germany, had a huge choir. See Reitemeier, *Pfarrkirchen*, 562.

168. Bartlett Russell Butler, "Liturgical Music in Sixteenth Century Nürnberg: A Socio-Musical Study" (PhD diss., University of Illinois, 1970), 47.

169. Reitemeier, *Pfarrkirchen*, 545–48.

170. *MPBL*, 34, 41, 42, 45, 49, 52, 58; *MPBS*, 8, 9, 12, 13, 14, 16–23, 26–33, 35–38.

171. Butler, "Liturgical Music," 48–49.

172. Compare with Milner, *Senses*, 100–101, 115–16.

173. *MPBL*, 44.

174. *MPBS*, 17.

175. Butler, "Liturgical Music," 58–63.

176. Wilhelm Bäumker, *Das katholische deutsche Kirchenlied in seinen Singweisen*, vol. 2 (Freiburg im Breisgau: Herder, 1883), 8–12; Joseph Herl, *Worship Wars in Early Lutheranism: Choir, Congregation, and Three Centuries of Conflict* (Oxford: Oxford University Press, 2004), 23–25.

177. The procurator of St. Lorenz also left a note on the performance of these four voices by an assembly of school boys, altar boys, and vicars, under the direction of the schoolmaster, though without indication of who sang which parts. See Schlemmer, *Gottesdienst*, 298–99.

178. Herl, *Worship Wars*, 24.

179. Ibid., 23–27. Philipp Harnoncourt, *Gesamtkirchliche und teilkirchliche Liturgie: Studien zum liturgischen Heiligenkalendar und zum Gesang im Gottesdienst unter besonderer Berücksichtigung des deutschen Sprachgebiets* (Freiburg: Herder, 1974), 297–301; Johannes Janota, *Studien zu Funktion und Typus des deutschen geistlichen Liedes im Mittelalter* (Munich: Beck, 1968), 43–44, 71–76.

180. Herl, *Worship Wars*, 69–86.

181. Reitemeier, *Pfarrkirchen*, 280–82.

182. Hampe, "Schreyer," 200.

183. Ibid., 203. Caesar, "Schreyer," 87.

184. Hampe, "Schreyer," 203.

185. Reitemeier, *Pfarrkirchen*, 570–71.

186. Ibid., 541–45.

187. Caesar, "Schreyer," 89.

188. Hermann Harrassowitz, "Geschichte der Kirchenmusik an St. Lorenz in Nürnberg," *MVGN* 60 (1973): 1–152, at 3–18.

189. Herl, *Worship Wars*, 25; Rudolf Pacik, "Zur Stellung der Orgel in der katholischen Liturgie des 16. Jahrhunderts," in *Orgel und Orgelspiel im 16. Jahrhundert*, vol. 2, edited by Walter Salmen (Innsbruck: Helbling, 1978), 120–43.

190. Schlemmer, *Gottesdienst*, 299.

191. See discussion, above.

192. Beginning with Alain Corbin, *Village Bells: Sound and Meaning in the Nineteenth-Century French Countryside*, trans. Martin Thom (New York: Columbia University Press, 1998). More recently, and in the sixteenth-century German context, see Hahn, "Soundscape."

193. Braun, *Altargerät*, 573–77.

194. Reitemeier, *Pfarrkirchen*, 250.

195. *MPBS*; *MPBL*. In St. Sebald, the fourth bell was left unidentified as a "great bell"; in St. Lorenz, the fourth bell was identified as the "Lorenz-bell" (consecrated in the name of the church's patron saint).

196. Reitemeier mentions both parish churches in Wesel, as well as churches in Windsheim, Rothenburg ob der Tauber, and Freiburg. See *Pfarrkirchen*, 285–86. Johan Eck's *Pfarrbuch* also documents multiple large bells. See *Ecks Pfarrbuch*, 143, 168, 179.

197. *MPBL*, 13.

198. Ash Wednesday, for example, paralleled this usage almost exactly. See *MPBS*, 12.

199. In St. Lorenz, the simultaneous ringing of all four bells is indicated eleven times (8.9 percent of feast days identified in the liturgical calendar). In St. Sebald, it is indicated thirty-six times (20 percent of feast days identified in the liturgical calendar). *MPBL*; *MPBS*.

200. *MPBL*; *MPBS*.

201. *MPBL*, 51–52, qtd. at 51.

202. *MPBS*, 16–20.

203. *MPBL*, 47–49.

204. Alfred Haverkamp, "Ohne Glocken keine Gemeinde—kommunale Organisationsformen im Europa des Mittelalters," *Wirtschaft und Wissenschaft* 3, no. 4 (1995): 21–29.

205. Reitemeier, *Pfarrkirchen*, 525–29, 537.

206. *MPBS*, 39.

207. Reitemeier, *Pfarrkirchen*, 250, 289.

Chapter 2. The Senses and Sacramentality in Late Medieval Intellectual Discourse

1. Johann Geiler von Kaysersberg, "Predigen Teütsch vnd vil gutter leeren des hochgeleerten Herrn Johan von Kaisersperg in der goetliche geschrifft doctor und prediger

zu dem hohen stifft vnser liebenfrauwen mynster der stat Stroßburg (Augsburg: Hans Otmar, 1508)," in *Johannes Geiler von Kaysersberg Sämtliche Werke*, vol. 2, ed. Gerhard Bauer (Berlin: De Gruyter, 1991), 234.

2. Sander de Boer, *The Science of the Soul: The Commentary Tradition on Aristotle's De anima, c.1260–1360* (Leuven: Leuven University Press, 2013).

3. For an extended introduction to the various moments in the process of sensation in late medieval intellectual culture, see Matthew Milner, *The Senses and the English Reformation* (Burlington, Vt.: Ashgate, 2011), 13–25.

4. On the paradox of the senses in medieval Christian thought, see Gabrielle Spiegel, "Paradoxes of the Senses," in *Rethinking the Medieval Senses: Heritage/Fascinations/Frames*, ed. Stephen Nichols (Baltimore, Md.: Johns Hopkins University Press, 2008), 186–93.

5. Charles Newhauser, "Peter of Limoges, Optics, and the Science of the Senses," *Senses and Society* 5, no. 1 (2010): 29–44.

6. See for example Marquard von Lindau (d. 1392), "De quinque sensibus," in MSWB, HS I 240 (ca. 1400), fols. 2v–9v, and the anonymous "Die Fünf Sinne," in Tübingen Universitätsbibliothek HS Md 277 (ca. 1501), fols. 1r–3r.

7. Carl Nordenfalk, "The Five Senses in Late Medieval and Renaissance Art," *Journal of the Warburg and Courtauld Institutes* 48 (1985): 1–22.

8. Kaysersberg, "Predigen," 235.

9. Ibid., 108. Johann Geiler von Kaysersberg, "Dis schön buch genant der seelen Paradiß von waren vnd volkummen tugenden sagend (Strasbourg: Schürer, 1510)," in *Sämtliche Werke* 3 (1995): 7, 203, 604, 773–74.

10. John Van Engen, "Multiple Options: The World of the Fifteenth-Century Church," *Church History* 77, no. 2 (June 2008): 257–84, at 279–80; Caroline Walker Bynum, *Wonderful Blood: Theology and Practice in Late Medieval Northern Germany and Beyond* (Philadelphia: University of Pennsylvania Press, 2007).

11. Biel, *Sermones* I, ed. Wendelin Steinbach (Tübingen: Johann Otmar, 1499), fol. f3v.

12. Heiko Oberman, *Harvest of Medieval Theology: Gabriel Biel and Late Medieval Nominalism* (Cambridge, Mass.: Harvard University Press, 1963), 57–59, 272n87. Here quoting from Biel, *Sermones* II. As Oberman points out, Biel was fond of using the expression "sensual coin of the devil" to talk about the problem of sin.

13. Notable contemporaries, including Nicholas Cusanus (d. 1464), Johannes von Auerbach (d. 1469), Heinrich Herpff (d. 1478), Konrad Grütsch (d. 1475), and Paul Wann (d. 1489), articulated the same position. See Cusanus, *Idiota de sapientiae* (1450), trans. Jasper Hopkins (Minneapolis: Banning, 1996), 497–99; Nicholas Cusanus, *De venatione sapientiae* (1463), trans. Jasper Hopkins (Minneapolis: Banning, 1998), 1282; Nicholas Cusanus, *De Beryllo* (1453), trans. Jasper Hopkins (Minneapolis: Banning, 1998), 823–24; Johannes von Auerbach, *Summa de confessionis et de sacramentis* (Augsburg: Zainer, 1469), fols. 21r–25r; Konrad Grütsch, *Quadragesimale Gritsch de tempore et de Sanctis* (Strasbourg, 1486), fol. g4r; Heinrich Herpff, *Sermones fratris Henrici herp . . . de tempore hyemales et festiuales* (Augsburg: Rynman, 1509), fols. s6v, s8r; Paul Wann, *Sermones de tempore* (Passau: Petri, 1491), fols. s7v–s8r.

14. Sense objects impressing themselves on the sense organs and souls of percipients were analogized to the impression of a seal into wax throughout medieval Europe. See

Mary Carruthers, *The Book of Memory: A Study of Memory in Medieval Culture*, 2nd ed. (Cambridge: Cambridge University Press, 2008), 69–76; Michael Camille, "Before the Gaze: The Internal Senses and Late Medieval Practices of Seeing," in *Visuality before and beyond the Renaissance*, ed. Robert Nelson (Cambridge: Cambridge University Press, 2000), 197–223; Suzannah Biernoff, *Sight and Embodiment in the Middle Ages: Ocular Desires* (New York: Palgrave, 2002), 13, 133–64; Katherine Tachau, "Seeing as Action and Passion in the Thirteenth and Fourteenth Centuries," in *The Mind's Eye: Art and Theological Argument in the Middle Ages*, ed. Jeffrey Hamburger (Princeton, N.J.: Princeton University Press, 2006), 336–59; Cordelia Warr, "Re-Reading the Relationship between Devotional Images, Visions, and the Body: Clare of Montefalco and Margaret of Citta di Castello," *Viator* 38, no. 1 (2007), 217–49.

15. Catherine Bell, *Ritual Theory, Ritual Practice* (Oxford: Oxford University Press, 2009), 130–40.

16. For overviews of competing Augustinian (Platonic) and Aristotelian theories of sensation in the Middle Ages, see Pekka Kärkäinnen, "The Senses in Philosophy and Science: Mechanics of the Body or Activity of the Soul?" in *A Cultural History of the Senses in the Middle Ages*, ed. Charles Newhauser (New York: Bloomsbury, 2014), 111–32.

17. For Hugh's influence on theories of public performance, see Carol Symes, *A Common Stage: Theater and Public Life in Medieval Arras* (Ithaca, N.Y.: Cornell University Press, 2007), 8–10. W. Tatarkiewicz, "*Theatrica*, the Science of Entertainment: From the XIIth to the XVIIth Century," *Journal of the History of Ideas* 26, no. 2 (1965), 263–72.

18. Hugh of St. Victor, *On the Sacraments of the Christian Faith*, trans. Roy Deferrari (Cambridge, Mass.: Medieval Academy of America, 1951), 155. Added emphases.

19. Ibid., 157.

20. Peter Dillard, "Removing the Mote in the Knower's Eye: Education and Epistemology in Hugh of St. Victor's Didascalion," *Heythrop Journal* 55, no. 2 (2014): 203–15, at 210–11.

21. Hugh of St. Victor, *Didascalicon: A Medieval Guide to the Arts*, trans. Jerome Taylor (New York: Columbia University Press, 1991), 64.

22. For a clear discussion of intromission and extramission, see Kärkäinnen, "Senses in Philosophy and Science," 111–32.

23. *On the Sacraments*, 164, 273–78, 315–21.

24. Ibid., 148–49.

25. Robert Scribner, *Religion and Culture in Germany, 1400–1800* (Leiden: Brill, 2001), 57; Caroline Walker Bynum, *Christian Materiality: An Essay on Religion in Late Medieval Europe* (New York: Zone, 2011).

26. *On the Sacraments*, 164.

27. Albertus Magnus, *Summa theologiae* vol. 31, ed. E. Borgnet (Paris: Vives, 1894), part 1, tract. 20, q. 80, m.1, p. 858, column b. For Aquinas's definition, see *Summa Theologiae*, part 3, question 60, article 4, in the Editio Leonina of his works, vol. 12 (1906), 7–8.

28. Durandus, *Rationale divinorum officiorum* (Lyon: Huguetan, 1508), book 1, chap. 9 (*de ecclesiae sacramentis*) (not paginated).

29. Ibid., book 4, chap. 1, no. 12.

30. Ibid., book 1, chap. 1, no. 24.

31. Citing from the fifteenth-century vernacular translation, edited by Gerhard Buijssen: *Durandus' Rationale im spätmittelhochdeutscher Übersetzung*, vol. 1 (Assen: Van Gorcum, 1966), 281.

32. For Aquinas, see Harm Goris, "Thomism in Fifteenth-Century Germany," in *Aquinas as Authority: A Collection of Studies Presented at the Second Conference of the Thomas Institut Utrecht*, ed. Paul van Geest (Utrecht: Peeters Leuven, 2001), 1–24. For Albert, see: Albert Zimmermann, ed., *Albert der Grosse: Seine Zeit, sein Werk, seine Wirkung* (Berlin: de Gruyter, 1981); Martin Grabmann, *Mittelalterliches Geistesleben: Abhandlungen zur Gescichte der Scholastik und Mystik*, vol. 2 (Munich: Hueber, 1936), 340–41, 356; Adolf Kolping, "Die Drucke der Albert dem Grossen zugeschriebenen Messerklärung," *Freiburger Zeitschrift für Philosophie und Theologie* 2 (1955): 197–205.

33. Henryk Anzulewicz, "The Systematic Theology of Albert the Great," in *A Companion to Albert the Great: Theology, Philosophy, and the Sciences*, ed. Irven Resnick (Leiden: Brill, 2013), 15–68, at 66; Adolf Kolping, "Die handschriftliche Verbreitung der Messerklärung Alberts des Grossen," *Zeitschrift für katholische Theologie* 82 (1960): 1–39; Erich Kleineidam, *Universitas Studii Erffordensis: Überblick über die Geschichte der Universität Erfurt*, vol. 1 (Leipzig: St. Benno, 1964); Katherine Park, "Albert's Influence on Late Medieval Psychology," in *Albertus Magnus and the Sciences: Commemorative Essays, 1980*, ed. James Weisheipl (Toronto: Pontifical Institute of Mediaeval Studies, 1980), 501–35, especially at 522–34.

34. The first was printed in Augsburg by Günter Zainer in 1477. The second appeared in Strasbourg at the press of Georg Husner in 1485.

35. Editions appear in Mainz (Fust & Schöffer: 1459), Augsburg (Zainer: 1470 and 1473), Strasbourg (Rusch: 1470; Husner: 1478, 1479, 1481, 1483, 1484, 1486, 1488, 1493, 1501; Prüß: 1486), Cologne (Zell: 1475), Ulm (Zainer: 1475), Speyer (Drach: 1476), Basel (Wenßler: 1476. Wenßler & Ruppel: 1477; Keßler: 1488), Nuremberg (Koberger: 1480, 1481, 1494), and Hagenau (1509 and 1519).

36. S. M. Holmes, "Reading the Church: William Durandus and the New Approach to the History of Ecclesiology," *Ecclesiology* 11 (2011), 29–49; Alselme Davril, "Les états successifs du texte du *Rationale* de Guillaume Durand et la preparation de l'édition critique," in *Guillaume Durand, Eveque de Mende*, ed. Pierre-Marie Guy (Paris: Centre National de la Recherche Scientifique, 1992), 137–42.

37. Davril, "Les états successifs," 137–42. In Germany, vernacular manuscripts survive in Munich, Nuremberg, and Vienna. For Munich, see BSB Cgm 1121 (excerpt of book 7, chap. 38), and Cgm 512 (books 5–6). Both Munich manuscripts were produced around 1475. In Vienna, see Österreichische Nationalbibliothek, Cod. 2765, 3045, 3046. In Nuremberg, the convent of St. Katherine's acquired a complete translation in the second half of the fifteenth century. It is divided into three manuscripts. See NSB Cent III, 85 (part 2); Cent IV, 80 (part 1), and Cent V, 29 (part 3).

38. Auerbach, *Summa*, fols. 21r–25r, qtd. at 24v–25r.

39. Konrad Grütsch, *Quadragesimale*, fol. g4r. On Grütsch's education, work, and popularity in southwestern Germany, see Hans Jürgen Rieckenberg, "Grütsch, Konrad," in *Neue Deutsche Biographie* 7 (1966), 206.

40. Herpff, *Sermones*, fols. s6v, s8r.

41. Cusanus, *De venetatione*, 1282. Cusanus, *De Beryllo*, 824.

42. Wann, *Sermones de tempore*, s7v–s8r. Here Wann singled out the practices of oral confession, devotional prayers, fasting, penance, hearing the word of God, and contemplating devotional images.

43. Compare with Milner, *Senses*, 53–92, on the relation of this theoretical view and religion in late medieval England. More focused works on the commentary tradition specifically agree that the discourse had wider purchase beyond the narrowly defined boundaries of natural philosophy. See De Boer, *Science of the Soul*, 2–4 and variously. See also Dominik Perler, "Introduction," in *Transformations of the Soul: Aristotelian Psychology, 1250–1650*, ed. Dominik Perler (Leiden: Brill, 2009), 1–9; Richard C. Dales, *The Problem of the Rational Soul in the Thirteenth Century* (Leiden: Brill, 1995); Simo Knuutila, "Aristotle's Theory of Perception in Medieval Aristotelianism," in *Theories of Perception in Medieval and Early Modern Philosophy*, ed. Knuutila and Pekka Kärkäinnen (Dordrecht: Springer Science, 2008), 1–22.

44. Gordon Rudy, *The Mystical Language of Sensation in the Later Middle Ages* (New York: Routledge, 2002).

45. George Reilly, "The Psychology of Albert the Great Compared with that of Saint Thomas" (PhD diss., Catholic University of America, 1934), 21; Georg Wieland, *Zwischen Natur und Vernunft: Alberts des Großen Begriff vom Menschen* (Münster: Aschendorffsche Verlagsbuchhandlung, 1999); Dag Nikolaus Hasse, "The Early Albertus Magnus and His Arabic Sources on the Theory of the Soul," in Perler, *Transformations of the Soul*, 10–30; Nicholas H. Steneck, "Albert on the Psychology of Sense Perception," in Weisheipl, *Albertus Magnus and the Sciences*, 263–90; David Twetten and Steven Baldner, "Introduction to Albert's Philosophical Work," in Resnick, *Companion to Albert the Great*, 165–72; Markus Führer, "Albert the Great and Mystical Epistemology," in Resnick, *A Companion to Albert the Great*, 137–61. Niklaus Largier, "Inner Senses—Outer Senses: The Practice of Emotions in Medieval Mysticism," in *Codierungen von Emotionen im Mittelalter/Emotions and Sensibilities in the Middle Ages*, ed. C. Stephen Jaeger (Berlin: de Gruyter, 2003), 3–15.

46. Park, "Albert's Influence," 522–34. Mieczyslaw Markowski shows that Cologne directly influenced the faculty at Krakow. See Markowski, "Albert und der Albertismus in Krakau," in Zimmermann, *Albert der Grosse*, 177–92.

47. Pekka Kärkäinnen, "Psychology and the Soul in Late Medieval Erfurt," *Vivarium* 47 (2009): 421–43; Götz-Rüdiger Tewes, "Die Erfurter Nominalisten und ihre thomistischen Widersacher in Köln, Leipzig und Wittenberg: Ein Beitrag zum deutschen Humanismus am Vorabend der Reformation," in *Die Bibliotheca Amploniana*, ed. Andreas Speer (Berlin: Walter de Gruyter, 1995), 447–88. Despite their antischolastic rhetoric, the theology faculty was enthusiastically consuming both Albert and Aquinas in the fifteenth century. See Kleineidam, *Universitas Studii Erffordensis*, 183.

48. Milner, *Senses*, 15–16.

49. Hundt, *Anthropologium de hominis dignitate et natura* (Leipzig: Stöckel, 1501). Reisch's *Margarita philosophica* was first printed in Heidelberg in 1496, and went through several editions around the turn of the century. As Gilbert Heß explains, the first complete edition was printed in Freiburg im Breisgau in 1503. See Gilbert Heß, "Reisch, Gregor," *Neue Deutsche Biographie* 21 (2003), 384–86. I cite here from the 1503 edition:

Margarita philosophica, totius philosophiae rationalis, naturalis, et moralis principia (Freiburg im Breisgau: Schott, 1503).

50. F. J. Burkhard, "Ein handschriftlicher Kommentar Gabriel Biels zum Traktat *De anima* des Pierre von Ailly," in *Alte Fragen und neue Wege des Denkens: Festschrift für Josef Stallmach*, ed. Norbert Fischer (Bonn: Bouvier, 1977), 82–91. The manuscript was actually a commentary upon a commentary written by the French theologian Pierre d'Ailly (1351–1420).

51. Ibid., 87.

52. Ibid., 86.

53. *Anthropologium*, fol. 114v.

54. *Margarita philosophica*, fol. 282v.

55. Ibid., fol. 262v.

56. Ibid., fol. 271v.

57. Heymerich van den Velde, *Problemata inter Albertum et Sanctum Thomam* (Cologne: Johann Landen, 1496), fol. h7r.

58. Ibid., fol. h6v.

59. Gerhard von Herrenberg, *Expositiones textuales dubiorum* (Cologne: Quentell, 1497), fols. A1r–D4v and e3v–g1r. The commentaries of von Mechlin and Harderwijck are both collected in *Textus trium librorum de anima Aristotelis cum commentario secundum doctrinam venerabilis domini Alberti Magni* (Cologne: Koelhoff, 1491). See especially f2v–f3r, which closely parallels the points made by van den Velde, above.

60. Olaf Pluta, "Materialism in the Philosophy of Mind: Nicholas of Amsterdam's *Quaestiones* de Anima," in *Mind, Cognition, and Representation: The Tradition of Commentaries on Aristotle's De anima*, ed. Paul Baker (Burlington, Vt.: Ashgate, 2007), 109–26; Olaf Pluta, "On the Matter of the Mind: Late Medieval Views on Mind, Body, and Imagination," in *Imagination in the Later Middle Ages and Early Modern Times*, ed. Lodi Nauta (Leuven: Peeters, 2004), 21–34; Olaf Pluta, "How Matter Becomes Mind: Late-Medieval Theories of Emergence," in *Forming the Mind: Essays on the Internal Senses and the Mind/Body Problem from Avicenna to the Medical Enlightenment*, ed. Henrik Lagerlund (Dordrecht: Springer, 2007), 149–67.

61. Magnus Hundt, *Introductionum in universalem Aristotelis physicen* (Leipzig: Stöckel, 1500), fol. 115v; Magnus Hundt, *Anthropologium*. In Leipzig, Hundt's colleagues Johannes Peilicke and Johannes Lintholtz von Müncheberg developed similar positions in their natural philosophical work. See Peilicke, *Philosophie naturalis Compendium* (Leipzig: Lotter, 1499). Lintholz von Müncheberg, *Textus trium librorum de anima* (Frankfurt an der Oder: Baumgarten, 1507). For Erfurt, see Bartholomäus Arnoldi von Usingen's *Exercitium de anima* (Erfurt, 1507), especially fols. B3v–E1r.

62. Scribner, *Religion and Culture*, 85–145.

63. Pekka Kärkkäinen, "Synderesis in Late Medieval Philosophy and the Wittenberg Reformers," *British Journal for the History of Philosophy* 20, no. 5 (2012): 881–901.

64. *Anthropologium*, fols. 15r, 115v, qtd. at 15r.

65. Ibid., fol. 15r.

66. Quoted in Michael Baylor, *Action and Person: Conscience in Late Scholasticism and the Young Luther* (Leiden: Brill, 1977), 99.

67. Peilicke, *Compendium*, fol. J6r.

68. Ibid, fols. O1v–O2r.

69. Compare with Prasad Theruvathu, *Ineffabilis in the Thought of Nicolas of Cusa* (Münster: Aschendorff Verlag, 2010).

70. Barbara Pitkin, "The Reformation of Preaching: Transformations of Worship Soundscapes in Early Modern Germany and Switzerland," *Yale Journal of Music and Religion* 1, no. 2 (2015): 5–20.

71. Hans-Jochen Schiewer, "German Sermons in the Middle Ages," in *The Sermon*, ed. Beverly Mayne Kienzle (Turnhout: Brepols, 2000), 861–961, at 886–89.

72. Schiewer, "German Sermons," 888.

73. Ibid., 888.

74. Maarten Hoenen, "Denys the Carthusian and Heymeric de Campo on the Pilgrimages of Children to Mont-Saint-Michel (1458)," *Archives d'histoire doctrinale et littéraire du moyen âge* 61 (1994), 387–418; Maarten Hoenen, "Academics and Intellectual Life in the Low Countries: The University Career of Heymeric de Campo," *Recherches de théologie ancienne et medieval* 61 (1994): 173–209; Anna Frederiksson Adman, "Heymericus de Campo, Dyalogus super Revelacionibus beate Birgitte: A Critical Edition with an Introduction" (PhD diss., Uppsala University, 2003).

75. As Nancy Caciola has admirably demonstrated in *Discerning Spirits: Divine and Demonic Possession in the Middle Ages* (Ithaca, N.Y.: Cornell University Press, 2003).

76. Hoenen, "Academics," 202; Hoenen, "Denys"; Adman, "Heymericus," 173–75.

77. Robert Scribner, "Popular Piety and Modes of Visual Perception in Late Medieval and Reformation Germany," *Journal of Religious History* 15 (1989): 448–69; Robert Scribner, "Zur Wahrnehmung des Heiligen in Deutschland am Ende des Mittelalters," in *Das Mittelalter: Unsere fremde Vergangenheit*, ed. Joachim Kuolt (Stuttgart: Helfant, 1990), 241–67.

78. Hans Belting, *Das Bild und sein Publikum im Mittelalter: Form und Funktion früher Bildtafeln der Passion* (Berlin: Gebrüder Mann, 1981); Camille, "Before the Gaze," 197–223.

79. Camille, "Before the Gaze," 210.

80. Biernoff, *Sight and Embodiment*, 143.

81. Qtd. in Adolph Franz, *Die Messe im deutschen Mittelalter: Beiträge zur Geschichte der Liturgie und des religiösen Volksleben* (Freiburg: Herder, 1902), 18.

82. Ibid., 32–33; Anton Mayer, "Die heilbringende Schau in Sitte und Kult," in *Heliige Überlieferung: Ausschnitte aus der Geschichte des Mönchtums und des heiligen Kultes: Festschrift für Ildefons Herwegen* (Münster: Aschendorf, 1938), 234–62; Peter Browe, "Die Elevation in der Messe," *Jahrbuch für Liturgiewissenschaft* 9 (1929), 20–67; Peter Browe, "Die Eucharistie als Zaubermittel im Mittelalter," *Archiv für Kulturgeschichte* 20 (1930): 134–54.

83. Qtd. in Miri Rubin, *Corpus Christi: The Eucharist in Late Medieval Culture* (Cambridge: Cambridge University Press, 1991), 292; See also Charles Zika, "Hosts, Processions, and Pilgrimages: Controlling the Sacred in Fifteenth-Century Germany," *Past and Present* 118 (1988): 25–64, at 32–35.

84. Fridolin, *Schatzbehalter der wahren Reichtümer des Heils* (Nuremberg: Koburger, 1491), fol. x1r. For background on Fridolin's popularity in the central German lands

between Mainz and Nuremberg-Bamberg, see Petra Seegets, *Passionstheologie und Passionsfrömmigkeit im ausgehenden Mittelaltar: Der Nürnberger Franziskaner Stephan Fridolin (gest. 1498) zwischen Kloster und Stadt* (Tübingen: Mohr Siebeck, 1998), 5, 24–44.

85. Willi Massa, *Eucharistiepredigt am Vorabend der Reformation: Eine materialkerygmatische Untersuchung zum Glaubensverständnis von Altarssakrament und Messe am Beginn des 16. Jahrhunderts als Beitrag zur Geschichte der Predigt* (Steyl: Steyler, 1966), 125–28. Temesvar's sermon collections were among the most purchased of the pre-Reformation era.

86. Ibid., 118–19, 122–31.

87. Guido de Monte Rocherii, *Manipulus curatorum* (Augsburg: Christmann Heyny, 1481), fols. 22r–v. Anne Thayer notes that the *Manipulus curatorum* was printed 120 times across Europe in the second half of the fifteenth century. See Thayer, "Learning to Worship in the Later Middle Ages: Enacting Symbolism, Fighting the Devil, and Receiving Grace," *Archiv für Reformationsgeschichte* 94 (2008): 36–65.

88. Franz Reichert, ed., *Die älteste deutsche Gesamtauslegung der Messe (Erstausgabe ca. 1480)* (Münster: Aschendorffsche Verlagsbuchhandlung, 1967), 99–100.

89. In Karl Bihlmeyer, ed., *Heinrich Seuse: Deutsche Schriften* (Stuttgart: Kohlhammer, 1907), 196–325, qtd. at 294, 296, 303.

90. Werner Williams-Krapp, "Frauenmystik und Ordensreform im 15. Jahrhundert," in *Literarische Interessenbildung im Mittelalter: DFG-Symposium 1991*, ed. Joachim Heinze (Stuttgart: Metzler, 1993), 301–13; Werner Williams-Krapp, "Observanzbewegungen, monastiche Spiritualität und geistliche Literatur im 15. Jahrhundert," *Internationales Archiv für Sozialgeschichte der deutschen Literatur* 20 (1995): 1–15.

91. Rubin, *Corpus Christi*, 63–82, 98–147. Zika, "Hosts."

92. Albrecht Dürer, "Die Entwürfe zu dem enzyklopädischen 'Werk Speis der Malerknaben,' in *Albrecht Dürer Schriften, Tagebücher, Briefe*, ed. Max Steck (Stuttgart: Kohlhammer, 1961), 204.

93. Charles Burnett, "Sound and Its Perception in the Middle Ages," in *The Second Sense: Studies in Hearing and Musical Judgment from Antiquity to the Seventeenth Century*, ed. Charles Burnett (London: Warburg Institute, 1991), 43–69.

94. Qtd. in Marjorie O'Rourke Boyle, *Erasmus on Language and Method in Theology* (Toronto: University of Toronto Press, 1977), 35. See also D. R. Woolf, "Hearing Renaissance England," in *Hearing History: A Reader*, ed. Mark M. Smith (Athens: University of Georgia Press, 2004), 112–35.

95. Erasmus, *De ratione studij, ac legendi, interpretandique auctores libellus aureus* (Strasbourg: Knobloch, 1521), fol. A2v.

96. Bruce Holsinger, *Music, Body, and Desire in Medieval Culture: Hildegard of Bingen to Chaucer* (Stanford, Calif.: Stanford University Press, 2002).

97. Burnett, "Sound and Its Perception"; D. P. Walker, "Ficino's *Spiritus* and Music," *Annales musicologues* 1 (1953): 131–50.

98. Qtd. in Walker, "Ficino's *Spiritus* and Music," 134n6.

99. Franz, *Messe*, 21–26.

100. Durandus, *Rationale*, 4:21.

101. Ibid., 4:64–65.

102. *Margarita philosophica*, fol. 97v.

103. Ibid. Compare with Boethius, *De institutione musica libri duo, De institutione musica libri quinque,* ed. Gottfried Friedlein (Leipzig: Teubner, 1867), 179–78.

104. Reisch, *Margarita philosophica*, fol. 97v.

105. Ibid. "Et Marsilius in eundem Concertus inquitur per aeream naturam in motu positam mouet corpus; per purificatum aerem concitat spiritum aereum/ anime corporiscum nodum; per affectum afficit sensum simul et animum; per significationem agit in mentem. Denique per ipsum subtilis aeris motum penetrat vehementer. Per contemporatorem lambit suauiter; per conformem qualitatem mira quadam voluptatem perfundit naturam tam spiritualemque materialem totumque simul rapit et sibi vendicat hominem."

106. Compare with Jacob M. Baum, "From Incense to Idolatry: The Reformation of Olfaction in Late Medieval German Ritual," *Sixteenth Century Journal* 44, no. 2 (2013): 323–44.

107. Aquinas, *Opera omnia,* vol. 12: *Summa theologica pars III quaestiones 60–90* (Rome: Commissio Leonina, 1906), 281.

108. Durandus, *Rationale*, 1:31–36.

109. Hundt, *Introductionum*, fol. 203v. Peilicke, *Compendium,* fol. M3v.

110. Herpff, *Sermones*, fol. s6v.

111. Hundt, *Introductionum*, fol. 226v.

112. Here cited from the 1515 manuscript owned by St. Katherine's Dominican convent in Nuremberg: NSB Cent VII 31. Qtd. here at fols. 64v–65v.

113. NSB Cent VII, 31, fols. 149v–150r.

114. Qtd. in Karl Josef Klinkhammer, *Adolf von Essen und seine Werke: Der Rosenkranz in der geschichtlichen Situtation seiner Entwicklung und in seinem bleibenden Anliegen* (Frankfurt: Knecht, 1972), 177.

115. MSWB HS I 322 (1454), fols. 85r–v, 87v, 89r, 90v–91v.

116. Baum, "Incense," 329–31.

117. Peilicke, *Compendium*, fols. M3v–M4r.

118. Hundt, *Introductionum*, fol. 225r.

119. Peilicke, *Compendium*, fol. M3v–M4r; Hundt, *Introductionum*, fol. 203v.

120. Hundt, *Introductionum*, 227r.

121. Richard Palmer, "In Bad Odour: Smell and Its Significance in Medicine from Antiquity to the Seventeenth Century," in *Medicine and the Five Senses*, ed. Roy Porter (Cambridge: Cambridge University Press, 1993), 61–68; In the German context, Renate Smollich, *Der Bisamapfel in Kunst und Wissenschaft* (Stuttgart: Deutscher Apotheker Verlag, 1983), identifies this phenomenon emerging in medical discourse more broadly in the fourteenth and fifteenth centuries. Dugan, *Ephemeral History*, 97–125, suggests early modern continuities with the medieval period in England.

122. Steinhöwel, *Büchlein der Ordnung der Pestilenz* (Ulm: Johann Zainer, 1473), fol. 4r.

123. *Anthropologium*, fol. 114v: "Differt spritus a vapore quo est corpus terrestre a calido sursum violenter eleuatum . . . Spiritum confortant cordalia de quibus Avicenna in de viribus cordis, vt sunt ambra, aurum, muscus, basilicon, camphora etc pille ex auro thure et mirrha. Nutrit etiam aere inspirato et confortatur odoribus aromaticis vt odore mente[mint] vini mellis pomorum, pirorum, calidi panis etc, vt latius scribit

Marsilius ficinus vir nostra etate clarus de vita longa dicentes. Quicumque vitam in corpore producere cupitis spiritum imprimis excolite hunc augete nutrimentis sanguinem temperantum atque clarum augentibus hunc aere spirito electo fouete quotidie suauibus odoribus alite. Sonis et cantibus oblectate. Et sicut odor est anime suauissimus cibum ita fetor malus et putridus corrumpit spiritum et inficit. Cetera licet vtilia, delectabilia, et honesta."

124. Hundt, *Introductionum*, fol. 226v.

125. Hundt, *Anthropologium*, fols. 113v–114r.

126. Ibid., fol. 114v.

127. Baum, "Incense," 327–28.

128. Hundt, *Introductionum*, fol. 229v.

129. *Compendium*, fol. M5v.

130. This idea was well established in learned culture by the end of the thirteenth century throughout Europe and, as Elizabeth Harvey has shown, endured well into the seventeenth century. See Elizabeth Harvey, "Introduction: The 'Sense of All Senses,'" in *Sensible Flesh: On Touch in Early Modern Culture*, ed. Elizabeth Harvey (Philadelphia: University of Pennsylvania Press, 2003), 1–21.

131. Peilicke, *Compendium*, fol. M3v. The point had been raised already in the thirteenth century by Albert the Great, who provided the Gospel example of Thomas's touching Christ's wounds after not being satisfied with seeing him. See Steneck, "Albert on the Psychology of Sense Perception," 287–90.

132. Hundt, *Introductionum*, fols. 229v–231r; Hundt, *Anthropologium*, fols. 50r, 80r.

133. Peilicke, *Compendium*, fol. M5v.

134. Largier, "Inner Senses"; Rudy, *Mystical Language*; Führer, "Albert the Great and Mystical Epistemology."

135. Largier, "Inner Senses," 14.

136. Ella Johnson, "To Taste (*Sapere*) Wisdom (*Sapientia*): Eucharistic Devotion in the Writings of Gertrude of Helfta," *Viator* 44, no. 2 (2013), 175–200; Ella Johnson, "In mei memoriam facietis': Remembering Ritual and Refiguring 'Woman' in Gertrude the Great of Helfta's *Spiritualia Exercitia*," in *Reading Memory and Identity in the Texts of Medieval European Holy Women*, ed. Bradley Herzog (New York: Palgrave, 2012), 165–96.

137. Johnson, "To Taste," 188–89, 194, 197.

138. *Büchlein der ewigen Weisheit*, in *Seuse: Deutsche Schriften*, 196–325, at 259–62. For the prominence of the language of "Einschlag," in Suso, see Edmund Colledge and J. C. Marlier, "'Mystical' Pictures in the Suso 'Exemplar' MS Strasbourg 2929," *Archivum fratrum praedicatorum* 54 (1984), 293–354.

139. *Büchlein der ewigen Weisheit*, 224–29.

140. Ibid., 294, 303.

141. A manuscript copy of the text from the second half of the fifteenth century can be found in NSB Cent VII, 32, fols. 83r–130r, qtd. here at 90v.

142. Craig Koslofsky, "The Kiss of Peace in the German Reformation," in *The Kiss in History*, ed. Karen Harvey (Manchester: Manchester University Press, 2005), 18–35. Thomas Lentes, "'Andacht' und 'Gebärde': Das religiöse Ausdrucksverhalten," in *Kulturelle Reformation: Sinnformationen im Umbruch, 1400–1600*, ed. Bernhard Jussen and Craig Koslofsky (Göttingen: Vandenhoeck & Ruprecht, 1999), 29–67, provides a fuller

account of how external gestures such as the kiss actually affected internal changes in the soul.

143. Durandus, *Rationale*, vol. 1, 328–29.

144. Ibid., 326.

145. Ibid., 315.

146. Ibid., 337.

147. On the dangerous sensuality of the dinner table, see Newhauser, "Peter of Limoges," 38–39.

148. His handbook, *Unser lieben Frawen Psalter, vonn den dreien rosenkrenntzen, wie man die ordnen vnnd peten sol mitt vil bewerten exempeln eyn vast nutzlichs büchlin*, appeared in several German editions in the late fifteenth and early sixteenth centuries, suggesting that it was fairly popular. Here, we draw on the Augsburg 1502, printed by Lucas Zeissenmair. Qtd. at fol. 4r. For an overview of printed rosary handbooks, see Anne Winston-Allen, *Stories of the Rose: The Making of the Rosary in the Middle Ages* (University Park: Pennsylvania State University Press, 1997). For the manuscript precursors of these printed works, see Klinkhammer, *Adolf von Essen*; Andreas Heinz, "Die Zisterzienser und die Anfänge des Rosenkranzes," *Analecta Cisterciensia* 33 (1977): 262–309. Andreas Heinz, "Eine spätmittelalterliche Exempelsammlung zur Propagierung des Trierer Karthäuser-Rosenkranzes," *Trierer Theologische Zeitschrift* 92 (1983): 306–18.

149. *Unser lieben Frawen Psalter*, fols. 6r, 8r.

150. This collection of tales was produced in a manuscript around the middle of the century in Bernkastel-Kues (about 50 km northeast of Trier). Printed in Heinz, "Exempelsammlung," 309–14.

151. Heinz, "Exempelsammlung," 312.

152. Markus von Weida, *Der Spiegel der hochloblichen Bruderschafft des Rosenkrantz Marie* (Leipzig: n.p., 1515), fol. 217r.

153. Ibid., 6v–9r.

154. *Deutsche Gesamtauslegung*, 99.

155. Ibid., 186.

156. MWSB HS I, 51, fols. 38r, 40v.

157. *Büchlein der ewigen Weisheit*, 303.

158. The prayers are edited and collected in *Johannes von Neumarkt: Bischof und Hofkanzler: Religiöse Frührenaissance in Böhmen zur Zeit Kaiser Karls IV*, ed. Joseph Klapper (Leipzig: St. Benno, 1964), 37–41, 71–74.

159. Fridolin, *Schatzbehalter*, fol. x1r.

160. Franz Posset, "The Sweetness of God," *American Benedictine Review* 44 (1993): 143–78. Franz Posset, "*Christi Dulcedo*: The 'Sweetness of Christ' in Western Christian Thought," *Cistercian Studies Quarterly* 30 (1995): 245–65; Edith Scholl, "The Sweetness of the Lord: *Dulcis* and *Suavis*," *Cistercisan Studies Quarterly* 27 (1992): 359–66.

161. Rachel Fulton, "'Taste and See That the Lord Is Sweet' (Ps. 33: 9): The Flavor of God in the Monastic West," *Journal of Religion* 86 (2006): 169–204; Mary Carruthers, "Sweetness," *Speculum* 81 (2006), 999–1013; Rosemary Drage Hale, "'Taste and See, for God Is Sweet': Sensory Perception and Memory in Medieval Christian Mystical Experience," in *Vox Mystica: Essays on Medieval Mysticism in Honor of Professor Valerie M. Lagorio*,

Valerie Marie Lagorio and Anne Clark Bennet (Cambridge: Cambridge University Press, 1995), 3–14; Ella Johnson, "To Taste"; Ella Johnson, "In mei memoriam facietis."

162. Carruthers, "Sweetness," 999.

163. Ann Astell, *Eating Beauty: The Eucharist and the Spiritual Arts of the Middle Ages* (Ithaca, N.Y.: Cornell University Press, 2006), especially her discussion of late medieval aesthetics at 1–4.

164. *Büchlein der ewigen Weisheit*, 303.

165. See the prayers of Johannes von Neumarkt in *Johannes von Neumarkt*, 140.

166. Otto von Passau, *Die vierundzwanzig Alten oder der goldene Thron* (Augsburg: Anton Sorg, 1480), fol. 62v.

167. Pseudo-Johannes von Kastl, *Ein nücz und schone ler von der aygen erkantnuß*, ed. Renata Wagner (Munich: Beck, 1972), 111: "man erkennet auch got in der begerung und in enpfindlicher sußikeit als vil slecht ainfeltig geistlich person, die der schrift nicht wissen und doch got erkennen in der lieb und im fleißicleich dinen, in gleicher weiße als unterscheid ist erkennen die sußikeit des honigs allein in dem gehör und in den worten und die selben sußikeit erkennen in dem versuchen und in der pekerung dest kostens."

168. Herpf, *Sermones*, fol. s6v.

169. Charles Burnett, "The Superiority of Taste," *Journal of the Warburg and Courtauld Institutes* 54 (1991): 230–38, qtd. at 230.

170. Hundt, *Introductionum*, fol 228v; Hundt, *Anthropologium*, 66v–67r. Peilicke, *Compendium*, fols. M3v–M4v.

171. Qtd. in Kenneth Albala, *Eating Right in the Renaissance* (Berkeley: University of California Press, 2002), 173.

172. *Anthropologium*, fol. 80v.

173. *Introductionum*, fol. 228v; Peilicke, *Compendium*, fols. M4v–M5r. For medieval Europe more broadly, see Fulton, "Taste and See."

174. Ortolf von Baierland, *Arzneibuch* (Nuremberg: Anton Koburger, 1477), fols. 17r, 23r, 26v–28r, 49v.

175. *Küchenmeisterei* (Augsburg: Johann Schaur, 1494), fol. D4r. The *Küchenmeisterei* was the most popular and frequently printed cookbook in late fifteenth century Germany. See Melitta Weiss Adamson, *Food in Medieval Times* (Westport, Conn.: Greenwood, 2004), xiv.

176. *Versehung eines Menschen Leib, Seel, Her und Gut* (Nuremberg: Wagner, 1489), fols. 5r, 57v–58r, 73v.

177. *Arzneibuch*, fol. 49v.

178. Paul Rozin, "Why We Eat What We Eat, and Why We Worry about It," *Bulletin of the American Academy of Arts and Sciences* 50, no. 5 (1997): 26–48; Jacob Steiner, "The Gustofacial Response: Observation on Normal and Anencephalic Newborn Infants," in *Fourth Symposium on Oral Sensation and Perception*, ed. J. Bosma (Bethesda, Md.: U.S. Department of Health, Education and Welfare, 1973), 254–78; Jacob Steiner, Judith Ganchrow, and Munif Daher, "Neonatal Facial Expression in Response to Different Qualities and Intensities of Gustatory Stimuli," *Infant Behavior and Development* 6 (1983): 189–200; Kent C. Berridge, "Measuring Hedonic Impact in Animals and Infants: Microstructure of Affective Reactivity Patterns," *Neuroscience and Biobehavioral Reviews* 24 (2000): 173–98.

179. Fulton, "Taste and See," 185–86, 201–2.

180. Massa, *Eucharistiepredigt*, 38, 118–31.

181. Von Paltz, *Coelifoedina* (Erfurt: Schenck, 1502), fol. M3r.

182. Bynum, *Christian Materiality*; Berndt Hamm, "Die Medialität der nahen Gnade im späten Mittelalter," in *Medialität des Heils im späten Mittelalter*, ed. Carla Dauven-van Knippenberg (Zurich: Chronos, 2009), 21–59; Berndt Hamm, "Typen spätmittelalterlichr Gnadenmedialität," in *Media salutis: Gnaden- und Heilsmedien in der abendländischen Religiosität des Mittelalters und der Frühen Neuzeit*, ed. Bernd Hamm (Tübingen: Mohr Siebeck, 2011), 43–83.

Chapter 3. The Senses and Religious Experience in Vernacular Theology

1. Tucher's diary is preserved in NSB Cent VI, 57, fols. 263r–292v. It has been edited and published by Ulla Williams and Werner Williams-Krapp as *Die "Offenbarungen" der Katharina Tucher* (Tübingen: Max Niemeyer, 1998). Qtd. here at 67.

2. For the most comprehensive overview of this history, see Gordon Rudy, *Mystical Language of Sensation in the Later Middle Ages* (New York: Routledge, 2002). See also Bernard McGinn, "The Changing Shape of Late Medieval Mysticism," *Church History* 65, no. 2 (1996): 197–219; Bernard McGinn, "The Language of Inner Experience in Christian Mysticism," *Spiritus: A Journal of Christian Spirituality* 1, no. 2 (2001): 156–71; Bernard McGinn, *The Harvest of Mysticism in Medieval Germany (1300–1500)* (New York: Crossroad, 2005), esp. 361–65. The editors of Tucher's diary, in their introduction to the text, make this point as well. See Ulla Williams and Werner Williams-Krapp, "Einleitung," in *Offenbarungen*, 1–27.

3. McGinn specifically dismisses this dimension of the diary as unimportant. See McGinn, *Harvest*, 361–65.

4. Vernacular theology been a crucial concept in late medieval and early modern English studies, taken up most often by scholars of literature. More recently, scholars of Italy have begun to deal with vernacular theology. See Nicholas Watson, "Censorship and Cultural Change in Late-Medieval England: Vernacular Theology, the Oxford Debate, and Arundel's Constitutions of 1409," *Speculum* 70, no. 4 (1995): 822–64; Eliana Corbari, "Lost and Found in Translation: The Heart of Vernacular Theology in Late Medieval Italy," *Franciscan Studies* 71 (2013): 263–79; Eliana Corbari, *Vernacular Theology: Dominican Sermons and Audience in Late Medieval Italy* (Berlin: de Gruyter, 2013).

5. Virginia Reinburg, *French Books of Hours: Making an Archive of Prayer, c. 1400–1600* (Cambridge: Cambridge University Press, 2012).

6. Alain Corbin emphasized the importance of ego-documents and other times of subjective accounts in the project of writing a complete history of the senses. See Corbin, *Time, Desire and Horror: Towards a History of the Senses*, trans. Jean Birrell (Oxford: Polity, 1995), 181–95.

7. John Van Engen, "Multiple Options: The World of the Fifteenth-Century Church," *Church History* 77, no. 2 (2008): 257–84; Caroline Walker Bynum, *Wonderful Blood: Theology and Practice in Late Medieval Northern Germany and Beyond* (Philadelphia: University of Pennsylavania Press, 2007); McGinn, surveying much of the specialist scholarship, attributes the problem to the sheer number of manuscripts produced in the

fifteenth century, and the difficulties of comprehensively mastering the source materials. See McGinn, *Harvest*, ix–x.

8. Catherine Bell, *Ritual Theory, Ritual Practice* (Oxford: Oxford University Press, 2009), 170.

9. Williams and Williams-Krapp, "Einleitung," 1–27; Anneke B. Mulder-Bakker, "The Age of Discretion: Women at Forty and Beyond," in *Middle-Aged Women in the Middle Ages*, ed. Sue Niebrydowski (Rochester, N.Y.: Brewer, 2011), 15–24; Deborah Rose-Lefmann, "'As It Is Painted': Reflections of Image-Based Devotional Practices in the 'Confessions' of Katharina Tucher," *Studia Mystica* 2 (1996): 185–204.

10. Williams and Williams-Krapp, "Einleitung," 13–14, 21–22.

11. Almost all of them remained in the convent library's collection and are now housed in the city library of Nuremberg. See Williams and Williams-Krapp, "Einleitung," 23–26, for the complete bibliography.

12. McGinn, *Harvest*, 362.

13. *Offenbarungen*, 70.

14. Ibid., 33.

15. Ibid., 46.

16. Ibid., 33.

17. Ibid., 70.

18. McGinn, *Harvest*, 362. Entry 8, McGinn notes, is exemplary in this regard.

19. *Offenbarungen*, 34–35, 43–44.

20. Ibid., 64.

21. McGinn, *Harvest*, 360–62.

22. Catherine of Siena's hagiography was preserved in NSB Cent IV, 14, fols. 205r–308r, although it is no longer extant. For Katharina's collection of lyrics and poetry, see NSB, Cent VI, 43d, fols. 80v–100v; NSB, Cent VI, 59, fols. 9r–41r; Berlin Staatsbibliothek, PKB, mgo. 137, fols. 151v–160r. Tucher's copy of Suso's *Little Book* is in NSB, Cent VI, 81, fols. 1r–248r.

23. They survive in the Nuremberg city library. See NSB Cent VI 430, 91, Will II, 19.8°.

24. NSB Cent VI, 91, fols. 117r–118v.

25. The prayers appear in NSB Will 19.8°, fols. 142v–143v.

26. Rudy, *Mystical Language*, 14.

27. This has been the position of Rudy, *Mystical Language*. McGinn specifically applies this interpretation to Tucher's diary in *Harvest*, 361–65, rejecting the notion that the practical dimensions of Eucharist piety were of significant concern. For this interpretation of female autobiography more broadly, see also Karen Greenspan, "Autohagiography and Medieval Womens' Spiritual Autobiography," in *Gender and Text in the Later Middle Ages*, ed. Jane Chance (Gainesville: University of Florida Press, 1996), 216–36.

28. Markus Führer, "Albert the Great and Mystical Epistemology," in *A Companion to Albert the Great: Theology, Philosophy, and the Sciences*, ed. Irven Resnick (Leiden: Brill, 2013), 137–61; Rachel Fulton, "'Taste and See That the Lord Is Sweet' (Ps. 33:9): The Flavor of God in the Monastic West," *Journal of Religion* 86 (2006): 169–204; Drage Hale, "'Taste and See, for God Is Sweet,'" 3–14; Niklaus Largier, "Inner Senses—Outer Senses: The Practice of Emotions in Medieval Mysticism," in *Codierungen von Emotionen im*

Mittelalter/Emotions and Sensibilities in the Middle Ages, ed. C. Stephen Jaeger (Berlin: de Gruyter, 2003), 3–15; Barbara Newman, "What Did It Mean to Say 'I Saw'"? The Clash between Theory and Practice in Medieval Visionary Culture," *Speculum* 80, no. 1 (2005): 1–43.

29. *Offenbarungen*, 64–65: on St. John's Day, 1420 (December 27), she was in church when Christ admonished her to stop drinking wine. Later that day, or sometime on the following day, Tucher reported kneeling in the Chapel of Our Lady, and hearing Mary forbid her from taking any other husband besides Christ. In total, fourteen entries for the particular feast day: Pentecost (1418), Corpus Christi (May 26, 1418), St. Lorenz Day (August 10, 1418), St. Sebald's Day (August 19, 1418), New Year's Day (1419), Good Friday (April 14, 1419), New Year's Day (1420), St. Andreas' Day (November 29, 1420), Christmas Eve (1420), St. John's Day (December 27, 1420), Feast of the Holy Innocents (December 28, 1420), New Year's Eve (1420), New Year's Day (1421), Feast of the Epiphany (Friday before January 4 and Sunday after January 13, 1421).

30. She also reported receiving the sacrament on New Year's Day, 1421. See *Offenbarungen* 39, 66, 83, qtd. at 39.

31. Ibid.

32. Ibid., 36.

33. Ibid., 42.

34. Mulder-Bakker, "Age of Discretion," 15.

35. Compare with Franz Xaver Haimerl, *Die mittelalterliche Frömmigkeit im Spiegel der Gebetbuchliteratur Süddeutschlands* (Munich: Zink, 1952), 1–38.

36. MSWB, HS II 230, (ca. 1500), fol. 24r.

37. Köln Erzbischöfliche Diözesan- und Dombibliothek (Hereafter KEDD), Cod. 1503, fol. 25r.

38. NSB Cent V, App 81, fol. 92v.

39. BSB, cgm. 4483, fol. 112r.

40. Ibid., fol. 111r.

41. Compare with Peter Saenger, "Books of Hours and the Reading Habits of the Later Middle Ages," in *The Culture of Print: Power and the Uses of Print in Early Modern Europe*, trans. Lydia Cochrane, ed. Roger Chartier (Cambridge: Polity, 1989), 141–73.

42. "Das Gebetbuch der Caritas Pirckheimer," in *Caritas Pirckheimer—Quellensammlung*, ed. Josef Pfanner (Landshut: Solanus-Druck, 1961), 24.

43. Frankfurt am Main Universitätsbibliothek (Hereafter FMU) Ms. Praed. 184, fol. 48v–49r.

44. Ibid., fols. 29v–30r: "O hemelsches broit du bist erne spyse der engel komm mych vnd mache ryne daz hertzs van allen flecken der sunden, O suysses hemelbroit mach mich gesont van allen smertzen der sunden, vff daz myne Hertzs keyns syssicheit entfynde . . . O licht schynendes broit du daz in dir haist alle woillusticheit vnd alle gesmack der suyssicheit. Du der vns alla zyt byst spysen vnd in dir nummer gebrechen Myne hertze muysse dich also essen dar myne sele myt suyssicheit dynes gesmackes werde erfolt."

45. Heidelberg Universitätsbiliothek (Hereafter HU) Cpg. 645, fols. 34v–35r: "O susser her ihu crist myn vnandechtiges kaltes hertz begeret dir hut vereyniget werden, darvmb

entzunde es mit dem feuer dyner lieb, Erlucht myn blindigkheit mit dyner waren gegenwertigkeit, der du bist der schon glantz veterlicher clarheit kere mir alle weltliche sussigkeyt Inn bitterkeyt, alle widderwertigkeyt in gedult . . . du myn trost dy myn lieb dy myn sussigkeyt vnd alles das gut, daz mir bestehen mag; mach mich die allein susß . . . in nÿssung diesßer himellischen spise verwandell mich also in dich." For biographical notes on Hanns, see Haimerl, *Mittelalterliche Frömmigkeit*, 114–15.

46. Rostock Universitätsbibliothek (Hereafter RU) Mss.theol.14, fols. 105v–106r.

47. Ibid., fols. 130v–131v.

48. Ibid., fols. 106r–v, 155v–156r. The floral and garden symbolism here clearly drew upon courtly literature of the fourteenth and fifteenth centuries, which was also deeply influential in contemporaneous Marian devotions. See Jeffrey Hamburger, *Nuns as Artists: The Visual Culture of a Medieval Convent* (Berkeley: University of California Press, 1997), 63–100.

49. NSB Cent VII 24, fol. 251r.

50. Ibid, fols. 141r–142r: "du bist süß am smacke lüstig in der enpfindligkeit, ein süsser auffhalter vnser trawrigkeit behüt vns besuch vns vernew vns mit ynniger andacht vnd lieb vnd beschirm vns vor aller schedlichen widerwertigkeÿt leibs vnd der sele, o xpe schönes lemlen du prun vnd lebe aller tugent der werlt . . . sihe vns an parmhertzigkliche vnd setige vns mit deinem heiligen leichnam krefftigklich vnd in deinem heiligen heÿlsamen hochedeln rosen farben blute trenck vns wasch vns von allen sünden vnd vnraynigkeit."

51. *Caritas Pirckheimer*, 49.

52. MSWB, HS I 427, fols 33r–v. For similar language from other women's prayer books from this region, see MSWB HS I 418, Hs I 422.

53. Compare with Susan Karant-Nunn, *Reformation of Feeling: Shaping the Religious Emotions in Early Modern Germany* (Oxford: Oxford University Press, 2010), for the notion of emotional scripts. Matthew Milner, "The Senses in Religion: Towards the Reformation of the Senses," in *A Cultural History of the Senses in the Renaissance*, ed. Hermann Roodenburg (New York: Bloomsbury, 2014), 87–106, suggests the portability of this concept into sensory history.

54. On the early monastic history of prayer books in the German-speaking world, see Jeffrey Hamburger, "A Liber Precum in Sélestat and the Development of the Illustrated Prayer Book in Germany," *Art Bulletin* 73, no. 2 (1991): 209–36. Gerard Achten, *Das christliche Gebetbuch im Mittelalter: Andachts- und Stundenbücher in Handschrift und Frühdruck* (Berlin: Preussischer Kulturbesitz, 1987).

55. Haimerl, *Mitteralterliche Frömmigkeit.* Other prayer books are identifiable with a particular religious community, such as the Dominican men of Frankfurt, or the Dominican women of Freiburg im Breisgauu. See FMU, MS. Praed. 185, fol. 8r (dated 1504). Freiburg im Breisgau Universitätsbibliothek (Hereafter FBU) HS 214 (dated 1479).

56. Collective biography, or 'prosopography,' has been a well-established methodology among social historians since the 1960s. It can be an especially useful tool in premodern contexts, when individual biographical information is often only partially available. For the classical articulation of prosopography as a critical tool of early modern social history, see Lawrence Stone, "Prosopography," *Daedalus* 100, no. 1 (1971): 46–79.

57. Corbari has demonstrated the profound influence of the Dominicans and Franciscans on urban piety in Italy. See Corbari, *Vernacular Theology*. In Germany, the evidence suggests the Dominicans played a similar leading role. Especially in Nuremberg and Strasbourg, the male and female houses proved effective in cultivating vernacular religious knowledge. See Barbara Steinke, *Paradiesgarten oder Gefängnis? Das Nürnberger Katherinenkloster zwischen Klosterreform und Reformation* (Tübingen: Mohr Siebeck, 2006).

58. NSB Cent IV 36 (Kochin), NSB Cent VI, 43n (Hoschlin).

59. NSB Cent VII 8.

60. MSWB Hs I 221.

61. NSB Cent VII 85.

62. GNM Hs 1737. The manuscript remained in the family into the nineteenth century, as indicated by the final entries by the books final named owner, Christoph von Schwarzenberg. See fols. 131v–134v.

63. Most notably, Caroline Walker Bynum developed this argument in *Holy Feast and Holy Fast: The Religious Significance of Food to Medieval Women* (Berkeley: University of California Press, 1987).

64. Interestingly, this shift occurred as the numbers of new female saints drastically declined. In the thirteenth and fourteenth centuries, the biographical and autobiographical narratives of these women's lives had been a central devotional focus for many. In the fifteenth century, however, Magdalena of Freiburg (ca. 1407–1485) was the only prominent new figure about whom a biography was written and circulated. See Greenspan, "Autohagiography."

65. Freiburg im Breisgau Erzbischöflisches Archiv (hereafter FBeA) Hs. 11, Hs. 13.

66. Steinke, *Paradiesgarten*, 54–58.

67. BSB, cgm. 9110. Images of the *Mass of St. Gregory* from this prayer book are available through the online *Gregorsmesse* database, curated by the University of Münster, http://gregorsmesse.uni-muenster.de.

68. FBU, Hs. 79. At folio 100r, Haffner dated the manuscript and indicated that he was its new owner.

69. FBeA Hs. 11, fols. 15v, 22v.

70. BSB, cgm 255. For descriptions of the Nuremberg manuscripts, see Haimerl, *Mittelalterliche Frömmigkeit*, 152–60.

71. Herzogin Anna Amalia Bibliothek (hereafter HAAB) Q 59. The chronicle appears on fols. 1r–v.

72. FMU, Ms. germ. oct. 3. Humbracht's prayer book includes exceptional miniatures of the *Mass of St. Gregory* (fol. 21r) and a Mary being pierced by seven swords (fol. 41r).

73. RU, Mss. Theol. 14.

74. BSB, cgm. 4483. The manuscript is dated to 1457. Käbitz identifies himself as "filius granatoris" in another manuscript (BSB, cgm. 811, fol. 20v.)

75. HU, Cpg. 640. As did his fellow Augsburger Leonhart Schielin, an artist. See F. H. Hofbibliothek Sigmaringen, Ms 52.

76. KeDD, Cod. 1503.

77. HU, Cpg. 645.

78. See for example the manuscripts of Elisa Bontin in Oberschaffshausen (1504), a housewife in Freiburg (1507–1518), and the wife of Heinrich Linck in Swabia (1496/97): FBU, Hs. 213, Hs. 477; Tübingen Universitätsbibliothek, Md 123. For the significance of housewives in fifteenth and sixteenth century urban culture, See Lyndal Roper, *The Holy Household: Women and Morals in Reformation Augsburg* (Oxford: Clarendon, 1989), 27–54.

79. Karin Schneider, "Die Bibliothek des Katharinenklosters in Nürnberg und die städtische Gesellschaft," in *Studien zum städtischen Bildungswesen des späten Mittelalters und der frühen Neuzeit*, ed. Bernd Moeller (Göttingen: Vandenhoeck & Ruprecht, 1983), 70–82; Werner Williams-Krapp, "Observanzbewegungen, monastische Spiritualität und geistliche Literatur im 15. Jahrhundert," *Internationales Archiv für Sozialgeschichte der deutschen Literatur* 20 (1995): 1–15; Steinke, *Paradiesgarten*, 6–9.

80. Schneider, "Bibliothek," 70–82. The library of St. Katherine's by the end of the century constituted the largest single collection of German-language manuscripts in all of Europe.

81. Werner Williams-Krapp, "Observanzbewegungen," 6; Max Burckhardt, "Bibliotheksaufbau, Bücherbesitz und Leserschaft im spätmittelalterlichen Basel," in *Bildgungswesen des späten Mittelalters und der frühen Neuzeit,* 33–52; Klaus Schreiner, "Bücher, Bibliotheken und 'gemeiner Nutzen' im Spätmittelalter und in der Frühneuzeit: Geistes und sozialgeschichtliche Beiträge zur Frage nach der 'utilitas librorum,'" *Bibliothek und Wissenschaft* 9 (1975): 202–49; Klaus Schreiner, "Laienbildung als Herausforderung für Kirche und Gesellschaft: Religiöse Vorbehalte und soziale Widerstände gegen die Verbreitung von Wissen im späten Mittelalter und in der Reformation," *Zeitschrift für historische Forschung* 11 (1984): 207–354.

82. For examples from northern German towns, see Bremen Staats- und Universitätsbibliothek, Msc. 0025 (ca. 1450–1500); Münster Diözesan-Bibliothek (hereafter MDB), Hs. G12 145 (ca. 1500–1550); Staatsarchiv Münster (hereafter StaM), Msc. AV (Dep.) 8. For the 1466 prayer book of Loren Orreum, of Prague, see HAAB, Oct. 76.

83. Werner Williams-Krapp, "Frauenmystik und Ordensreform im 15. Jahrhundert," in *Literarische Interessenbildung im Mittelalter: DFG-Symposium 1991*, ed. Joachim Heinze (Stuttgart: Metzler, 1993), 301–13.

84. Hamburger, *The Visual and the Visionary: Art and Female Spirituality in Late Medieval Germany* (New York: Zone, 1998), 460–61; Bynum, *Holy Feast and Holy Fast*, 55–56, 64–65, 161–80, 270, 276; Bynum, *Wonderful Blood*, 6, 14–15, 164.

85. Jeffrey Hamburger, "Medieval Self-Fashioning: Authorship, Authority, and Autobiography in Seuse's *Exemplar*," in *Christ among the Medieval Dominicans: Representations of Christ in the Texts and Images of the Order of Preachers*, ed. Kent Emery (Notre Dame, Ind.: Notre Dame University Press, 1998), 430–61; Hans-Jochen Schiewer, "Auditionen und Visionen einer Beginne: Die 'Selige Scherern,' Johannes Müllberg und der Baseler Beginenstreit: Mit einem Textabdruck," in *Die Vermittlung geistlicher Inhalte im deutschen Mittelalter: Internationales Symposium, Roscrea 1994*, ed. Timothy Jackson (Tübingen: Mohr Siebeck, 1996), 289–317. Judith Theben, *Die mystische Lyrik des 14. Und 15. Jahrhunderts: Untersuchungen-Texte-Repertorium* (Berlin: de Gruyter, 2010).

86. Reinburg, *Books of Hours*, 6.

87. Ibid., 23.
88. Ibid., 2.
89. HU, Cpg. 645, fols. 193r–194r.
90. HU, Cpg. 640, fol. 75r.
91. Ibid., fols. 75r–85v. The date 1494 is indicated at 85v.
92. Reinburg, *Books of Hours*, 5.
93. HAAB, Oct. 76, fols. 30r, 32r.
94. Bynum, *Wonderful Blood*, 6, 14–15. See also Hamburger, *Visual*, 460–61.
95. StaM, Msc. AV (Dep.) 8, fols. 280r–338v. Quoted at 308v.
96. BSB, cgm. 4483, fol. 109v.
97. Ibid., fols. 109v–110r.
98. HU, Cpg. 640, fol. 72r.
99. Ibid., fols. 71v–75r.
100. FBU, Hs. 213, fol. 162v. The manuscript dates to 1504.
101. Caciola, *Discerning Spirits*, 274–314.
102. Qtd. in Steinke, *Paradiesgarten*, 33.
103. Hamburger, *Visual*, 386–417.
104. Carl Nordenfalk, "The Five Senses in Late Medieval and Renaissance Art," *Journal of the Warburg and Courtauld Institutes* 48 (1985): 1–22.
105. Carina Johnson, "Idolatrous Cultures and the Practice of Religion," *Journal of the History of Ideas* 67, no. 4 (2006): 597–621; Carina Johnson, *Cultural Hierarchy in Early Modern Europe: The Ottomans and Mexicans* (Cambridge: Cambridge University Press, 2011).
106. Cusanus, *De pace fidei*, trans. Jasper Hopkins (Minneapolis: Banning, 1994), 669.
107. Ibid., 666–69.
108. Johnson, "Idolatrous Cultures," 605–6.
109. For an overview of Erasmus's views on this point, see Niall Atkinson, "The Social Life of the Senses: Architecture, Food, and Manners," in *Cultural History of the Senses*, 19–41.
110. Compare with Mark Smith, "Producing Sense, Consuming Sense, Making Sense: Perils and Prospects for Sensory History," *Journal of Social History* 40, no. 4 (2007): 841–58; Mark Smith, *Sensing the Past: Seeing, Hearing, Smelling, Tasting, and Touching in History* (Berkeley: University of California Press, 2007), 4–5, 118–25. For a complementary, anthropological, perspective on sensory production and consumption, see David Howes, "Can These Dry Bones Live? An Anthropological Approach to the History of the Senses," *Journal of American History* 95, no. 2 (2008): 442–51.
111. Qtd. from Milner, "Senses in Religion," 92.
112. Charles Zika, "Hosts, Processions and Pilgrimages: Controlling the Sacred in Fifteenth-Century Germany," *Past and Present* 118 (1988): 25–64. See also Robert Scribner, "Popular Piety and Modes of Visual Perception in Late-Medieval and Reformation Germany," *Journal of Religious History* 15, no. 4 (1989): 448–69.
113. David Howes, *Sensual Relations: Engaging the Senses in Culture and Social Theory* (Ann Arbor: University of Michigan Press, 2003), 20–21, 48–57.
114. See chapter 2.

115. Smith, "Producing Sense," 841–58; Smith, *Sensing the Past*, 4–5, 118–25.

116. See especially Robert Scribner's late work, especially *Religion and Culture in Germany, 1400–1800* (Leiden: Brill, 2000), 85–145.

117. For an overview of these issues in the historiography of the German Reformation, see Susan Karant-Nunn, "Changing One's Mind: Transformations in Reformation History from a Germanist's Perspective," *Renaissance Quarterly* 58, no. 4 (2005): 1101–27.

118. Geertz, *The Interpretation of Cultures* (New York: Basic, 1972), 412–53.

Chapter 4. The Reformation of the Senses in Early Evangelical Culture

1. For an overview of this position for early modern Europe in general, see the contributions in Herman Roodenburg, ed., *A Cultural History of the Senses in the Renaissance* (New York: Bloomsbury, 2014). The most comprehensive statement of the continuity hypothesis as it relates to religion specifically, albeit in the English context, can be found in Matthew Milner, *The English Reformation and the Senses* (Burlington, Vt.: Ashgate, 2011).

2. Reychart, *Ein christenlich Gesprächsbüchlein von zweien Weibern* (Augsburg: Steiner, 1523), fol. A2r–v. For biographical details on Reychart, see Martin Arnold, *Handwerker als theologische Schriftsteller: Studien zur Flugschriften der frühen Reformation* (Göttingen: Vandenhoeck & Ruprecht, 1990), 304–6.

3. Compare with Duffy, *The Stripping of the Altars: Traditional Religion in England, 1400–1580*, 2nd ed. (New Haven, Conn.: Yale University Press, 2005).

4. Luther, WA 6: 484–574, qtd. at 512.

5. Luther, WA 6: 349–78, qtd. at 355.

6. Franz Posset, "Sensing God with the 'Palate of the Heart' according to Augustine and Other Spiritual Authors," *American Benedictine Review* 49, no. 4 (1998): 356–86, qtd. at 381. For sermons given at Nuremberg during the Advent season of 1516, which condemn outward ceremony, see Staupitz, *Ein nutzbarliches büchlein von der entlichen volziehung ewiger fürsehung* (Nuremberg: Peypus, 1517), especially fols. D2v–D3r.

7. See chapter 3.

8. Franz Posset, "The Sweetness of God," *American Benedictine Review* 44, no. 2 (1993): 143–78, at 155–67.

9. Ibid. See also Steven Ozment, *Mysticism and Dissent: Religious Ideology and Social Protest in the Sixteenth Century* (New Haven, Conn.: Yale University Press, 1973), for the importance of mysticism among thinkers of Staupitz's generation, as well as the first generation of evangelical dissidents.

10. Marcia B. Hall, "Introduction," in *The Sensuous in the Counter-Reformation Church*, ed. Marcia Hall and Tracy Cooper (Cambridge: Cambridge University Press, 2013), 1–20. Carlos M. Eire, *The War against the Idols: The Reformation of Worship from Erasmus to Calvin* (Cambridge: Cambridge University Press, 1986), 28–53.

11. Posset, "Sweetness," 155–67. Staupitz preached in the Augustinian church in Tübingen starting in 1498 and during the first few years of the sixteenth century. He preached in Salzburg in 1512, in Nuremberg during Advent in 1516, at Advent in the following year at Munich, and then in Salzburg from 1520 to his death in 1524.

12. Ibid.

13. Harold J. Grimm, "The Role of Nuremberg in the Spread of the Reformation," in *Continuity and Discontinuity in Church History: Essays Presented to George Huntston Williams*, ed. Forrester Church and Timothy Georg (Leiden: Brill, 1979), 182–97; Gerald Strauss, *Nuremberg in the Sixteenth Century: City Politics and Life between Middle Ages and Modern Times* (Bloomington: Indiana University Press, 1976), 160–61.

14. James Kittelson, "Humanism and the Reformation in Germany," *Central European History* 9, no. 4 (1976): 303–22; Paula S. Datsko Barker, "Caritas Pirckheimer: A Female Humanist Confronts the Reformation," *Sixteenth Century Journal* 26, no. 2 (1995): 259–72.

15. Robert Scribner, "Oral Culture and the Diffusion of Reformation Ideas," *History of European Ideas* 5, no. 3 (1984): 237–56.

16. Linck, *Ein heilsame Lere, wie das Herz . . . durch die sieben Seligkeit . . . auff das Wort Gottes gebauet wird* (Nuremberg: n.p., 1519), fol. B2r.

17. Lazarus Spengler, *Schützred und christenliche antwurt ains erbarn liebhabers götlicher warhait der hailigen geschrifft, auf etlicher widersprechen* (Augsburg: Otmar, 1519), fol. B1r.

18. Ibid.

19. Robert Scribner, *For the Sake of the Simple Folk: Popular Propaganda for the German Reformation* (Oxford: Clarendon, 1994), 5.

20. Mark U. Edwards, *Printing, Propaganda, and Martin Luther* (Berkeley: University of California Press, 1994), 17.

21. Bernd Moeller, "Die Rezeption Luthers in der frühen Reformation," in *Reformationstheorien: Ein kirchenhistorischer Disput über Einheit und Vielfalt der Reformation*, ed. Berndt Hamm (Göttingen: Vandenhoeck & Ruprecht, 1995), 9–29; Hans-Jürgen Goertz, "Eine 'bewegte' Epoche: Zur Heterogenität reformatorischer Bewegungen," in *Wegscheiden der Reformation: Alternatives Denken vom 16. bis zum 18. Jahrhundert*, ed. Günter Vogler (Weimar: Böhlau, 1994), 23–56; Susan Karant-Nunn, "What Was Preached in the German Cities in the Early Years of the Reformation? *Wildwuchs* versus Lutheran Unity," in *The Process of Change in Early Modern Europe*, ed. Philipp Bebb (Athens: Ohio University Press, 1988), 81–96; Miriam Usher Chrisman, *Conflicting Visions of Reform: German Lay Propaganda Pamphlets, 1519–1530* (Atlantic Highlands, N.J.: Humanities, 1996); Paul Russell, *Lay Theology in the Reformation: Popular Pamphleteers in Southwest Germany, 1521–1525* (Cambridge: Cambridge University Press, 1986).

22. "Die wittembergisch Nachtigall, die man jetz höret überall," in *Hans Sachs: Werke in zwei Bänden*, vol. 1: *Gedichte*, ed. Karl Martin Schiller (Berlin: Aufbau, 1966), 123–39 qtd. at 9–10: "Tage vnd Nacht in Kirchen pleren . . . mit Wachen, Fasten, langen Bet/ mit Gertenhauen, Kreuzweisliegen,/ mit Knien, Neigen, Bücken, Biegen,/ mit Glockenlauten, Orgelschlagen . . . mit Heiltum, Kerzen, Fanen tragen . . . mit Räuchern und mit Glockentaufen,/ mit Lampenschüren, Gnadverkaufen,/ mit Kirchen-, Wachs-, Salz-, Wasserweihen; / und desgleichen auch die Laien: / mit Opfern und den Lichtleinbrennen,/ mit Wallfahrt und den Heilig denen,/ den Abend fasten, den Tag feiren/ und beicht nach der alten Leiren,/ mit Bruderschaft und Rosenkränzen,/ mit Ablaßlesen, Kirchenschwenzen,/ mit Pacemküssen, Heiltumschauen, mit großem Kost die Altar zieren,/ Tafel auf die welschen Monieren,/ sammate Meßgewand, Kellich gülden,/ mit Monstranzen und silbren Bilden,/ in Klöster schaffen Rent und Zinst-/ dies alles heißt der Papst Gottesdienst."

23. Peter Matheson, *The Rhetoric of Reformation* (Edinburgh: Clark, 1998), 122–23.

24. For elaboration of hyperaesthesia as an anthropological concept, see David Howes, "Hyperaesthesia; or, The Sensual Logic of Late Capitalism," in *Empire of the Senses: The Sensual Culture Reader*, ed. David Howes (New York: Berg, 2005), 281–303.

25. Stuart Clark, *Thinking with Demons: The Idea of Witchcraft in Early Modern Europe* (Oxford: Oxford University Press, 1997), 31–68, qtd. at 36, 50. See also Craig Koslofsky, *Evening's Empire: A History of the Night in Early Modern Europe* (Cambridge: Cambridge University Press, 2011), 19–90, esp. 62. For narrower readings of this phenomenon in Luther's early works, and its theological underpinnings, see Andrew Pettegree, *Reformation and the Culture of Persuasion* (Cambridge: Cambridge University Press, 2005), 20, and C. Scott Dixon, *Protestants: A History from Wittenberg to Pennsylvania, 1517–1740* (Oxford: Wiley, 2010), 1–8.

26. Hans Joachim Köhler has compiled the definitive, although incomplete, bibliography of printed pamphlets in Germany in the first three decades of the sixteenth century. See Köhler, ed., *Bibliographie der Flugschriften des 16. Jahrhunderts*, 3 vols. (Tübingen: Bibliotheca Academica, 1991, 1992, 1996). The volumes span all authors, organized alphabetically, through those with the last name S. Anonymous pamphlets are included as well. The final volume, including authors T-Z, has not been published. The bibliography details 4382 entries in total, including anonymously authored pamphlets. Here I have focused strictly on German-language materials in the years 1518–1525 to narrow the scope of materials, which was then narrowed still further by title keyword searches. Titles identifying ritual-specific topics, such as "ceremonies," "good works," or "mass," were included in the sample for analysis. Other criteria used to identify relevant sources were titles indicating some kind of binary distinction between traditional and evangelical Christianity: distinctions between "flesh" and "spirit," "law" and "gospel," "light" and "dark," "works" and "faith," "old" and "new" religion, "night" and "day," "evangelical" and "Roman," "papal," or "popish," as well as dialogues claiming to present both sides of the argument are commonplace in the pamphlet literature. Beyond this, well-known works such as Sachs's *Nightingale*, as well as works by important early evangelical leaders like Luther, Huldrych Zwingli, Philipp Melanchthon, and Martin Bucer, were also analyzed. Virtually all of the materials in Köhler's bibliography have been digitized and are accessible online via the *Central Index of Digital Prints* (*Zentrales Verzeichnis Digitalisierter Drucke*), http://www.zvdd.de.

27. "Mich wunder das kein geld im land ist (1524)," qtd. in *Johann Eberlin von Günzburg: Sämtliche Schriften*, vol. 3, ed. Ludwig Enders (Halle: Niemeyer, 1902), 174–75: Sich das haus an, wie weyt, wie hoch, wie ein thurn als ein bergschlos, wie lange fenster, wie wol gepflastert, wie vnterschiedlich chor vnd kirche, wie kostliche venedisch gemalt glaßwerck, wie vil huepscher bild an die wend gemalt, wie vil eißen vnd bley kompt zum thurn vnd zum gantzen hauß, ya mehr dan stro zu eim paurnhauß, wie huepsch gestiel ym chor fur die schwetzigen vollen pfaffen . . . Darnach kostlich stein zu vilen altaren, schoene tucher darauff, vnd schoene gulden teflein, zinen vnd messing leuchter, pulpret drauff, gitter darfur. Sovil stangen, fanen, leisten, kostlich thueren vnd andere schlos daran . . . muß man haben meßbucher, gsangbucher, kreutz, monstrantzen von silber oelbuchßlein, sacrament heußlen, tauffstein, vnd vberauß zirliche kleider, chorreck vnd alben, von subtiler leinwat, samet vnd seiden, damast etc . . . muß man haben altar

kendtlen, engel fur die altar, das sie die kertzen haltn vil oel in die lampen vnd wachs zu kertzen . . . silbern, auch gulden kelch, vnd patenen, sameten corporaltaschen, berlen pacem, galler leinwat zu corporalen . . . vnd vil tuch, kannen, becken . . . mussen wir haben ein friemesser, ein pfarrer, ein custer, chorschuler, etc, vnd vil glocken.

28. Matthäus Hitzschold, *Ein sermon vom recht christlichen Leben* (Erfurt: Knappe, 1522), fol. A4r.

29. Erasmus Alberus, *Ein schöner dialogus Martino Luther und der geschickten Botschaft aus der Hölle* (Augsburg: Ramminger, 1523), fol. B2r.

30. Theobald Billican, *Von der Mess gemayn Schlußred* (Augsburg: Ulhart, 1524), fols. A2r–v.

31. Martin Bryßgauer, *Wie man christlicher weysz beychten, Sacrament emtpfahen, Mesz halten vnd das Sacrament anbetten sol* (Strasbourg: Schwann, 1524), fol. D4r.

32. Johann Sonnentaller, *Ursach, Warumb der vermeint geystlich huff mit yren patronen das Evangelion nit annimpt sunder schend det lester und verfolget mit kurtzer Contrafactur der pfafferey Müncherey Nonnerey* (Strasbourg: Prüß, 1524), fol. C2v: "Haben sy doch platen kutten/ sindt beschoren/ tragen lang reck/ besunder farben/ geystlich kleydung/ sindt mit oel gesalbt/ haben wiss korreck/ halten mess/ singen hoch vnd lessen nider/ bucken sich hyn vnd wider/ orgeln pfiffen/ lueten glocken/ wihen kertzen/ reuechen wyrauch/ sprengen wasser/ tragen cruetz/ fanen/ gulden kelch vnd silbern monstranz."

33. Leo Jud, *Ein christenlich Widerfechtung wider Matthis Kretzen falsche Meß* (Zurich: Hager, 1524), fol. B4r; Gallus Korn, *Warum die kirch vier evangelisten hat* (Zwickau: Schönsperger, 1524), fol. C1r; Martin Reinhart, *Vnderrichte wie sich ein frumer Christ bey den Papistischen Messen/so yetz noch vil gehalten werden . . . halten soll* (Augsburg: Ulhart, 1524), fol. A2v; Michael Keller, *Etlicher Sermones von dem Nachtmahl Christi* (Augsburg: Ulhart, 1525), fol. F2r; Philipp Melhofer, *Offenbarung der allerheimlichsten Heimlichkeit der jetzigen Baalpriester* (Augsburg: Ulhart, 1525), fol. Q3v.

34. Urbanus Rhegius, *Wie man christlich feyern sol* (Augsburg: Ramminger, 1522), fol. C2r. Urbanus Rhegius, *Von Kirchenweyhe* (Augsburg: Ramminger, 1522), fols. A2r–v; Urbanus Rhegius, *Vom hochwürdigen Sakrament des Altars: Unterricht* (Augsburg: Ulhart, 1523), fols. A3v, B1v.

35. Jakob Strauß, *Ein kurz christenlich Unterricht des großen Irrtums, so im Heiligtum zu Ehren gehalten* (Erfurt: Buchfürer, 1523), fols. A4r, B2v.

36. Jakob Strauß, *Ein schöner, lieblicher Unterricht, zu bedenken und empfangen den Leib Christi, und sein roßenfarbes plut zu nyessen* (Augsburg: Schönsperger, 1524), fols. B5v–C1r.

37. Joachim von Watt, *Das Büchlein ist genant vom alten und neüwen Got, Glauben vnd Leer* (Strasbourg: Beck, 1521), fols. f1r–f3. Watt's utterance about "cats in heat" occurs at f2r.

38. Ibid., fol. f3v.

39. Hans Greiffenberger, *Ein kurzer Begriff von guten Werken* (Augsburg: Ramminger, 1524), fol. 3v.

40. Hans Herbst, *Eyn Brüderliche und Christenliche Heyliger geschrifft gegrundte ermanung* (Nuremberg: Höltzel, 1524), fol. A2v.

41. Utz Rychssner, *Eine schöne Unterweyssung daß wir in Christo alle Brueder und Schwestern sind* (Augsburg: Steiner, 1524), fols. D1r–v. Utz Rychssner, *Ein hübsch Ge-*

prächsbüchlein von einem Pfaffen und einem Weber (Augsburg: Steiner, 1524), fols. B1v, D2r, qtd. at D2r.

42. Hans Schwalb, *Beklagung eines Laien über viel Mißbrauch christlichen Lebens* (Augsburg: Ramminger, 1521), fols. A2r–v.

43. Luther, WA 6: 355. See also n5, above.

44. Heinrich Kettenbach, *Eyn gesprech Bruder Hainrich von Kettenbach mit aim frommen alte mutterlin von Vlm* (Augsburg: Ramminger, 1523), fols. A2r, A4v.

45. Ibid., fol. A4v. For a brief discussion of the dialogue, see Philip Hahn, "Sensing Sacred Space: Ulm Minster, the Reformation, and Parishioners' Sensory Perception, c. 1470 to 1640," in *Archiv für Reformationsgeschichte* 105 (2014): 55–91, at 65–66.

46. Kettenbach, *Eyn gesprech*, fol. A2r.

47. Johann Fritzhans, *An ein ehrbarn, ehrsamen, weisen Rat und ganze christliche Gemein der Stadt Magdeburg, Gottes Wort belangende* (Wittenberg: Lufft, 1523), fol. A4v; Erasmus Alberus, *Absag oder Fehdschrift des höllischen Fürsten Lucifers* (Speyer: Schmidt, 1523), fol. A2v; Wenceslaus Linck, *Sermon von dem Außgang der Kinder gottes auß des Entichrists gefengknuß* (Nuremberg: Hergot, 1524), fols. B1v–D2v; Diepold Peringer, *Ein Sermon geprediget von der Abgötterey: geprediget zu Kitzing im Franckenland auff vnsers Herren Fronleychnams tag* (Nuremberg: Hergot, 1524), fol. C3r. Rychssner, *Gesprächsbüchlein*, fol. D2r.

48. Urbanus Rhegius, *Das Blatten, Kutten, Kappen, Schern, Schmern/ Saltz/ Schmaltz vnd aller dergleichen Gott abschewlich seindt* (Worms: Schöffer, 1524), fol. A2v.

49. Watt, *Büchlein*, fol. F2v.

50. Philipp Melanchthon, and Martin Luther, *Figur des antichristlichen Papsts und seiner Synagog* (Wittenberg: Rhau-Grunenberg, 1523), fol. A3v. For more extended gender analysis of this image, Christiane Andersson, "Popular Imagery in German Reformation Broadsheets," in *Print and Culture in the Renaissance: Essays on the Advent of Printing in Europe*, ed. Gerald Tyson and Sylvia Wagonheim (Newark: University of Delaware Press, 1986), 120–50, and Ulinka Rublack, *Reformation Europe* (Cambridge: Cambridge University Press, 2005), 1–3.

51. Ulrich von Hutten, *Clag vnd vormanung gegen dem übermässigen vnchristenlichen gewalt des Bapsts zu Rom* (Strasbourg: Schott, 1520); Ulrich Bossler, *Dialogus oder gesprech des Appostolicums angelica und anderer Specerey der Appoteken antreffen Doctor M. Lutterers ler und sine anhanck* (Augsburg: Nadler, 1521); Johann Lonicer, *Von ererbyteung und anrüffung der Heiligen, so ferr die göttlich schrifft zeügknüsß gibt* (Strasbourg: Schott, 1523), fol. G2r; Alberus, *Absag oder Fehdschrift*, fol. A2v; Linck, *Außgang*, fols. B2v–D2r; Balthasar Hubmaier, *Summ eines gantzen christenlichen Lebens* (Augsburg: Ramminger, 1525), fol. A2r.

52. Scribner, *Simple Folk*, 38, 96–97; Andersson, "Popular Imagery."

53. The admittedly short list of female evangelical authors analyzed in the sample includes: Argula von Grumbach, *Eine christenliche Schrifft ainer Erbarn Frawen* (Munich: Schobser, 1523); Argula von Grumbach, *Wie ein christliche Frau des Adels in Bayern die Hoheschul zu Ingolstadt strafet* (Augsburg: Ulhart, 1523); Florentina von Oberweimar, *Ein Geschicht wie Gott einer ehrbarn Klosterjungfrauen ausgeholfen hat* (Wittenberg: Cranach & Döring, 1524); Ursula Weyda, *Wyder das vnchristlich schreyben vnd Lesterbuech des Apts Simon zuo Pegaw vnn seiner Brueder* (Zwickau: Schönsperger, 1524); Katharina Zell,

Den leidenen christglaubigen weybern der gemain zu Rentzingen (Strasbourg: Knöpfel, 1524).

54. Lyndal Roper, *The Holy Household: Women and Morals in Reformation Augsburg* (Oxford: Oxford University Press, 1989); Susan Karant-Nunn, "Kinder, Küche, Kirche: Social Ideology in the Sermons of Johannes Mathesius," *Germania Illustrata: Essays on Early Modern Germany Presented to Gerald Strauss*, ed. Andrew Fix and Susant Karant-Nunn (Kirksville, Mo.: Truman State University Press, 1992), 121–40; Susan Karant-Nunn, "Fragrant Wedding Roses: Lutheran Wedding Sermons and Gender Definition in Early Modern Germany," *German History* 1 (1999): 25–40; Allison P. Coudert, "The Myth of the Improved Status of Protestant Women: The Case of the Witchcraze," *The Politics of Gender in Early Modern Europe*, ed. Jean Brink, Allison Coudert, Maryanne Horowitz (Kirksville, Mo.: Truman State University Press, 1989), 61–90.

55. Roper, *Holy Household*, 5.

56. On the feminization of sensory iconography, see Carl Nordenfalk, "The Five Senses in Late Medieval and Renaissance Art," *Journal of the Warburg and Courtauld Institutes* 48 (1985): 1–22.

57. The centrality of the concern with orderly gender relations among the early evangelicals is further demonstrated by the fact that many of the most prominent polemicists of the *Wildwuchs* continued to write on the topic well beyond the 1520s and saw it as a crucial component of their life's work as religious reformers. Among those analyzed here who fit this description are Erasmus Alberus, Johann Brenz, Johannes Bugenhagen, Martin Luther, and Urbanus Rhegius. See Scott Hendrix, "Masculinity and Patriarchy in Reformation Germany," *Journal of the History of Ideas* 56, no. 2 (1995): 177–93; Julius Hoffmann, *Die "Hausväterliteratur" und die "Predigten über den christlichen Hausstand": Lehre vom Hause und Bildung für das häusliche Leben im 16., 17. und 18. Jahrhhundert* (Weinheim: Beltz, 1959).

58. Konrad Adler, *Ein Sermon von der Schul Christi* (Augsburg: Grimm, 1523). A copy of this pamphlet appears to have been owned by Lazarus Spengler and is located in StadtAN E1/1731, nr. 44. Pagination marks added later run from the numbers 794–815, qtd. at 802.

59. Carina Johnson, "Idolatrous Cultures and the Practice of Religion," *Journal of the History of Ideas* 67, no. 4 (2006): 597–621; Carina Johnson, *Cultural Hierarchy in Sixteenth-Century Europe: The Ottomans and Mexicans* (Cambridge: Cambridge University Press, 2011), esp. 48–56, 64–70, 135–49.

60. Ibid. See also Stephanie Leitch, *Mapping Ethnography in Early Modern Germany: New Worlds in Print Culture* (New York: Palgrave Macmillan, 2010); Renate Pieper, *Die Vermittlung einer neuen Welt: Amerika im Nachtrichtennetz des Habsburgischen Imperiums, 1493–1598* (Mainz: Philipp von Zabern, 2000); Christine Johnson, *The German Discovery of the World: Renaissance Encounters with the Strange and Marvelous* (Charlottesville: University of Virginia Press, 2008), 19–46; Lee Palmer Wandel, *The Reformation: Towards a New History* (Cambridge: Cambridge University Press, 2011), 39–62.

61. Rhegius, *Wie man christlich feyern sol*; Fritzhans, *Weisen Rat*, fol. B2r; Zwingli, *Von erkiesen und freyheit der speisen* (Basel: Petri, 1522); Kettenbach, *Ein sermon vom fasten*

vnd feyern (Wittenberg: Rhau-Grunenberg, 1522); Kettenbach, *Ain sermon oder predig von der christlichen kirchen* (Augsburg: Otmar, 1522), fols. A3v, C1r, C3v; Wenceslaus Linck, *Hie auff gottes wort allain als auff ainen bestendigen felsen* (Augsburg: Steiner, 1523), fol. B1v; Jud, *Widerfechtung*, fol. B3r. Circumcision, too, was an important element in these comparisons.

62. Melanchthon, *Figur*, fol. B2r; Pamphilus Gengenbach, *Der Laienspiegel Sancti Pauli des alten Glaubens wider den neuen* (Basel: Gengenbach, 1522), fol. C4r; Kettenbach, *Ein Sermon Bruoder Heinrichs zu der loblichen statt Vlm* (Bamberg: Erlinger, 1523), fol. A2r. Strauß, *Unterricht*, fols. B2v–C1r.

63. With respect to Islam, the rhetoric most frequently referenced (Ottoman) Turks specifically. See Thomas Kaufmann, *Türckenbüchlein: Zur Christlichen Wahrnehmung "Türkischer Religion" in Spätmittelalter und Reformation* (Göttingen: Vandenhoeck & Ruprecht, 2008).

64. For analysis of this title page border, see Joseph Koerner, *Reformation of the Image* (Chicago: University of Chicago Press, 2005), 94–96; Leitch, *Mapping Ethnography*, 164–76.

65. Cuntz von Oberndorf, *Dialogus oder ein Gespräche wider Doktor Ecken Büchlein* (Leipzig: Stöckel, 1520), fol. 380r.

66. Watt, *Büchlein*, fol. F1v.

67. Kettenbach, *Vergleychung der Bäpst satzung, gegen der leer Christi Jhesu* (Strasbourg: Beck, 1523), fols. A2v–A3r, C1v.

68. Jakob Strauß, *Ain trostliche verstendige leer über das wort sancti Pauli, der mensch soll sich selbs probieren, und also von dem brot essen, vnd von dem kelch trincken* (Augsburg: Otmar, 1522), fols. A3r, B2r; Jakob Strauß, *Kurtz und verstendig leer, uber das wort S. Pauli, zu den Römer* (Erfurt: Stürmer, 1523), fols. A2r. Wenceslaus Linck, *Artickel vnd posiciones* (Grimma: Widemar, 1523), A3r; Wenceslaus Linck, *Eyn Sermon von anrueffunge der heyligen* (Wartburg: Gutknecht, 1523); Simon Reuter, *Antwort wider die Baalspfaffen* (Bamberg: Erlinger, 1523).

69. Linck, *Artickel*, A3r.

70. Carina Johnson, "Idolatrous Cultures." Carina Johnson, *Cultural Hierarchy*, 48–56, 64–70.

71. Zwingli, *Der Hirt* (Zurich: Froschauer, 1524), fol. C4v; Ludwig Hätzer, *Urteil Gottes, unsers Ehegemahls, wie man sich mit allen Götzen und Bildnissen halten soll* (Augsburg: Steiner, 1523), fol. C1r; Anton Firn, *Supplication eines Pfarrers und der Pfarrkinder zu St. Thoman* (Augsburg: Ulhart, 1524), fol. 8r–v. Stephan Agricola, *Ein Bedencken, wie der wahrhaftig Gottesdienst möcht widerum aufgericht werden* (Eilenburg: Widemar, 1524), fol. C1r; Georg Spalatin, *Ceremonien vnd vngegründete mißbreuche y Gottisdienst abzuostellen* (Wittenberg: Weiss, 1525).

72. Spalatin, *Ceremonien*, fols. C2r–C3v. N.b. this was well before the confessional disputes of the second half of the sixteenth century made this an important element of a specifically Calvinist worldview, it had firmly rooted itself in the mental equipment of the early evangelical community more broadly. On this trope in later sixteenth century Calvinist culture, see Graeme Murdock, "The Importance of Being Josiah: An Image of Calvinist Identity," *Sixteenth Century Journal* 29, no. 4 (1998): 1043–59.

73. Luther, WA 6, 457.

74. Sascha Salatowsky, *De anima: Die Rezeption der aristotelischen Psychologie im 16. Und 17. Jahrhundert* (Amsterdam: Grüner, 2006), 69–75.

75. Watt, *Büchlein*, fols. B2r–v, G1r–v, H4r–v, I3r–v. Niklaus Manuel, *Eyn Faß Nacht spyl vom Bapst vnd siner priesterschafft* (Zurich: Froschauer, 1522), n.p.; Balthasar Stanberger, *Ein dialogus oder gesprech zwischen einem Prior, Leyenbruder und Bettler das wort gottes belanget* (Erfurt: Buchfürer, 1522), fols. B1v–B2r; Fritzhans, *Weisen Rat*, fols. A3r–A4r; Fritzhans, *Wie man das klar hell Gotteswort predigen soll* (Zwickau: Gastel, 1524), fol. A3v; Kettenbach, *Ein Sermon bruoder Heinrichs*, fols. A3v–A4v; Lonicer, *Von ererbyteung* (1523), fol. B3r; Theobald Billican, *Ain Sermon über das wort Christi* (Strasbourg: Knobloch, 1524), fols. A2r–v.

76. Stanberger, *Ein dialogus*, fol. B1v.

77. Lonicer, *Von ererbyteung*, fol. B3r.

78. Fritzhans, *Gotteswort*, fol. A4r.

79. Idem, *Weisen Rat*, fol. A3r.

80. Watt, *Büchlein*, fol. I1r.

81. Kettenbach, *Vergleychung*, fol. B2r.

82. Ibid, fol. B4v. On the use of accusations of sodomy to gender and discredit opponents in early Reformation discourse, see Helmut Puff, *Sodomy in Reformation Germany and Switzerland, 1400–1600* (Chicago: University of Chicago Press, 2003), 107–24, 140–66.

83. Paul Freedman, "Health, Wellness and the Allure of Spices in the Middle Ages," *Journal of Ethnopharmacology* 167, no. 5 (2015): 47–53.

84. Johnson, *German Discovery*, 123–65.

85. Ibid., 124.

86. Ibid., 127–31.

87. Philip Broadhead, "Contribution of Hans Sachs to the Debate on the Reformation in Nuremberg: A Study of the Religious Dialogues of 1524," in *Hans Sachs and Folke Theatre in the Late Middle Ages*, ed. Robert Aylett (Lewiston, N.Y.: Edwin Melln, 1995), 43–62, at 44–46; Günther Vogler, *Nürnberg 1524/25: Studien zur Geschichte der reformatorischen und sozialen Bewegung in der Reichsstadt* (Berlin: VEB Deutscher Verlag der Wissenschaften, 1982).

88. Johnson, *German Disovery*, 133, 136–39.

89. Ibid., 144.

90. Ibid., 141.

91. Ibid., 142.

92. Broadhead, "Contribution," 44–46.

93. Johnson, *German Discovery*, 144.

94. Luther, WA 6, 422.

95. Kettenbach, *Ein Sermon bruoder Heinrichs*, fol. A4v. Kettenbach, *Eyn gesprech*, fol. A2r–v; Lonicer, *Ererbyetung*, fol. B3r; Hubmaier, *Achtzehn Schlußrede* (Augsburg: Ramminger, 1524), fol. A3r; Watt, *Büchlein*, fols. G1r, H4r; Niklaus Manuel, *Eyn Faßnacht spyl*; Billican, *Wort Christi*, fol. A2r–v; Fritzhans, *Gotteswort*, fols. A3v, C1r–v.

96. Jud, *Widerfechtung*, fol. B4r.

97. Günzburg, *Klag und Antwort von lutherischen und päpistischen Pfaffen über die Reformation, zu Regensburg ausgangen* (Nuremberg: Höltzel, 1524), fol. B1r.

98. Günzburg, "Mich wunder das kein geld im land ist."

99. Compare with Hayden White, *Content of the Form: Narrative Discourse and Historical Representation* (Baltimore, Md.: Johns Hopkins University Press, 1987).

100. Scott Hendrix, "Rerooting the Faith: The Reformation as Re-Christianization," *Church History* 69, no. 3 (2000): 558–77.

101. Compare with Peter Matheson, *The Imaginative World of the Reformation* (Edinburgh: Clark, 2000), 7, for the pervasiveness of the trope of the "clear and pure" Word in early Reformation culture.

102. Hubmaier, *Summ*, fol. A2r. For Hubmaier's place in the context of the so-called "radical reformation," see George Huntston Williams, *The Radical Reformation*, 3rd ed. (Kirksville, Mo.: Truman State University Press, 1995).

103. Lee Palmer Wandel has recently suggested that Anabaptists were responsible for the radicalization of the early evangelical community as a whole during these formative years, but on the issue of contrariety between evangelical Word and traditional ceremony, the positions staked out from the very beginning were unequivocally radical. See *Towards a New History*, 95–97.

104. Luther, WA 6, 511–12.

105. For a critical appraisal of the great divide theory from the perspective of sensory history, see Mark Smith, *Sensing the Past: Seeing, Hearing, Smelling, Tasting, and Touching in History* (Berkeley: University of California Press, 2007), 8–13.

106. Peter Blickle, "Die Reformation vor dem Hintergrund von Kommunalisierung und Christianisierung: Eine Skizze," in *Kommunalisierung und Christianisierung: Voraussetzungen und Folgen der Reformation, 1400–1600*, ed. Peter Blickle (Berlin: Duncker, 1989), 9–28.

107. John Bossy, *Christianity in the West, 1400–1700* (Oxford: Oxford University Press, 1985), 97–104; Ulinka Rublack, "Grapho-Relics: Lutheranism and the Materialization of the Word," *Past and Present*, supp. 5 (2010): 144–66. Koerner, *Reformation*, 252–307. Wandel, *Towards a New History*, 63–88. Bridget Heal, "The Catholic Eye and the Protestant Ear: The Reformation as a Non-Visual Event?" in *The Myth of the Reformation*, ed. Peter Opitz (Göttingen: Vandenhoeck & Ruprecht, 2013), 321–55.

108. Qtd. in Alister McGrath, *Reformation Thought: An Introduction*, 2nd ed. (Oxford: Blackwell, 1993), 140.

109. Rublack, *Reformation Europe*, 193.

110. Koerner, *Reformation*, 38–43.

111. Ibid., 43.

112. Luther had already stated this position in the *Babylonian Captivity*. Zwingli argued for visual mimesis in Eucharist performance most systematically in his treatise *Action oder Brauch des Nachtmals Gedechtnus oder Dancksagung Christi* (Zurich: Frochauer, 1525), and *Ein klare underrichtung vom nachtmal Christi* (Zurich: Hager, 1526). See Lee Palmer Wandel, "Envisioning God: Image and Liturgy in Reformation Zurich," *Sixteenth Century Journal* 24, no. 1 (1993): 21–40.

113. Bossy, *Christianity*, 100. See also Koerner, *Reformation*, 38–43.

114. Fritzhans, *Gotteswort*, fol. A4r.

115. Bryßgauer, *Wie man christlicher weysz*, fol. D1r.

116. Watt, *Büchlein*, fols. Fv–F3r, H2r–v; Schwalb, *Beklagung*, fol. A3r. Wenceslaus Linck, *Die letzsten drey Psalmen von Orgelen, Paucken, Glocken, und der gleychen eüsserlichen Gotßdienst, ob und wie Got darynnen gelobt wyrdt* (Zwickau: Gastel, 1523), fols. A3v–A4r; Reuter, *Antwort*, fol. A1r; Wolfgang Russ, *Ein Sermon, in welcher Mensch gereizt und ermahnt wird zu Lieb der evangelischen Lehre* (Zwickau: Schönsperger, 1523), fol. A4v–B1r; Fritzhans, *Gotteswort*, fol. C1r–v; Rhegius, *Underricht wie sich ain Christen mensch halten sol das er frucht der Meß erlang* (Augsburg: Grimm & Wirsung, 1522), fols. A2r–A3r.

117. Schwalb, *Beklagung*, fols. A2r, A3r.

118. Rhegius, *Wie man christlich feyern sol*, fol. C2r.

119. Rhegius, *Sakrament*, fol. B1v.

120. Melhofer, *Offenbarung*, fol. Q3v.

121. Johannes Bugenhagen, *Von der evangelischen mess* (1524), quoted in Amy Nelson Burnett, *Karlstadt and the Origins of the Eucharistic Controversy: A Study in the Circulation of Ideas* (Oxford: Oxford University Press, 2011), 45.

122. Rublack, *Reformation Europe*, 46.

123. Richard Newhauser, "Peter of Limoges, Optics, and the Science of the Senses," *Senses and Society* 5, no. 1 (2010): 28–44; see especially 37–38.

124. Dürer, "Die Entwürfe zu dem enzyklopädischen 'Speis der Malerknaben,'" in *Albrecht Dürer: Schriften, Tagebücher, Briefe*, ed. Max Steck (Stuttgart: 1961), 204.

125. Klaus Leder, *Kirche und Jugend in Nürnberg und seinem Landgebiet 1400–1800* (Neustadt an der Aisch: Degener, 1973), 7–20.

126. Berndt Hamm developed the concept of "normative centering" in a variety of works, mostly in German. See Berndt Hamm, "Reformation als normative Zentrierung von Religion und Gesellschaft," *Jahrbuch für Biblische Theologie* 7 (1992): 241–79; Berndt Hamm, "Von der spätmittelalterlichen reformatio zur Reformation: Der Prozess normativer Zentrierung von Religion und Gesellschaft in Deutschland," *Archiv für Reformationsgeschichte* 84 (1993): 7–82. Milner has made a similar argument for the English context.

127. On the concern with emotional appeal in early Lutheran preaching, see Susan Karant-Nunn, *The Reformation of Feeling: Shaping the Religious Emotions in Early Modern Germany* (Oxford: Oxford University Press, 2010), 73–100.

128. Bossy, *Christianity*, 98.

129. Luther, WA 6, 217.

130. Spengler, "Verantwortung und Auflösung vermeinter Argumente, die zu Widerstand und Unterdruckung des Wortes Gottes gebraucht werden (1523)," in *Lazarus Spenglers Schriften* vol. 1: *Schriften der Jahre 1509 bis Juni 1525*, ed. Berndt Hamm (Gütersloh: Gütersloher Verlagshaus, 1995), 354–95, at 377.

131. Wandel, *Towards a New History*, 78.

132. Andreas Karlstadt made this point in his call to iconoclasm, *Abtuung der Bilder* (Wittenberg: Schirlentz, 1522), fols. A2v, C3v.

133. Fritzhans, *Weisen Rat*, fol. A3v.

134. Bryßgauer, *Wie man christlicher weysz*, fol. D1v.

135. Wenceslaus Linck, *Außgang*, fol. B1v.

136. Oecolampadius, *Ain predig und ermanung . . . von wirdigen Ereenbietung dem Sacrament des fronleichnam Christi* (Augsburg: Grimm & Wirsung, 1521), fols. 3v–4r.

137. Ibid., fol. 6v.

138. Ibid., fols. 10v–11r.

139. Gerd Schwerhoff, "Wie gottlos waren die 'gottlosen maler': Zur Rekonstruktion des Nürnberger Verfahrens von 1525 und seiner Hinergründe," in *Die gottlosen Maler von Nürnberg: Konvention und Subversion in der Druckgrafik der Beham-Brüder*, ed. Jürgen Müller (Nuremberg: Albrecht Dürrer Haus, 2011), 33–44.

140. The key documents for this case have been collected in Gerhard Pfeiffer, ed., *Quellen zur Nürnberger Reformationsgeschichte: Von der Duldung liturgischer Änderungen bis zur Ausübung des Kirchenregiments durch Rat (Juni 1524-Juni 1525)* (Nuremberg: Verein für bayerische Kirchengeschichte, 1968), 38–43, 200–203; and in Walter Fellmann, ed., *Hans Denck Schriften*, 3 vols. (Gütersloh: Gütersloher, 1956–1960).

141. Qtd. in Volker Leppin, "Kirchenausstattungen in territorialen Kirchenordnungen bis 1548," in *Ordnungen für die Kirche, Wirkungen auf die Welt: Evangelische Kirchenordnungen des 16. Jahrhunderts*, ed. Sabine Arend (Tübingen: Mohr Siebeck, 2015), 137–156, at 139.

142. There was one episode of iconoclasm that predated the Wittenberg riots, but little is known about it. In early 1521, it seems that subjects in the Pomeranian town of Treptow (today Trzebiatow) broke into a chapel and destroyed several images on an altar, claiming inspiration from the evangelical movement. See Sergiusz Michalski, "Die Ausbreitung des reformatorischen Bildersturms, 1521–1537," in *Bildersturm: Wahnsinn oder Gottes Wille?*, ed. Peter Jezler (Bern: NZZ, 2000), 46–51.

143. Carl Christensen, *Art and the Reformation in Germanyu*(Columbus,: Ohio State University Press, 1979), 40–41.

144. Karlstadt, *Abtuung der Bilder*, fols. C3v, D1r.

145. Qtd. and translated in Christensen, *Art*, 25.

146. Ibid., 29.

147. Qtd. and trans. in Koerner, *Reformation*, 83.

148. He laid this out in his famous *Invocavit* sermons, given March 9–16, in the parish church. See WA 10 (III), 1–13.

149. Edwards, *Printing, Propaganda*, 29.

150. Ibid., 16; Pettegree, *Culture of Persuasionu*159.

151. Edwards, *Printing, Propaganda*, 40.

152. Qtd. in Edwards, *Printing, Propaganda*, 14.

153. Pettegree, *Culture of Persuasion*, 162–65.

154. For demographic figures, see Christian Pfister, "Population," in *Germany: A New Social and Economic History*, vol. 1: *1450–1630*, ed. Robert Scribner (London: Arnold, 1996), 33–62, at 39–43. These measurements are based on the 1914 borders of Germany which, incorporating Prussia's eastern territories, was a considerably larger geographic entity than the Holy Roman Empire of the sixteenth century. Further, with respect to the urban population, the figure of 16 percent is an estimate of inhabitants in towns of five

thousand or more. The largest towns, where most of the evangelical print culture was produced, would have represented an even smaller number of the overall population, and therefore, perhaps even more lopsided ratios of pamphlets to people.

155. Scribner, *Simple Folk*, 196–217.

156. Adolf Diehl, ed., *Dionysius Dreytweins Esslingische Chronik (1548–1564)* (Tübingen: Litterarischen Verein Stuttgart, 1901), 5–6. He later notes that it was this preaching specifically that motivated peasants to loot the valuables in monasteries and churches in the city (p. 20).

157. Karl Gustav Veesenmeyer, ed., *Sebastian Fischers Chronik, besonders von Ulmischen Sachen* (Ulm: Nübling, 1896), 14–18.

158. Compare with Mary Douglas, *Implicit Meanings: Selected Essays in Anthropology*, 2nd ed. (New York: Routledge, 1999), 3–7, for an overview of the concept.

159. Anton Schilling edited the original manuscript in the late nineteenth century. See Schilling, "Die religiösen und kirchlichen Zustände der ehemaligen Reichsstadt Biberach unmittelbar vor Einführung der Reformation," *Freiburger Diözesan Archiv* 19 (1887), 1–191, qtd. at 11.

160. The most important of these was Witzel's monumental five-volume *Typus Ecclesiae Catholicae*, which he constantly revised. It was printed many times in Mainz and Cologne in the 1540s and 1550s, the most complete edition appearing in 1559: *Typus Ecclesiae Catholicae*, 5 vols. (Cologne: Quentel and Calenius, 1559). His liturgical works were very numerous, and here we include only a small sampling of the most important: *Von den Eucharisty oder Meß, nach Answeisung der Schrift und der ältesten schrifterständigen h. Lehrer* (Leipzig: Schumann, 1534); *De Ceremoniis antiquae Ecclesiae* (Mainz: Behem, 1542); *Der heiligen Messen Brauch, wie er in der alten Kirchen vor tausend Jahren gewesen* (Mainz: Behem, 1541); *De traditione apostolica et ecclesiastica, daß die katholische Kirche Christi nicht allein was in der h. Schrift steht, sondern auch was sie bei den heiligen Vätern und ältesten Concilien göttlichs und löblichs funden, zu Gottes Dienst und Ehre ordentlich brauchen und beständiglich behalten möge* (Cologne: Quentel, 1549).

161. Georg Witzel, *Typus Ecclesiae Catholicae*, fol. F1v.

Chapter 5. Implementing the Reformation of the Senses in Practice

1. Luther, *Wider die himelischen Propheten, von den bildern vnd Sacrament* (Augsburg: Ulhart, 1525); Luther, *Sermon von dem Sacrament des leybs und bluts Christi, wider die Schwermgeyster* (Nuremberg: Gutknecht, 1526), not paginated.

2. Charles Garside, *Zwingli and the Arts* (New Haven, Conn.: Yale University Press, 1966), 159–60.

3. Carl Christensen, *Art and the Reformation in Germany* (Columbus: Ohio State University Press, 1979), 79–102; Carlos Eire, *War against the Idols: The Reformation of Worship from Erasmus to Calvin* (Cambridge: Cambridge University Press, 1986), 73–94. Lee Palmer Wandel, *Voracious Idols and Violent Hands: Iconoclasm in Reformation Zurich, Strasbourg, and Basel* (Cambridge: Cambridge University Press, 1994).

4. Ernst Walter Zeeden, *Konfessionsbildung: Studien zur Reformation, Gegenreformation, und katholischen Reform* (Stuttgart: Klett-Cotta, 1985), 113–91.

5. Christoph Strohm, "Lutherische und reformierte Kirchenordnungen im Vergleich," in *Ordnungen für die Kirche, Wirkungen auf die Welt: Evangelische Kirchenordnungen*

des 16. Jahrhunderts, ed. Sabine Arend and Gerald Dörner (Tübingen: Mohr Siebeck, 2015), 1–28.

6. Johannes Pfarrkirchner, "Bericht über die 'Götzenverehrung' in Betzensteiner Hüll," in *Kirchenvisitation im Landgebiet der Reichsstadt Nürnberg 1560/61*, ed. Gerhard Hirschmann (Neustadt an der Aisch: Degener, 1994), 131–36, qtd. at 132.

7. Ibid., 134.

8. Ibid., 135–36.

9. Ibid., 136: "Quare magistratui liceat curare ac efficere, ut impia dogmata et idolatriae tollantur ex ecclesia, testator exemplum Hiskiae, regis Juda, qui per sacerdotes curavit restaurari verso cultus dei et omnia idolatria altaria destrui et concremari et aliorum exemplorum etc."

10. Ibid., 137, 141–46.

11. Hirschmann, *Kirchenvisitation*, 144–45.

12. Bridget Heal, *The Cult of the Virgin Mary in Early Modern Germany: Protestant and Catholic Piety, 1500–1648* (Cambridge: Cambridge University Press, 2007), 112.

13. Heal, *Cult*, 112.

14. Zeeden, *Konfessionsbildung*, 113–91. For a key early work on this subject in English, see Christensen, *Art*. For a recent overview of the scholarship in this field, with concise bibliographic references to both German- and English-language materials, see Bridget Heal, "Visual and Material Culture," in *The Oxford Handbook of the Protestant Reformations*, ed. Ulinka Rublack (Oxford: Oxford University Press, 2017), 601–20.

15. Christopher Ocker has recently argued that more work needs to be done on church property more broadly. See Ocker, *Church Robbers and Reformers in Germany, 1525–1547: Confiscation and Religious Purpose in the Holy Roman Empire* (Leiden: Brill, 2006), esp. 1–13.

16. The treatment of these materials has a venerable tradition in German scholarship, going back to paradigmatic studies in the late nineteenth and early twentieth centuries. The first example was Aemilius Ludwig Richter's edition of early evangelical church ordinances, published as *Die evangelischen Kirchenordnungen des sechzehnten Jahrhunderts: Urkunden und Regesten zur Geschichte des Rechts und der Verfassung der evangelischen Kirche in Deutschland* (Weimar: Verlag des Landes-Industriecomptoirs, 1846 [reprint: Nieuwkoop: De Graf, 1967]). Above all, the work of Karl Pallas on visitations and Emil Sehling on ordinances laid the foundations for much of the social history of the reformation that developed in the late twentieth century. Both Pallas and Sehling undertook the painstaking work of compiling editions of these sources. See Karl Pallas, ed., *Die Registraturen der Kirchenvisitationen im ehemaligen sächsischen Kurkreise*, 6 vols. (Halle: Hendel, 1906–1918); Emil Sehling, *Die evangelische Kirchenordnungen des XVI. Jahrhunderts*, 22 vols. (Tübingen: Mohr Siebeck, 1902–2017). Sehling completed volumes 1–5 in his lifetime. The project was revived from 1955 to 1980 with the support of the German evangelical church and German Research Society. Twelve volumes appeared during these years. In 2002 the Heidelberg Academy of Sciences took over the project and continues to publish volumes. As of 2017, twenty-two volumes have been published. For the sake of uniformity and brevity, this resource will hereafter be referred to as *EKO*.

17. As we saw in chapter 1, a variety of materials aimed at outlining liturgical practice in communities across Germany.

18. Peter Thaddäus Lang, "Würfel, Wein und Wettersegen: Klerus und Gläubige im Bistum Eichstätt am Vorabend der Reformation," in *Martin Luther: Probleme seiner Zeit*, ed.Volker Press (Stuttgart: Klett-Cotta, 1986), 219–42.

19. Lang, "Würfel," 222.

20. Although, after his expulsion, he would increasingly advocate that Christians were duty bound to destroy images if authorities were not willing to do so. See Eire, *War*, 62–73.

21. Christensen, *Art*, 39–41.

22. Joseph Koerner, *Reformation of the Image* (Chicago: University of Chicago Press, 2005), 83.

23. Bettina Seyderhelm, "Die 'bewahrende Kraft des Luthertums' gegen die Beseitigung vorreformatorischer Kirchenausstattungen: Von der Erhaltung mittelalterlicher Goldschmiedearbeiten und anderer Kirchenausstattungen in mitteldeutschen evangelischen Kirchen," in *Kirchliche Kunst in Sachsen: Festgabe für Hartmut Mai zum 65. Geburtstag*, ed. Jens Bulisch (Beucha: Sax, 2002), 32–51, at 32–37. Evidence of this point was also already in circulation in the early sixteenth century: Frederick had published an illustrated catalog of his relics and the spiritual benefits that might accrue to pilgrims visiting the castle church. The catalogue was illustrated by Lucas Cranach the elder and has been published in a modern edition. See Cranach, *Wittenberger Heiltumsbuch: Faksimile-Neudruck der Ausgabe Wittenberg 1509* (Unterschneidheim: Uhl, 1969).

24. Christensen, *Art*, 38–41. Natalie Krentz, *Ritualwandel und Deutungshoheit: Die frühe Reformation in der Residenzstadt Wittenberg (1500–1533)* (Tübingen: Mohr Siebeck, 2014), 66–83; Seyderhelm, "Bewahrende Kraft," 32–37; Günter Wartenberg, "Bilder in den Kirchen der Wittenberger Reformation," in *Die bewahrende Kraft Luthertums: Mittelalterliche Kunstwerke in evangelischen Kirchen*, ed. Johann Michael Fritz (Regensburg: Schnell & Steiner, 1997), 19–33. Volker Leppin, "Kirchenausstattungen in territorialen Kirchenordnungen bis 1548," in *Ordnungen für die Kirche*, 137–56, at 143–44.

25. Eire, *War*, 66–68. Koerner, *Reformation*, 153–54.

26. For the narrative in Zürich, see Eire, *War*, 76–86; Wandel, *Voracious Idols*, 51–101.

27. Luther, *Ordenung gottis dienst*, in WA 12, 35.

28. WA 12, 205–6.

29. Ibid., 207.

30. Eire, *War*, 69.

31. Ocker, *Church Robbers*, 58–66; Leppin, "Kirchenausstattungen," 146–47.

32. WA 19, 113.

33. See chapter 4.

34. *Wider die himmlischen Propheten*.

35. Qtd. in Christensen, *Art*, 46.

36. As Christopher Boyd Brown shows, fetish of the aural Word, and the judgments about other external practices it made possible, became a keynote in sixteenth-century Lutheran culture. See Brown, *Singing the Gospel: Lutheran Hymns and the Success of the Reformation* (Cambridge, Mass.: Harvard University Press, 2005), 91.

37. See, most recently in English, the work of Bridget Heal, "'Better Papist than Calvinist': Art and Identity in Later Lutheran Germany," *German History* 29, no. 4 (2011): 584–609. See also her recent *A Magnificent Faith: Art and Identity in Lutheran Germany* (Oxford:

Oxford University Press, 2017). For images as adiaphora in the early Lutheran tradition, see also Joseph Koerner, *Reformation*, 159–60. In German, the major point of reference is Fritz, *Die bewahrende Kraft*. For other recent contributions, see Thomas Kaufmann, *Konfession und Kultur: Lutherischer Protestantismus in der zweiten Hälfte des Reformationsjahrhunderts* (Tübingen: Mohr Siebeck, 2006), 157–203. Thomas Lentes, "Zwischen Adiaphora und Artefakt: Bildbestreitigung in der Reformation," in *Handbuch der Bildtheologie*, vol. 1: *Bild-Konflikte*, ed. Reinhard Hoeps (Paderborn: Schöningh, 2007), 213–40.

38. Recently, Caroline Walker Bynum has challenged scholars to think about the technical classification of theological indifference as it relates to material culture more broadly. See Bynum, "Are Things 'Indifferent'? How Objects Change Our Understanding of Religious History," *German History* 34, no. 1 (2016): 88–112.

39. They are his general ordinance for services, written for the city council of Leisnig, an ordinance on the maintenance of the communal chest (also for Leisnig city council), both of which were written at the beginning of 1523, and his *Formula missae*, written near the end of the year, outlining the practice of the Mass as it was developing in Wittenberg. These materials can be found in EKO 1, 2–3, 598–604, as well as WA 12, 1–38, 197–221. See also Bodo Nischan, *Lutherans and Calvinists in the Age of Confessionalism* (Burlington, Vt.: Ashgate, 1999), V, 1–27; Philip Hahn, "The Reformation of the Soundscape: Bell-Ringing in Early Modern Lutheran Germany," *German History* 33, no. 4 (2015): 525–45, for detailed analyses of the elevation, images, and the use of bells specifically.

40. WA 12, 206–7.

41. This is usually embodied in the hermeneutic contrast between Law and Gospel, central to Protestant identity, and a well-trodden topic in theological scholarship. Recently, C. Scott Dixon has suggested the contrast frames and defines the entire history of Protestantism in the early modern era. See Dixon, *Protestants: A History from Wittenberg to Pennsylvania, 1517–1740* (Oxford: Wiley, 2010). Philippe Buc has observed that the contrast was central to the modern construction of ritual as a category of analysis. See Buc, *The Dangers of Ritual: Between Early Medieval Texts and Social Scientific Theory* (Princeton, N.J.: Princeton University Press, 2001), 164–179.

42. Sergiusz Michalski, *Reformation and the Visual Arts: The Protestant Image Question in Western and Eastern Europe* (New York: Routledge, 1993), 37. Michalski makes this point specifically for images.

43. WA 12, 214.

44. For an overview, see William Cavanaugh, "Eucharistic Sacrifice and the Social Imagination in Early Modern Europe," *Journal of Medieval and Early Modern Studies* 31, no. 3 (Fall 2001): 585–605; Jonathan Sheehan, "Altars of the Idols: Religion, Sacrifice, and the Early Modern Polity," *Journal of the History of Ideas* 67, no. 4 (2006): 648–74.

45. WA 12, 213.

46. Craig Koslofsky, "The Kiss of Peace in the German Reformation," in *The Kiss in History*, ed. Karen Harvey (Manchester: University of Manchester Press, 2005), 25–27.

47. WA 12, 213–14.

48. "Ordnung eines gemeinen kastens. Radschlag wie die geistlichen guter zu handeln sind," in EKO 1, 598–604.

49. EKO 1, 598–600.

50. Ibid.

51. Citing here from Nuremberg 1528 edition: Melanchthon, *Unterricht der Visitatoren an die Pfarrherrn im Kurfürstenthum zu Sachsen* (Nuremberg: Peypus, 1528). At fols. E3r–v.

52. Ibid, fols. E4r, F1v–F2r, F4r–v. G2r, G4r.

53. Ibid, fols. F2v, G2v.

54. On these points, Buc has analyzed both the *Confession* and the related *Apology for the Confession*. See *Dangers of Ritual*, 164–70.

55. EKO 1, 174–75 (John the Constant's proclamation), 175–77 (ordinance).

56. Seyderhelm, "Bewahrende Kraft," 44.

57. Sebastian Schlick, *Ordnung, wie es soll mit den Gottesdienst und desselben dienern in der Stadt Elbogen gehalten werden* (Augsburg: Steiner, 1523).

58. "Messordnung," in StadtAN E1/1731, Familienarchiv Spengler, nr. 47 (not paginated).

59. EKO 11, 44–45, 46–50 (Nuremberg). EKO 19, 124–29, 130–33 (Worms). Additionally, treatises by the leading evangelical pastors in Nuremberg and Strasbourg, Andreas Osiander and Martin Bucer, respectively, justify the need for liturgical reform in stark, unambiguous terms and build on the story of sensory reformation. See Osiander, "Grund und Ursach (1524)," in *Andreas Osiander Gesamtausgabe*, vol. 1, ed. Gottfried Seebaß (Gütersloh: Gütersloher Verlagshaus, 1975), 175–266. Bucer, *Grund und Ursach* (Strasbourg: Koepfel, 1524), esp. fols. E2r–H3r.

60. Gerald Dörner, "'Weil auff Erden nichts schöners ist dann solche Versammlungen in den Kirchen, die ein Bild und Gleichnuß sind der ewigen Versammlungen im Himmel': Ein Blick auf die oberdeutschen Agenden," in *Ordnungen für die Kirchen*, 53–74.

61. Richter, *Kirchenordnungen*, 1:28–30.

62. EKO 17, part 1, 46–53.

63. Ordinances for Heilbronn (1530) and Reutlingen (1531) closely follow the pattern set by Brenz, beginning with stories of the iconoclastic kings of the Old Testament, but outlining a policy of ritual adiaphora. See EKO 17, part 1, 273–77, 283–85 (Heilbronn), EKO 17, part 4, 38–44 (Reutlingen). Similar patterns prevailed in nearby Hesse from 1526 through the 1530s. See Leppin, "Kirchenausstattungen," 144–46.

64. EKO 6, part 1, 348–455. Compare with Jürgen Diestelmann, "Verkündigung des Evangeliums und Volksfrömmigkeit in der Braunschweiger Kirchenordnung von 1528," in *Die Reformation in der Stadt Braunschweig: Festschrift 1528–1978*, ed. Hermann Kuhr (Braunschweig: Braunschweiger Kirchenverband, 1989), 93–302.

65. Richter, *Kirchenordnungen*, vol. 1, 127–33 (Hamburg), 145–49 (Lübeck). For the Pomeranian visitation protocols, see Helmut Heyden, ed., *Protokolle der Pommerschen Kirchenvisitationen*, 3 vols. (Cologne: Böhlau, 1961, 1963, 1964).

66. EKO 11, 102–278. See also *Osiander Gesamtausgabe*, vols. 3–4, for further evidence.

67. EKO 11, 131.

68. Ibid., 134, 136–37.

69. For editions of the ordinance, see EKO 11, 279–310. See also *Osiander Gesamtausgabe* 5:63–177. For the broader context and impact of the ordinance on Lutheran liturgical policy, see C. Scott Dixon, *The Reformation and Rural Society: The Parishes*

of Brandenburg-Ansbach-Kulmbach (Cambridge: Cambridge University Press, 2002), 31–32; Eike Wolgast, "Die Reformation im Herzogtum Mecklenburg und das Schicksal der Kirchenausstattungen," in *Bewahrende Kraft*, 54–70.

70. EKO 3 (Brandenburg), 38–42, 45, 51–53, 67–68, 155–56, 194–95, 209, 240, 334, 366, 440; EKO 6, part 1 (Wolfenbüttel, Lüneburg), 13, 22, 50, 66–67, 522, 527, 586, 591–92; EKO 6, part 2 (Calenberg-Göttingen, as well as other large cities, such as Hannover and Northeim), 733–37, 788–93, 799, 852–53, 868–70, 911, 925–26, 944–50, 1004–10.

71. Bridget Heal, "Kirchenordnungen und das Weiterbestehen religiöser Kunstwerke in lutherischen Kirchen," in *Ordnungen für die Kirchen*, 157–74; Wolgast, "Herzogtum Mecklenburg," 60–67.

72. Osiander, "Gutachten über die Zeremonien," in *Osiander Gesamtausgabe* 2:267–68.

73. Joseph Herl, *Worship Wars in Early Lutheranism: Choir, Congregation, and Three Centuries of Conflict* (Oxford: Oxford University Press, 2004), 215–45. "Early modern" here is defined according to the chronological limits of his survey, which encompasses ordinances from 1523 to 1747.

74. Bodo Nischan, "The Fractio Panis: A Reformed Communion Practice in Late Reformation Germany," *Church History* 53, no. 1 (1984): 17–29.

75. Herl, *Worship Wars*, 215–45.

76. Amy Nelson-Burnett, "The Social History of Communion and the Reformation of the Eucharist," *Past and Present* 211 (May 2011): 77–119, esp. 98–105.

77. See Richter, *Kirchenordnungen* 1, 17–18.

78. A year later, a similar ordinance appeared for the northern German city of Stralsund. See Richter, *Kirchenordnungen* 1, 22–27.

79. EKO 1, 712–13.

80. EKO 1, 678.

81. EKO 1, 678, 711–13.

82. EKO 1, 515 (Altenburg).

83. Compare with *Reformation in Württemberg: Ausstellung zur 450-Jahr-Feier der Evangelische Landeskirche, Württembergische Landesbibliothek Stuttgart, 15 May bis 22 July 1984* (Stuttgart: Calwer, 1984), 276–92.

84. Leppin, "Kirchenausstattungen," 151–53.

85. Heyden, *Protokolle*, vol. 1 (1961), 12, 18, 25–27, 44, 47–48, 120, 162–63, 167, 284, 293–96; vol. 2, 40–41, 131–32, 142, 273, 322.

86. EKO 1, 282–83.

87. EKO 1, 262; EKO 6, part 1, 19–20, 76–77; EKO 6, part 2, 811, 858.

88. EKO 6, part 1, 445–46; Richter, *Kirchenordnungen* 1, 131, 147.

89. EKO 3, 28–32, 180–81. See also visitation protocols published in 1542 in Victor Herold, ed., *Die brandenburgischen Kirchenvisitations-Abschiede und- Register des XVI. und XVII. Jahrhunderts*, vol. 1 (Berlin: Gsellius, 1928), 243–44.

90. Johann Götz, *Die Glaubenspaltung im Gebiete der Markgraffschaft Ansbach-Kulmbach in den Jahren 1520–1535* (Freiburg im Breisgau: Herder, 1907), 140–59. For the 1536 protocol mandating the communal chest, see Karl Schornbaum, "Zur zweiten brandenburgischen Kirchenvisitation 1536," *Jahresbericht des historischen Vereins für Mittelfranken* 53 (1906): 1–22, at 15.

91. Götz, *Glaubenspaltung*, 143–50.

92. Karl Kayser, ed., *Die reformatorischen kirchenvisitationen in den welfischen Landen, 1542–1544* (Göttingen: Vandenhoeck & Ruprecht, 1897), 254. Similar examples abound in the visitation records from this region. See entries for the villages of Alfeld, Gandersheim, Bockenheim, and various monastic institutions in lower Saxony, at 50, 54, 58–59, 74, 79, 90–91.

93. Compare with Heal, "Visual and Material Culture," for an overview of the scholarship.

94. Bynum, "Are Things 'Indifferent.'"

95. Michael Fritz, "Die bewahrende Kraft des Luthertums: Mittelalterliche Kunstwerke in evangelischen Kirchen," in *Die bewahrende Kraft*, 9–18.

96. Wolgast, "Herzogtum Mecklenburg," 54–70.

97. Fritz, "Die bewahrende Kraft," 17.

98. Zeeden, *Konfessionsbildung*, 133–34, 136–39; Christensen, *Art*; Gottfried Seebaß, "Mittelalterliche Kunstwerke in evangelisch gewordenen Kirchen Nürnbergs," in *Die bewahrende Kraft*, 34–53.

99. Heal, "Sacred Image and Sacred Space in Lutheran Germany," in *Sacred Space in Early Modern Europe*, ed. Andrew Spicer (Cambridge: Cambridge University Press, 2005), 39–59.

100. Nischan, *Lutherans and Calvinists*, V, 1–27.

101. Heal, *Cult*, 74–76.

102. Heal, "Sacred Space," 50.

103. Leppin, "Kirchenausstattungen," 144–46.

104. Wolgast, "Herzogtum Mecklenburg," 61–64.

105. Heal, "Kirchenordnungen," 161–162. Heal, *Cult*, 274–76.

106. Art. XX: "De bonis operibus," in *Corpus Reformatorum: Opera Omnia Philippi Melanthonis*, vol. 26, ed. Heinrich Bindseil (Braunschweig, 1858), 284–85.

107. *Osiander Gesamtausgabe* 2:261, 3:156.

108. EKO 11, 169.

109. EKO 1, 600–601.

110. Qtd. in Heal, "Sacred Image," 48.

111. Ibid., 48–50.

112. Ibid., 54–55.

113. Carl Christensen, "Iconoclasm and the Preservation of Ecclesiastical Art in Reformation Nuremberg," *Archiv für Reformationsgeschichte* 61 (1970): 205–21, at 220.

114. StAN, Rep. 44e, SIL 131, nr. 22, fols. 2r–8r, 17r–24r.

115. Seebaß, "Mittelalterliche Kunstwerke," 41–42. Heal, *Cult*, 71.

116. Arnd Reitemeier, *Pfarrkirchen in der Stadt des späten Mittelalters: Politik, Wirtschaft und Verwaltung* (Stuttgart: Franz Steiner, 2005), 242.

117. Malte Prietzel, "Alterleute und Kastenherren: Die Rechnungen der Kirche St. Jacobi in Göttingen von 1523/24 und 1534," *Göttinger Jahrbuch* 41 (1993): 61–95., at 82–85.

118. Nischan, *Lutherans and Calvinists.*

119. Ibid., 145; Kaufmann, *Konfession und Kultur*, 157–203; Holger Reimers, *Ludwig Münstermann: Zwischen protestantischer Askese und gegenreformatorischer Sinnlichkeit* (Marburg: Jonas, 1993).

120. Koerner, *Reformation.*

121. For examples in Lutheran and Catholic territories alike, see Pallas, *Registraturen*, vols. 1–6; Kayser, *Kirchenvisitationen*; Herold, *Brandenburgischen Kirchenvisitations-Abschiede*, vol. 1; Gerhard Zimmermann, ed., *Die brandenburgischen Kirchenvisitations-Abschiede*, vol. 2: *Das Land Ruppin* (Berlin: De Gruyter, 1963); Heyden, *Protokolle*, vols. 1–3; Karl Eder, ed., *Die landesfürstliche Visitation von 1544/1545 in der Steiermark: Ein Beitrag zur Reformationsgeschichte Innerösterreichs* (Graz: Selbstverlag der Landeskomission, 1955); Reiner Braun, ed., *Die bayerischen Teile des Erzbistums Salzburg und des Bistums Chiemsee in der Visitation des Jahres 1558* (Ottilien: St. Ottilien, 1991). Anton Landersdorfer, ed., *Das Bistum Freising in der Bayerischen Visitation des Jahres 1560* (Ottilien: Erzabtei St. Ottilien, 1991).

122. Qtd. in Nischan, *Lutherans and Calvinists*, V, 7.

123. Ibid., 8.

124. "Aus dem Intinerar des Wolfgang Musculus," in *Analecta Lutherana: Briefe und Aktenstücke zur Geschichte Luthers*, ed. Theodor Kolde (Gotha: Perthes, 1883), 216–30, qtd. at 217.

125. Musculus's account of the Mass he attended at Wittenberg, edited by Kolde, has recently been translated into English by Joseph Herl. See *Worship Wars*, 195–96.

126. Nischan, *Lutherans and Calvinists*, V, 9–10.

127. *Osiander Gesamtausgabe* 4:219–56.

128. Klaus Keyser, "Einleitung: Ratschlag zur Elevation, 1538, Januar 3," in *Osiander Gesamtausgabe* 6:434–36.

129. Jacob M. Baum, "Opening a Window to the Devil: Religious Ritual as Baroque Spectacle in Early Modern Germany," in *German Visual Culture*, vol. 2: *Spectacle*, ed. Thomas Haakenson and Jennifer Creech (Oxford: Peter Lang, 2015), 13–40.

130. "Predigtbericht des Achatius Parsberger," in *Osiander Gesamtausgabe* 6:466–468, qtd. at 467, 468.

131. Nischan, "Fractio."

132. Herl, *Worship Wars*, 215–45. The number changes to 8.7 percent when taking into account the full chronological scope of Herl's survey, from 1523 to 1747.

133. Ibid., 224.

134. Ibid., 215–45.

135. Qtd. in Nischan, *Lutherans and Calvinists*, V, 24.

136. Koerner, *Reformation*, 405–7.

137. WA 49, 588–615.

138. Koerner, *Reformation*, 407–12.

139. Ibid., 419. Dieter Grossmann, "Die Bedeutung der Schlosskapellen für den protestantischen Kirchenbau," in *Renaissance in Nord-Mitteleuropa* vol. 1, edited by Georg Ulrich Grossmann (Munich: Deutscher Kunstverlag, 1990), 127–47; Hans-Joachim Krause, "Zur Ikonographie der Protestantischen Schlosskapellen des 16. Jahrhunderts," in *Von Macht der Bilder: Kunst und Reformation*, ed. Ernst Ulmann (Leipzig: Akademie, 1983), 385–412.

140. Koerner, *Reformation*, 405–19.

141. WA 49, 613–14.

142. Ibid. See also Koerner's analysis in *Reformation*, 409–10.

143. Qtd. in Koerner, *Reformation*, 410.

144. Ibid.

145. For a small sample from the Saxon territories, see, for example: Philipp Wagner, *Einweihung des nawen chürfürstlichen Hauses die Augustusburgk genant* (Dresden: Stöckel, 1572), fols. B3r–v; Siegfried Sack, *Von Christlicher Einweihung der Kirchen aus dem Exempel Salomonis . . . in der newen Kirchen in der Newenstadt Magdeburg . . .* (Magdeburg: Roß, 1585), fols. C4v–D1v; Martin Mirus, *Encaenia oder Renovalia der Stifft-Kirchen zu Halberstadt* (Jena: Richtzenhan, 1591), fols. A2r–v; Gregor Strigenitz, *Esrae Predigtstül* (Leipzig: Schnellboltz, 1597), fols. G2r–H2v; Simon Gedicke, *Encaenia oder Einweihung . . . dreyer Kirchen im löblichen Ertzstift Magdeburg* (Magdeburg: Kirchner, 1597); Erhart Lauterbach, *Zwo Einweihungs Predigten . . .* (Leipzig: Lamberg, 1608), fols. A2r–v; Adam Siegfried, *Einweihung der . . . newerbawten Asseburgischen Schloßkirchen zu Walhausen* (Eisleben: Gaubisch, 1616), fols. A2r–v; Balthasar Opitius, *Eine Christliche Predigt/ zur einweihung des neuen Tempels auff S. Georgenthal* (Leipzig: Am Ende, 1613), fols. B1r.

146. For supermusicality, see above, chapter 1.

147. Barbara Pitkin, "The Reformation of Preaching: Transformations of Worship Soundscapes in Early Modern Germany and Switzerland," *Yale Journal of Music and Religion* 1, no. 2 (2015): 5–20.

148. Ibid. See also Beth Kreitzer, "The Lutheran Sermon," in *Preachers and People in the Reformations and Early Modern Period*, ed. Larissa Taylor (Leiden: Brill, 2001), 35–64; Hans-Bernhard Meyer, *Luther und die Messe: eine liturgiewissenschaftliche Untersuchung über das Verhältnis Luthers zum Messwesen des späten Mittelalters* (Paderborn: Bonifatius, 1965).

149. Kreitzer, "Lutheran Sermon."

150. Herl, *Worship Wars*, 215–45.

151. Ibid.; Susan Karant-Nunn, *Reformation of Ritual: An Interpretation of Early Modern Germany* (New York: Routledge, 1997), 125–30.

152. Pitkin, "Reformation of Preaching," 11; Lee Palmer Wandel, *The Eucharist in the Reformation: Incarnation and Liturgy* (Cambridge: Cambridge University Press, 2006), 94–108; Volker Leppin, "Martin Luther," and Thomas Schattauer, "From Sacrifice to Supper: Eucharistic Practice in the Lutheran Reformation," in *A Companion to the Eucharist in the Reformation*, ed. Lee Palmer Wandel (Leiden: Brill, 2013), 39–57, 205–30; Kreitzer, "Lutheran Sermon," 41–42.

153. This was a common refrain in the instructions issued by Nuremberg visitors to the parish churches in its rural hinterlands. Occasionally, visitors even commented on the "dark voices" of bad pastors, or their "monkish accents." See Hirschmann, ed., *Kirchenvisitation*, 66, 70, 84, 94, 198. See also Karant-Nunn, *Reformation of Ritual*, 125–30.

154. Kreitzer, "Lutheran Sermon," 48–51.

155. John Frymire, *The Primacy of the Postils: Catholics, Protestants, and the Dissemination of Ideas in Early Modern Germany* (Leiden: Brill, 2010), 25–75, 77–98, 148–52, 157–224.

156. Herl, *Worship Wars*, 215–45.

157. There is a vast specialized literature on the historical musicology of the Lutheran tradition. Often regarded as the first modern study is Friedrich Blume, *Geschichte der*

evangelischen Kirchenmusik, 2nd ed. (Kassel: Bärenreiter, 1965). For the most comprehensive, up-to-date bibliography in English, See Herl, *Worship Wars*.

158. Herl, *Worship Wars*, 6–7, 217.

159. Ibid, 8–10, 217–18.

160. Ibid., 219–33: Herl identifies them: Strasbourg (1530), Württemberg (1536, 1553, 1565), Augsburg (1537 and 1545), Albertine Saxony (1540), Nördlingen (1544), Braunschweig (1550), Mecklenburg (1552), Eisfeld (1554) and the Palatinate (1554, 1563), Prussia (1558, 1568), Steuerwald (1561), Thüngen (1564), Hesse (1566), Andorff (1567), Ritzebüttel (after 1570), Hohenlohe (1571, 1578), as well as the rural territories under the jurisdiction of cities like Schönburg (1542), Nuremberg and Schwäbisch-Hall (1543), and Wittenberg (1559).

161. Ibid., 218–19.

162. Ibid., 219–233. The major exception to this trend was electoral Brandenburg, which at midcentury still required almost the entire Mass to be sung in Latin.

163. "Itinerar des Wolfgang Musculus." Translated in Herl, *Worship Wars*, 195–96.

164. Ibid.

165. The letter is addressed to the Duke of Norfolk and dated March 14, 1532. In Henry Ellis, ed., *Original Letters Illustrative of English History*, 3rd series, vol. 2 (London: Bentley, 1846), 192.

166. Ibid.

167. "Excerpt from the minutes of the colloquium between Jacob Andreae and Theodore Beza, held at Mömpelgard in 1586," in Herl, *Worship Wars*, 196–98.

168. *Original Letters*, 192.

169. Herl, *Worship Wars*, 195. On defenders of polyphony, see Boyd Brown, *Singing*, 35–36.

170. Herl, *Worship Wars*, 112–23.

171. Gottfried Seebaß, "Mittelalterliche Kunstwerke," 43–44. Bartlett Russell Butler, "Liturgical Music in Sixteenth-Century Nürnberg: A Socio-Musical Study," (PhD diss., University of Illinois, 1970), 107–8, 474.

172. Butler, "Liturgical Music," 434–39.

173. Ibid., 492–505.

174. See Boyd Brown, *Singing*, 36–38.

175. Herl, *Worship Wars*, 117–18. Ulm, which in 1531 broke for a reformed variety of Protestantism, initially went through a radical phase of iconoclasm that included the wholesale elimination of polyphony and organ music. The city only slowly transitioned to Lutheranism in the next generation, beginning around 1570. See Philip Hahn, "Sensing Sacred Space."

176. Herl, *Worship Wars*, 48.

177. Ibid., 130–51.

178. "Aus dem Itinerar," 217.

179. Herl, *Worship Wars*, 130.

180. Butler, "Liturgical Music," 107–8, 474–91.

181. Ibid., 491–92.

182. Qtd. in Herl, *Worship Wars*, 197.

183. Qtd. in Hahn, "Soundscape," 529.

184. Ibid., 530.

185. Hahn identifies the primary uses as summoning parishioners to prayer services and the sermon, and ringing out during funerals. Beyond religious services, the ringing of these large bells as a form of apotropaic magic against natural and supernatural threats continued much as it had in the later Middle Ages. Quotidian uses of the bell were largely the same.

186. Qtd. in Herl, *Worship Wars*, 195.

187. StAN Rep. 44 SIL 131, nr. 22.

188. Compare with Milner, *Senses*, 291–92.

189. Hahn, "Sensing Sacred Space," 71–72.

190. Ibid.

191. Koerner, *Reformation*, 425–29.

192. Ibid., 415.

193. Jacob M. Baum, "From Incense to Idolatry: The Reformation of Olfaction in Late Medieval German Ritual," *Sixteenth Century Journal* 44, no. 2 (2013): 323–44.

194. Prietzel, "Altarleute," 68, 83–91.

195. StAN, Rep. 44e, SIL 131, nr. 22.

196. Heyden, *Protokolle*, 1:46, 283–303; 2:97–104.

197. StAN, Rep. 44e, SIL 112, nr. 12, not paginated.

198. *Corpus Reformatorum* 1, 713. See Bartlett, "Liturgical Music," 128–32, on the influence of Melanchthon's policy in Nuremberg.

199. Rauscher, *Hundert außerwelte, grosse, unverschempte, feiste, wolgemeste, erstunkene Papistische Lugen* (Regensburg: Geißler, 1562), fol. N1v.

200. Compare with Heal, "Art and Identity," and Hahn, "Soundscape," and visual and aural culture, respectively.

201. Taurer, *Hochnothwendigster Bericht wider den newen bildstürmischen carlstadtischen Geist im Fürstenthum Anhald* (Eisleben: Gaubisch, 1597), no pagination.

202. This was a Europe-wide phenomenon. See Richard Palmer, "In Bad Odour: Smell and Its Significance in Medicine from Antiquity to the Seventeenth Century," in *Medicine and the Five Senses*, ed. Roy Porter (Cambridge: Cambridge University Press, 1993), 61–68. In the German-speaking world, the policy was recommended by the most prominent physicians of the sixteenth century, regardless of confessional affiliation. See, for example, Johann Winter von Andernach, *Bericht/ Regiment/ vnd Ordnung wie bei disen sterbenden leüffen/ die Pestilenz vnnd Pestilenzische Fieber züerkennen/ wes sich inn sollichen zeitten zuo curieren vnd zu heylen seye. Ausz beuelch eines Ersamen Rahts/ der statt Straßburg* (Strasbourg: Rihel, 1564), fol. 2r; Johannes Crato von Krafftheim, *Ordnung der preservation/ wie man sich wider die erschreckliche seuche der pestilenz verwahren/ auch rath wie die erkant vnd curiert werden sol/ Mit einer lehr von dem vorsorg der geschwir/ etc* (Breslau: Scharffenberg, 1555), fol. A2v; Caspar Kegler, *Ein nützliches vnd tröstlichs Regiment wider dy Pestilenz* (Leipzig: Schumann, 1529), fols. G1r–G3r; Matthias Unzer, *Kurtzer und einfältiger doch nützlicher und nothwendiger Bericht von der Pestilenz . . .* (Halle: Hynitzsch, 1607), fols. A4v–B1r.

203. His sermons were collected and published a year after his death. See Pankratius, *Fünfzehn Predigten von der schrecklichen Plage der Pestilenz* (Hof: Pfeilschmidt, 1577).

204. Ibid., fol. Dd2r.

205. Ernst Mummenhoff, *Die öffentliche Gesundheits- und Krankenpflege im alten Nürnberg, unveränderter Nachdruck aus 'Festschrift zur Eröffnung des neuen Krankenhauses der Stadt Nürnberg, s. 1–122' (1898)* (Neustadt an der Aisch: Verlag für Kunstreproduktion Christoph Schmidt, 1986), 4–10, 27, 54.

206. Compare with Baum, "Incense to Idolatry."

207. Leppin, "Kirchenausstattungen," 147–51.

208. Koslofsky, "Kiss of Peace."

209. Ibid. On the fraction, see Nischan, "Fractio."

210. David Sabean, *Power in the Blood: Popular Culture and Village Discourse in Early Modern Germany* (Cambridge: Cambridge University Press, 1984), 37–60; John Bossy, *Christianity in the West, 1400–1700* (Oxford: Oxford University Press, 1985), 66–72; Karant-Nunn, *Reformation of Ritual*, 130–34.

211. Jesse Spohnholz, "Multiconfessional Celebration of the Eucharist in Sixteenth-Century Wesel," *Sixteenth Century Journal* 39, no. 3 (2008): 705–29.

Chapter 6. Thinking with the Senses in the Second Reformation

1. Gedicke, "Calvinische Abendmahl gehalten zu Cölln an der Spree in der Domkirche, genannt zue Heiligen Dreyfaltigkeit, Anno Chri. 1613 am Heiligen Christtage," UB Göttingen, Cod.MS.hist.189.I: 10–11. Cited and quoted in Bodo Nischan, *Lutherans and Calvinists in the Age of Confessionalism* (Burlington, Vt.: Ashgate, 1999), IV, 22.

2. Bodo Nischan, in his later work, has done more than anyone else to develop the idea of this era as a Second Reformation. See especially his *Prince, People, and Confession: The Second Reformation in Brandenburg* (Philadelphia: University of Pennsylvania Press, 1994), and his collected essays in *Lutherans and Calvinists.*

3. In this regard, much of the scholarship derives from Scribner's fundamental insights in his essay "Ritual and Reformation," first published in *Popular Culture and Popular Movements in Reformation Germany* (London: Hambledon, 1987), 103–22.

4. Nischan, *Lutherans and Calvinists*, II, 142–58; IV, 31–50.

5. This in many respects goes back to the earlier work of Ernst Walter Zeeden, who drew attention to the many *katholische Überlieferungen* (Catholic traditions/hold-overs) in the sixteenth-century Lutheran churches. See Zeeden, *Konfessionsbildung: Studien zur Reformation, Gegenreformation, und katholischen Reform* (Stuttgart: Klett-Cotta, 1985), 113–91. See also Johann Michael Fritz, ed., *Die bewahrende Kraft des Luthertums: Mittelalterliche Kunstwerke in evangelischen Kirchen* (Regensburg: Schnell & Steiner, 1997); Holger Reimers, *Ludwig Münstermann: Zwischen protestantischer Askese und gegenreformatorischer Sinnlichkeit* (Marburg: Jonas, 1993).

6. Vera Isaiasz, "'Architectona Sacra': Feier und Semantik städtischer Kirchweihen im Luthertum des 16.und 17. Jahrhunderts," in *Stadt und Religion in der frühen Neuzeit: Soziale Ordnungen und ihre Representationen*, ed. Vera Isaiasz (Frankfurt: Campus, 2007), 125–46; Bridget Heal, "'Better Papist than Calvinist': Art and Identity in Later Lutheran Germany," *German History* 29, no. 4 (2011): 584–609.

7. Werner Freitag, "Berühren, Bekleiden, Niederknien: 'Wunderthätige Gnadenbilder' im Zeitalter der Konfessionalisierung," in *Die Bildlichkeit symbolischer Akte: Symbolische*

Kommunikation und gesellschaftliche Wertesysteme vom Mittelalter bis zur französischen Revolution, ed. Barbara Stollberg-Rilinger (Münster: Rhema, 2010), 200–221; Susan Karant-Nunn, *Reformation of Ritual: An Interpretation of Early Modern Germany* (New York: Routledge, 1997), 133.

8. Heal, "Art and Identity." Heal identifies the expression with Polycarp Leyser, Lutheran court preacher in Dresden from 1594 to 1610.

9. For the most part, this is a conclusion drawn from the lack of engagement with the Calvinist side of the debate, although Susan Karant-Nunn has recently argued more explicitly for a more general "de-sensualization" or "suppression" of both senses and emotions within the Protestant tradition, culminating with Calvinist or reformed views. See Karant-Nunn, "'Gedanken, Herz und Sinn': Die Unterdrückung der religiösen Emotionen," in *Kulturelle Reformation: Sinnformationen im Umbruch, 1400–1600*, ed. Bernhard Jussen and Craig Koslofsky (Göttingen: Vandenhoeck & Ruprecht, 1999), 69–96. More recently, see Karant-Nunn, *Reformation of Feeling: Shaping the Religious Emotions in Early Modern Germany* (Oxford: Oxford University Press, 2010), 101–7.

10. Mia Mochizuki, *The Netherlandisch Image after Iconoclasm: Material Religion in the Dutch Golden Age* (Burlington, Vt.: Ashgate, 2008), esp. 1–3.

11. *Corpus Reformatorum: Philippi Melanthonis Opera quae supersunt omnia*, vol. 11, ed. Karl Gottlieb Bretschneider (Halle: Schwetschke, 1843), 281.

12. Sasha Salatowsky, *De anima: Die rezeption der aristotelischen Psychologie im 16. und 17. Jahrhundert* (Amsterdam: Grüner, 2006), 114–16. See also *Corpus Reformatorum* 3:493, for Melanchthon's own comments on improving Aristotle in light of the new scientific advances.

13. *Corpus Reformatorum* 13, 128.

14. Brief biographies of these men can be found in the *Neue Deutsche Biographie*, a periodical now searchable online: https://www.deutsche-biographie.de.

15. Quoting from Otto Heinrich's reform statutes of 1558, in August Thorbecke, ed., *Statuten und Reformationen der Universität Heidelberg vom 16. bis 18. Jahrhundert* (Leipzig: Duncker & Humblot, 1891), 99. Similar statutes were passed under Ludwig VI in 1580, and his successor Johann Casimir, in 1588. See Thorbecke, *Statuten*, 161, 200, 220.

16. Strigel, *Jn Philippi Melanchthonis Libellum de anima notae breves et ervditae* (Leipzig: Wipprecht, 1590). Strigel was professor of ethics at Leipzig and Jena before coming to Heidelberg in 1568.

17. Sebastian Leonhart, *Kurtze vnd einfeltige Beschreibung totivs cvrricvli vitae* (Dresden: n.p., 1592), fol. 8v.

18. Franz Hüttner, ed., "Selbstbiographie des Stadtpfarrers Wolfgang Ammon (d. 1634)," *Archiv für Kulturgeschichte* 1 (1903), 50–98, at 72.

19. Friedrich Wilhelm Cuno, "Scultetus, Abraham," *Allgemeine Deutsche Biographie* (1891), 492–96. Scultetus also left behind an autobiography which provides an invaluable record of this perspective on his development as an intellectual, as well as his involvement in the momentous political events of the early seventeenth century. See Scultetus, *De curriculo vitae, inprimis vero de actionibus Pragensibus Abrahami Sculteti, Professoris nuper Theologi, in florentissima tunc Academia Heidelbergensi, narratio apologetica* (Emden: Petreus, 1625). It was first translated into German by one Andreas Palatinus, appearing

in 1628 under the title *Historische Erzehlung von dem Lauff des Lebens, insonderheit aber von den Pragerischen Handlungen D. Abraham Sculteti, gewesenen Professoris Theologiae, in der Fürtrefflichen Academi zu Heidelberg* (Emden: Kallenbach, 1628). A modern edition of this translation has been published by Gustav Benrath as *Die Selbstbiographie des Heidelberger Theologen und Hofpredigers Abraham Scultetus (1566–1624)* (Karlsruhe: Evangelischer Presseverband, 1966).

20. Scultetus, *De sensu et sensibilibus assertiones physicae, cum discussione problematum quorundam opticorum et astronomicorum* (Heidelberg: Smesmannus, 1591).

21. Scultetus, *Ethicorum libri duo, eiusdem studio laelli peregrine philosophi romani de noscendis et emendandis animi affectionibus* (Oberursel: Sutor, 1603). David Sytsma has devoted some attention to this piece of Scultetus's oeuvre. See Sytsma, "The Logic of the Heart: Analyzing the Affections in Early Reformed Orthodoxy," in *Church and School in Early Modern Protestantism: Studies in Honor of Richard A. Muller on the Maturation of Theological Tradition*, ed. David Sytsma (Leiden: Brill, 2013), 471–88.

22. Sytsma, "Logic," 474–83.

23. Scultetus, *Ethicorum*, 26–38, 129–165, esp. 132–34, 154.

24. Ibid., 134.

25. Clyde Manschrek, "The Role of Melanchthon in the Adiaphora Controversy," *Archiv für Reformationsgeschichte* 48 (1957), 165–81; Thomas Kaufmann, *Das Ende der Reformation: Magdeburgs "Herrgotts Kanzlei" (1548–1551/2)* (Tübingen: Mohr Siebeck, 2003); Thomas Kaufmann, "Our Lord God's Chancery" in "Magdeburg and Its Fight against the Interim," *Church History* 73, no. 3 (2004): 566–82; Luka Ilić, *Theologian of Sin and Grace: The Process of Radicalization in the Theology of Matthias Flacius Illyricus* (Göttingen: Vandenhoeck & Ruprecht, 2014), 87–131; Anja Moritz, *Interim und Apokalypse: Die religiösen Vereinheitlichungsversuche Karls V im Spiegel der magdeburgischen Publizistik, 1548–1551/52* (Tübingen: Mohr Siebeck, 2011); Nathan Baruch Rein, "Faith and Empire: Conflicting Visions of Religion in a Late Reformation Controversy—The Augsburg *Interim* and its Opponents, 1548–50," *Journal of the American Academy of Religion* 71, no. 1 (March 2003): 45–74; Luise Schorn-Schütte, ed., *Das Interim 1548/50: Herrschaftskrise und Glaubenskonflikt* (Gütersloh: Gütersloher Verlagshaus, 2005).

26. Nischan, *Lutherans and Calvinists* 2:144–45. See also Tom G. A. Hardt, "The Saliger Sacramental Controversy," *Lutheran Quarterly* 4 (1990): 405–18.

27. *Corpus Reformatorum* 7, 29.

28. Ibid., 40–44.

29. Matthew Milner, *The Senses and the English Reformation* (Burlington, Vt.: Ashgate, 2011), 283–341; Matthew Milner, "The Senses and Religion: Towards the Reformation of the Senses," in *A Cultural History of the Senses in the Renaissance*, ed. Hermann Roodenburg (New York: Bloomsbury, 2014), 87–105, at 104–5.

30. For Flacius, see Marina Miladinov, "Mittelding or Idolatry? Veneration of Saints in Matthias Flacius Illyricus (1520–1575)," in *Matija Vlačić Ilirik: Zbornik radova s Drugog međunarodnog znanstvenog skupa Matija Vlačić Ilirik*, ed. Marina Miladinov (Labin: Grad Labin, 2008), 75–107. See also Nikolaus Gallus, *Eine Disputation von Mitteldingen, vnd von itzigen verenderungen in kirchen, die Christlich vnd wol geordnent sind* (Magdeburg: Rödinger, 1550).

31. Westphal, *Verlegung des gründlichen Berichts der Adiaphoristen* (Magdeburg, 1551), fols. C4r–D2r.

32. Heller had been city astronomer since the mid-1540s, had run his own printing press, served as city mathematician and rector of the school of St. Egidien. He came to trial before the city council in 1562 and early 1563, but it seems that a sizable Gnesio-Lutheran faction had been in the city for quite some time before this. The language often came up in the course of evening gatherings held at other Gnesio-Lutherans' homes in the city, according to Heller's account. The records of the trial can be found in StAN Rep. A-Akten, SIL 182, Nr. 2. For further analysis of the case, see Jacob M. Baum, "Opening a Window to the Devil: Religious Ritual as Baroque Spectacle in Early Modern Germany," in *German Visual Culture*, vol. 2: *Spectacle*, ed. Thomas Haakenson and Jennifer Creech (Oxford: Peter Lang, 2015), 13–40.

33. Lyndal Roper, "Martin Luther's Body: The 'Stout Doctor' and His Biographers," *American Historical Review* 115, no. 2 (2010): 351–84.

34. Qtd. in Miladinov, "Mittelding," 85.

35. See chapter 4 for an overview of Witzel.

36. Hermann Ehmer, ed., *Leben des Jakob Andreae, Doktor der Theologie, von ihm selbst mit großer Treue und Auftrichtigkeit beschrieben, bis auf das Jahr 1562* (Stuttgart: Calwer, 1991), 31.

37. Ibid., 33.

38. Ibid., 49.

39. Ibid., 35.

40. Karl Gustav Veesenmeyer, ed., *Sebastian Fischers Chronik, besonders von Ulmischen Sachen* (Ulm: Nübling, 1896), 137.

41. Ibid., 139.

42. Ibid., 159.

43. Ibid., 159.

44. Westphal, *Zwo Schrifften M. Joachimi Westphali, Pfarherrn zu Hamburg*. . . (Magdeburg: Rödinger, 1550), fol. A3v.

45. Gallus, *Disputation*, fol. F3r.

46. Pfeffinger, *Grüntlicher und warhafftiger Bericht der vorigen und jetzigen für und nach dem Kriege ergangen Handlungen von den Adiaphoris oder Mitteldingen* (Leipzig: Bapst, 1550), fols. A3r–v, E4r–v, G4r–v, G6v.

47. Westphal, *Zwo Schrifften*, fol. A2r.

48. Westphal, *Kurtzer begriff der Argument und Beweisungen, durch welche die Dienstbarkeit in Caeremonien von den Papisten und ihren Dienern zu leiden aufgelegt, verworffen, und verlegt wird* (Magdeburg: n.p., 1549), fol. A3v.

49. Ibid., fol. B1r.

50. Westphal, *Vier Predigten, das man den tewren schatz Göttlichs worts, unnd des rechten Gottesdiensts bewaren sol, widder die Papisten, Interimisten und Adiaphoristen* (Magdeburg: Lotter, 1550), fol. A4v.

51. Flacius, *Ein Buch, von waren und falschen Mitteldingen* (Magdeburg: Rödinger, 1550), fol. K2r. Flacius, *Erklerung der schendlichen Suonde der jenigen die durch das Concilium Interim vnd Adiaphora von Christo zu Antichrist fallen* (Magdeburg: Rödinger, 1550), fols. B4r–C1r.

52. Amsdorf, *Horas canonicas in Klöstern und Stifften singen und gebotene Adiaphora halten, ist eben so wol Abgötterey, als die schentlichste Opffermesse* (Jena: Rhebart, 1563), fol. B2v.

53. Ibid.

54. "Heller an Schöber," in StAN, Rep. 15a. A–Akten, SIL 182 (unnumbered item).

55. Ibid.

56. During Heller's trial, the city council ordered a comprehensive investigation of his personal library, which documented the presence of these books, as well as several letters from Matthias Flacius and Nikolaus Gallus. See "Reliquiae Bibliothek Regiomontanae," in StAN, Rep. 15a. A–Akten, SIL 182 (unnumbered item).

57. Gallus, *Disputation*, fol. C4r.

58. Westphal, *Vier predigten*, fol. C4v.

59. Flacius, *Christlicher vnd bestendiger Grundt/ von der Waren/ Wesentlichen/ Eusserlichen gegenwart vnd muendlicher niessung deß Leibs vnd Bluts Christ/ im H. Abendmal* (n.p., 1575), fols. 43v, 47v.

60. Ibid., preface (unpaginated).

61. Ibid., fols. 25r–v.

62. Ibid., fols. 27r–30v.

63. Ibid., fols. 6v–7r.

64. Ibid., fol. 42v.

65. Compare with Milner, *Senses*, 202–3.

66. Flacius, *Niessung*, fols. 37v–38r: daß er [der mensch] moege nit allein von vnseren seelen durch den glauben/ sondern auch von vnserm Leib durch die sinne/ vnd sonst auff andere weise/ wie im gefallen/ begriffen werden . . . [further] die Natur oder eigenschafft deß menschen/ welcher nit allein eine Seele/ sondern auch ein Leib hat/ vnd sich nur viel nach dem leib oder fleisch vnd seinen sinnen richten vnd regiren muß/sonderlich aber/ seider oder nach dem jammerlichen fall/ ja auch geistlichen tod der Seele/ so sich im Paradiß durch die verführung vnnd ermordung deß Satans zugetragen hat . . .

67. The peripatetic axiom is often observed in scholarship on Aquinas's treatments of sense perception. For an overview with relevant bibliographic references, see Pekka Kärkäinnen, "The Senses in Philosophy and Science: Mechanics of the Body or Activity of the Soul?" in *A Cultural History of the Senses in the Middle Ages*, ed. Charles Newhauser (London: Bloomsbury, 2014), 111–32.

68. Flacius, *Niessung*, fol. 38v.

69. Ibid., fol. 25r–v.

70. Ibid., fol. 25r.

71. Ibid., fol. 36r.

72. Ibid., fol. 36r.

73. "Concordien-formel (1577), Epitome, article VII, no. 6," Das evangelische Archiv im Internet, accessed July 5, 2017, http://www.glaubensstimme.de/doku.php?id=bekenntnisse:concordienformel.

74. Chemnitz, *Die Reine gesunde Lehre von der wahren gegenwertigkeit des Leibs vnd Bluts Christi in seinem abendmal* (Leipzig: Vögelin, 1561), 20–21.

75. Ibid., 22.

76. Ibid., 29. See also Nikolaus Selnecker, *Libellvs brevis et vtilis, de Coena Domini editus* (Strasbourg: Mylius, 1561), 58; Nikolaus Selnecker, *Paedagogia christiana: continens capita et locos doctrinas christianae* (Frankfurt: Brubach, 1565), 689–91; Nikolaus Selnecker, *Bericht von der waren gegenwertigkeit des leibs vnd bluts vnsers Herrn* (Heidelberg: Mayer, 1565), fols. 72v–74v, 80r–v, 82r; Cyriacus Spangenberg, *Wider die Verleugner der Gegenwäartigkeit des Leibes Christi im Sacrament* (Ursel: Heinrich, 1583), fols. A5r, B7r–B8r.

77. Selnecker, *Paedegogia*, 689–91.

78. Selnecker, *Bericht*, fols. 72v–73r.

79. Alister McGrath, *Reformation Thought: An Introduction*, 2nd ed. (Oxford: Blackwell, 1993), 121. Glenn Most, *Doubting Thomas* (Cambridge, Mass.: Harvard University Press, 2007), 140–49.

80. Scultetus, *Neue Zeitung aus Berlin in zweyen christlichen Gesprächen zweyer wandersleut/ Hans Knorren/ vnd Benedict Haberecht/ von dem jetzigen Zustand zu Berlin* (Pfirt: Knobloch, 1614), 36–37.

81. Gunnoe, *Thomas Erastus and the Palatinate: A Renaissance Physician in the Second Reformation* (Leiden: Brill, 2011), 8–20, 139–40; Volker Press, "Die 'Zweite Reformation' in der Kurpfalz," in *Die reformierte Konfessionalisierung in Deutschland*, ed. Heinz Schilling (Gütersloh: Gütersloher Verlagshaus, 1986), 104–29.

82. Kaspar Olevianus, *Summ vnd jnnhalt vier predigten vom H. Abendmahl vnsers Heilands Jesu Christi: Darinn allein auß Gottes wort vnd nicht auß der vernunfft noch menschlichen Lehr, der rechte einfältige verstandt . . . wirdt fürgetragen* (Heidelberg: Mayer, 1564), fol. 3r.

83. Gunnoe, *Erastus*, 61–70.

84. Heshusius, *Das Jesu Christi warer Leib vnd Blut im heiligen Abendmal gegenwertig sey/ wider den Rottengeist zu Bremen/ Doct. Albert Hardenberg* (Magdeburg: Kirchener, 1560), fol. C4r.

85. Heshusius, *Treue Warnung für den Heidelbergischen Calvinischen Catechismum* (Eisleben: Gaubisch, 1564), fol. 54v.

86. Ibid., fol. 57v.

87. Heshusius, *Jesu Christi*, fol. L2v.

88. Ibid., fols. F4r–v, K1v–K2r; Heshusius, *Warnung*, fols. 24v–25r.

89. Heshusius, *Treue Warnung*, 23r, 24v–25r.

90. Karant-Nunn, *Reformation of Feeling*, 97–99.

91. Heshusius, *Trostbüchlein, in hohen geistlichen Anfechtungen vnd schwermütiger Trawrigkeit* (Jena: Ernst von Gera, 1572), 56: "vnter des wil auch noetig sein, das die Christen so in anfechtung sind/ offt zum Tisch des Herrn gehn. Denn solche speise hat der Son Gottes dazu verordnet/ das wir vnser mattes vnd schier verschmachtes Gewissen/ damit laben vnd erquicken sollen, vnd Gott will durch vleißige betrachtung vnser empfangner Tauffe/ auch stete niessung des Leibs vnd Bluts Christi in vns Krefftig sein/ vnser Gewissen versigeln/ den Glauben stercken/ der anfechtung stewren/ den Geist geben/ vnd seine gaben in vns vermehren."

92. Heshusius, *Jesu Christi*, fols. E1v, E3v, L2r–v; Heshusius, *Warnung*, fols. 47v–49r.

93. Heal, "'Better Papist than Calvinist,'" esp. 603–8; Kaufmann, *Konfession und Kultur*, 157–99; Reimers, *Ludwig Münstermann*.

94. Heshusius, *Warnung*, fols. 25v–26r.
95. Flacius, *Niessung*, fols. 26v–27r.
96. Ibid., fol. 35v.
97. Ibid., fols. 36r–v.
98. Willing, *Ettliche Christliche predigten/ so in werendem Reichsztag zu Augspurg/ anno domini 1566* (Heidelberg: Agricola, 1567), fol. 164r–v.
99. Ibid., fols. 165r–v.
100. Ibid., fol. 167r.
101. Ibid., fol. 176v.
102. *Katechismus oder christlicher Underricht, wie der in Kirchen und Schulen der Churfürstl. Pfaltz getrieben wirdt* (Heidelberg: Mayer, 1563). For useful background, see Lyle Bierma, Charles Gunnoe, and Karin Maag, eds., *An Introduction to the Heidelberg Catechism: Sources, History, and Theology* (Grand Rapids, Mich.: Baker Academic, 2005).
103. Gunnoe, *Thomas Erastus*.
104. Ursinus, *Gründtlicher bericht vom heiligen Abendmal unsers Herren Jesu Christi* (Heidelberg: Mayer, 1564), fol. 8r.
105. Ibid., fols. 10r–v.
106. *Katechismus*, 44–45.
107. Ibid., 50–51.
108. Ibid., 19–20.
109. On these traditional associations, see Victoria von Hoffmann, *From Gluttony to Enlightenment: The World of Taste in Early Modern Europe* (Urbana: University of Illinois Press, 2016), 39–72.
110. Arnold Huijgen, *Divine Accommodation in John Calvin's Theology: Analysis and Assessment* (Göttingen: Vandenhoeck & Ruprecht, 2014). Milner has made the connection between accommodation and sensibility in the English context, although only in passing (see *Senses*, 225). In the German-speaking world, it appears to have been much more central to Calvinist patterns of thinking with the senses.
111. Qtd. in Huijgen, *Accommodation*, 134.
112. Qtd. in Huijgen, *Divine Accommodation*, 134. Huijgen argues that the basis of Calvin's sacramental theology originates with this problem.
113. Thomas Erastus, *Gründtlicher Bericht, wie die wort Christi Das ist mein leib etc zuuersthen seien* (Heidelberg: Lück, 1562), 1–5; Thomas Erastus, *Erzelung etlicher vrsachen, warumb das hochwirdig Sacrament des Nachtmals vnsers Herren vnd Heylandts Jhesu Christi, nicht solle ohne das brodbrechen gehalten werden* (Heidelberg: Mayer, 1563), 1. Olevianus, *Summ*. Ursinus, *Bericht*, fol. 19v.
114. Erastus, *Bericht*, 1–5.
115. Ursinus, *Bericht*, fol. 10r.
116. Ibid., fols. 13v–14r.
117. Erastus, *Bericht*, 9.
118. Gunnoe, *Erastus*, 97–98, 156.
119. Erastus, *Bericht*, 10.
120. Ibid.
121. Ibid., 11.
122. Ibid., 19–20.

123. Erastus, *Brodbrechen*, 11, 13–15.

124. Erastus, *Bericht*, 50.

125. Ursinus, *Bericht*, fols. 7v–8r.

126. Ibid., fols. 11r, 13v.

127. Ibid., fols. 15r, 16v.

128. Olevianus, *Summ*, fol. 3r.

129. Harm Klueting, "Pezel, Christoph," *Neue deutsche Biographie* 20 (2001): 287.

130. Pezel, *Auffrichtige Rechenschafft von Lehr vnd Ceremonien, so jnn euangelischen Reformierten Kirchen/ anch der Richtschnur Goettliches Worts angestellet* (Bremen: Peters, 1592), fols. A3r–v.

131. Ibid., 43, 66–68.

132. Ibid., 69–140.

133. Amling, *Bericht und lehre Göttliches Wort/was von den Ceremonien unnd eusserlichen Kirchenbreuchen . . . zu halten sey* (Zerbst: Schmidt, Bonaventura & Zanach, 1596), 27–28;

134. David Pareus, *Summarische Erklärung, der wahren Catholischen Lehr, so in der Chur Pfaltz bey Rhein, vnd andern vom Bäpstlichen Sawerteyg geseuberten Kirchen bestendig vnd einmütiglich aus Gottes wort geübet wirdt* (Heidelberg: Harnisch, 1593); Johann von Münster, *Christliche und wohlgegründte Antwort des edlen und Ernvehsten Junckhern Johan von Münster zu Vortlage: auff den Schmeichel und recht nach Scorpions Art an ihn gestelten brief Petri Michaelis Brillenmachers Jesuiten Mönchs zu Münster* (Bremen: Peters, 1591).

135. Olearius, *Wider den Caluinischen Grewel der Verwüstung jn des Fürstenthumb Anhalt* (Halle: Gräber, 1597), 77–80.

136. Olearius, *Vorzeichnis mehr denn Zwey hundert Caluinischer Jrrthumb* (Halle: Gräber, 1597), fol. 104v.

137. Leyser, *Christianismus, Papismus, et Calvinismus: Das ist drei unterschiedliche Auslegungen des catechism Luthers* (Dresden: Stöckel, 1602).

138. Pezel, *Ceremonien*, 159.

139. Pezel, *Ceremonien*, 160. Amling, *Bericht*, 70–71, 74.

140. Scultetus, *Kurtzer, aber schrifftmäßiger Bericht von den Götzen Bilder* (Heidelberg: Vögelin, 1620), fol. B2v.

141. Ibid., fols. B2r–v.

142. Pezel, *Ceremonien*, 33–41; Pezel, *Christliche vnd einfeltige Erklerung der notwendigen Lere vom heiligen Abendmal vnsers Herrn Jesu Christi* (Ursel: Nikolaus Henricus, 1578), fols. B2r–B3v, D3r–v, D5r–D6r; Amling, *Bericht*, 74, 84–89, 98–103.

143. Pezel, *Ceremonien*, 37.

144. Ibid., 38.

145. Amling, *Bericht*, 103.

146. On the links between Pareus, Scultetus, and Johann Sigismund of Brandenburg, see Nischan, *Prince*; Nischan, "The Second Reformation in Brandenburg: Aims and Goals," *Sixteenth Century Journal* 14, no. 2 (1983): 173–87.

147. Pareus, *Christlich vnd gründlich Bedencken vom Brot vnnd Brotbrechen im H. Abendmal des Herren* (Amberg: Forster, 1598).

148. Ibid., 82.
149. Ibid., 82–83.
150. Ibid., 83–85.
151. Ibid., 82–89.
152. Ibid., 90–92.
153. Ibid., 92.
154. Scultetus, *Neue Zeitung*, 50, 57–59.
155. Ibid., 29, 44, 56.
156. Ibid., 50. See also 69–70.
157. See Salomon Finck, *Gründliche und Nothwendige Antwort auff die ohn langsten ausgesprengte Berlinische newe Zeitungen oder Gesprechen/ Hansen Knorren/ und Benedict Haberechten/ etc. Wie auch Auff die zween Sacramentspiegel/ so unter dem Namen Salomo Fincken/ Lutherischen Spital Prediger zu Königsberg in Preussen* (Wittenberg: Helwig, 1614). Salomon Finck, *Sacramentspiegel, darinnen zusehen/ wie die alten Schmeißvögel nach der Apostelzeit das Sacrament des Abendmals mit Aberglauben vnnd Menschentandt besudelt vnd solches ohne einigen grundt Göttliches Worts biß auff den heutigen Tag vortheidigen*, 2 vols. (Frankfurt an der Oder: Hartman, 1615–16).
158. Ibid., 57–58.
159. Ibid., 59.
160. Ibid., 50.
161. Ibid., 45.
162. Scultetus, *Selbstbiographie*, 13–14.
163. Ibid., 19.
164. Ibid., 20.
165. Ibid., 21.
166. Qtd. and trans. in Karant-Nunn, *Reformation of Feeling*, 210.

Conclusion

1. For England, see Matthew Milner, *The Senses and the English Reformation* (Burlington, Vt.: Ashgate, 2011).
2. See chapter 5 for Zeeden's notion of "catholic survival" in practice.
3. Again, see Milner, *Senses*, for England.

Bibliography of Primary Sources

Manuscript and Archival Sources

Bayerische Staatsbibliothek, Munich (BSB):
  Cgm. 29, 165, 255, 357, 811, 4483, 9110
Berlin Staatsbibliothek, Preussischer Kulturbesitz (PKB):
  Mgo. 137, 628
Bremen Staats- und Universitätsbibliothek:
  Msc. 0025
Frankfurt am Main Universitätsbibliothek (FMU):
  Ms. Praed. 184, 185
  Ms. germ. oct. 3
Freiburg im Breisgau Augustinermuseum (FBAugustiner):
  Inv. Nr. 11741
Freiburg im Breisgau Erzbischöfliches Archiv (FBeA):
  Hs. 11, 13.
Freiburg im Breisgau Stadtarchiv (FBStadtA):
  B1 Nr. 126
Freiburg im Breisgau Universitätsbibliothek (FBU):
  Hs. 79, 209, 213, 214, 477
Fürstlich Hohenzollernsche Hofbibliothek Sigmaringen (FHHS):
  Ms. 23, 52, 442
Germanisches Nationalmuseum, Nuremberg (GNM):
  Hs 1733, 1734, 1737, 22403, 158088
  HS Merkel 100
Heidelberg Universitätsbibliothek (HU):
  Cpg. 640, 645
Herzogin Anna Amalia Bibliothek, Weimar (HAAB):
  Q 59
  Oct. 76

Köln Erzbischöfliche Diözesan- und Dombibliothek (KeDD)
Cod. 1503
Köln Historisches Archiv der Stadt (HAStK):
7020 72
Landeskirchliches Archiv Nürnberg (LkAN):
Fen. IV 90 12°
Münster Diözesan-Bibliothek (MDB):
Hs. G12 145
Rostock Universitätsbibliothek (RU):
Mss.theol.14
Staatsarchiv Münster (StaM):
Msc. AV (Dep.) 8
Staatsarchiv Nürnberg (StAN):
Rep. A-Akten, SIL 182.
Rep. 44e, Losungamt SIL 112, nr. 12
Rep. 44e, Losungamt SIL 130, Nrs. 6, 7
Rep. 44e, Losungamt SIL 131, Nrs. 2, 7, 7a, 10, 13, 22
Rep. 44e, Losungamt SIL 133, nr. 9
Rep. 59, Nürnberger Salbücher, Nrs. 1, 2, 3
Stadtarchiv Nürnberg (StadtAN)
E1/1731, nrs. 44, 47.
Stadtbibliothek Nürnberg (NSB):
Cent III 85
Cent IV 36, 80
Cent V 29, App 81
Cent VI 43d, 43n, 43o, 57, 59, 81, 82, 85, 91
Cent VII 7, 8, 24, 31, 32, 34, 60, 62, 67, 85
Will II 19.8°
Will 7, 1447
Trier Bistumsarchiv (TbA):
Hs. 529
Tübingen Universitätsbibliothek (TU):
HS Md 123, 277
Wissenschaftliche Stadtbibliothek Mainz (MWSB):
HS I, 51, 82, 221, 240, 322, 418, 422, 427, 434a
HS II 230, 283

Printed Primary Sources

Adler, Kaspar. *Ein Sermon von der Schul Christi*. Augsburg: Grimm, 1523.

Agricola, Johannes. *Eyn kurtze anred zu allen missgünstigen Doctor Luthers vnd der Christenlichen freyheit*. Augsburg: n.p., 1522.

Agricola, Stephan. *Ein Bedencken, wie der wahrhaftig Gottesdienst möcht widerum aufgericht werden*. Eilenburg: Widemar, 1524.

Alberus, Erasmus. *Absag oder Fehdschrift des höllischen Fürsten Lucifers*. Speyer: Schmidt, 1523.

———. *Ein schöner dialogus Martino Luther und der geschickten Botschaft aus der Hölle*. Augsburg: Ramminger, 1523.

Amandus, Georg. *Wye ein geistlicher christlicher ritter und gottes heldt in diser Welt streytten sall*. Zwickau: Gastel, 1524.

Amling, Wolfgang. *Bericht und lehre Göttliches Worts/was von den Ceremonien unnd eusserlichen Kirchenbreuchen zu halten sey*. Zerbst: Schmidt, Bonaventura & Zanach, 1596.

Amsdorf, Nikolaus. *Horas canonicas: In Klöstern und Stifften singen und gebotene Adiaphora halten, ist eben so wol Abgötterey, als die schentlichste Opffermesse*. Jena: Rhebart, 1563.

Andernach, Johann Winter von. *Bericht/ Regiment/ vnd Ordnung wie bei disen sterbenden leüffen/ die Pestilenz vnnd Pestilenzische Fieber züerkennen/ wes sich inn sollichen zeitten zuo curieren vnd zu heylen seye. Ausz beuelch eines Ersamen Rahts/ der statt Straßburg*. Strasbourg: Rihel, 1564.

Aquinas, Thomas. *Opera omnia*. Vol. 12. Rome: Commissio Leonina, 1906.

Auerbach, Johannes von. *Summa de confessionis et de sacramentis*. Augsburg: Zainer, 1469.

Baierland, Ortolf von. *Arzneibuch*. Nuremberg: Koburger, 1477.

Bauer, Gerhard, ed. *Johannes Geiler von Kaysersberg Sämtliche Werke*. 3 vols. Berlin: de Gruyter, 1989–1995.

Bechler, Hans. *Ein Gespräch eines Fuchs und Wolfs*. Augsburg: Ramminger, 1524.

Benrath, Gustav, ed. *Die Selbstbiographie des Heidelberger Theologen und Hofpredigers Abraham Scultetus (1566–1624)*. Karlsruhe: Evangelischer Presseverband, 1966.

Biel, Gabriel. *Sermones* I. Edited by Wendelin Steinbach. Tübingen: Otmar, 1499.

Bihlmeyer, Karl, ed. *Heinrich Seuses: Deutsche Schriften*. Stuttgart: Kohlhammer, 1907.

Billican, Theobald. *Ain Sermon über das wort Christi*. Strasbourg: Knobloch, 1524.

———. *An die christelich kirch versamlung der Stat Weyl*. Augsburg: Ramminger, 1522.

———. *Von der Mess gemayn Schlußred*. Augsburg: Ulhart, 1524.

Boethius. *De institutione musica libri duo, De institutione musica libri quinque*. Edited by Gottfried Friedlein. Leipzig: Teubner, 1867.

Bossler, Ulrich. *Dialogus oder gesprech des Appostolicums angelica und anderer Specerey der Appoteken antreffen Doctor M. Lutterers ler und sine anhanck*. Augsburg: Nadler, 1521.

Braun, Reiner, ed. *Die Bayerischen Teile des Erzbistums Salzburg und des Bistums Chiemsee in der Visitation des Jahres 1558*. Ottilien: St. Ottilien, 1991.

Brenz, Johannes. *Ein sermon zu allen Christgläubigen menschen von der kirchen*. Augsburg: Ramminger, 1523.

Bretschneider, Karl, et al., eds. *Corpus Reformatorum: Opera Omnia Philippi Melanthonis*. 28 vols. Halle: Schwetschke, 1834–1860.

Brunfels, Otto. *Von dem evangelischen anstosz*. Strasbourg: Schott, 1523.

Bryßgauer, Martin. *Wie man christlicher weysz beychten, Sacrament emtpfahen, Mesz halten vnd das Sacrament anbetten sol*. Strasbourg: Schwann, 1524.

Bucer, Martin. *Dialogus, das ist ein Gespräch oder Rede zwischen zweien, einem Pfarrer und einem Schultheiß*. Basel: Wolff, 1521.

———. *Grund und Ursach*. Strasbourg: Köpfel, 1524.

Bugenhagen, Johannes. *Antwort über ein Frage vom hochwürdigen Sakrament*. Erfurt: Loersfeld, 1525.

———. *Etliche christliche Bedenken von der Meß und andern Zeremonien*. Leipzig: Blum, 1525.

———. *Von der evangelischen Meß*. Augsburg: Steiner, 1524.

Buijssen Gerhard, ed. *Durandus' Rationale im spätmittelhochdeutscher Übersetzung*. 4 vols. Assen: Van Gorcum, 1966–1983.

Bulheym, Stefan von. *Ein brüderliche warnung an meister Mathis Pfarrherren zu Sanct Lorentzen im Münster zu Strassburg*. Strasbourg: n.p., 1523.

Burchardi, Ulrich. *Ein Dialogus oder Gespräch von dem christlichen Glauben*. Augsburg: Ramminger, 1524.

———. *Ein schöner, lustiger Dialogus von dem rechten, wahren Glauben*. Augsburg: Ulhart, 1525.

Capito, Wolgang. *Von drei Straßburger Pfaffen und den geäußerten Kirchengütern*. Strasbourg: Köpfel, 1525.

Chemnitz, Martin. *Die Reine gesunde Lehre von der wahren gegenwertigkeit des Leibs vnd Bluts Christi in seinem abendmal*. Leipzig: Vögelin, 1561.

"Concordien-formel (1577), Epitome, article VII, no. 6." Das evangelische Archiv im Internet. Accessed July 5, 2017. http://www.glaubensstimme.de/doku.php?id=bekenntnisse:concordienformel.

Cranach, Lucas. *Wittenberger Heiltumsbuch: Faksimile-Neudruck der Ausgabe Wittenberg 1509*. Unterschneidheim: Uhl, 1969.

Cronberg, Hartmut von. *Ein christliche Schrift und Vermahnung an alle Stände des Römischen Reichs*. Zwickau: Gastel, 1523.

Culmann, Leonhard. *Wie iunge und alt leut recht petten sollen: Ein schlecht einfeltige underrichtung*. Nuremberg: Jobst Gutknecht, 1537.

Cusanus, Nicolas. *De Beryllo* (1453). Translated by Jasper Hopkins. Minneapolis: Banning, 1998.

———. *De pace fidei*. Translated by Jasper Hopkins. Minneapolis: Banning, 1994.

———. *De venatione sapientiae* (1463). Translated by Jasper Hopkins. Minneapolis: Banning, 1998.

———. *Idiota de sapientiae* (1450). Translated by Jasper Hopkins. Minneapolis: Banning, 1996.

Diehl, Adolf, ed. *Dionysius Dreytweins Esslingische Chronik (1548–1564)*. Tübingen: Litterarischen Verein Stuttgart, 1901.

Diepold, Johann. *Ein nützlicher Sermon zu allen Christenmenschen von der rechten evangelischen Meß*. Augsburg: Steiner, 1522.

Dietrich, Veit. *Summaria Christlicher lehr, für das junge volck, was auss eim yeden Sontags Euangelio u mercken sey*. Nuremberg: Berg & Neuber, 1555.

Distelmaier, Konrad. *Ein Gesprächbüchlein von eim Gsodschneider und eim Holzhauer*. Augsburg: Froschauer, 1523.

Drübel, Eckhart zum. *Ein demütige Ermahnung an ein ganze gemeine Christenheit.* Augsburg: Ramminger, 1523.

Durandus, William. *Rationale divinorum officiorum.* Lyon: Huguetan, 1508.

Ellis, Henry, ed. *Original Letters Illustrative of English History.* 3rd series, vol. 2. London: Bentley, 1846.

Eder, Karl, ed. *Die landesfürstliche Visitation von 1544/1545 in der Steiermark: Ein Beitrag zur Reformationsgeschichte Innerösterreichs.* Graz: Selbstverlag der Landeskomission, 1955.

Ehmer, Hermann, ed. *Leben des Jakob Andreae, Doktor der Theologie, von ihm selbst mit großer Treue und Auftrichtigkeit beschrieben, bis auf das Jahr 1562.* Stuttgart: Calwer, 1991.

Elbogen, Sebastian Schlick von. *Ordnung, wie es soll mit dem Gottesdienst und desselben dienern in der Stadt Elbogen gehalten werden.* Augsburg: Steiner, 1523.

Erasmus, Desiderius. *De ratione studij, ac legendi, interpretandique auctores libellus aureus.* Strasbourg: Knobloch, 1521.

Erastus, Thomas. *Erzelung etlicher vrsachen, warumb das hochwirdig Sacrament des Nachtmals vnsers Herren vnd Heylandts Jhesu Christi, nicht solle ohne das brodbrechen gehalten werden.* Heidelberg: Mayer, 1563.

———. *Gründtlicher Bericht, wie die wort Christi Das ist mein leib etc zuuersthen seien.* Heidelberg: Lück, 1562.

Evangelischer Oberkirchenrat Württemberg, eds. *Reformation in Württemberg: Ausstellung zur 450-Jahr-Feier der Evangelische Landeskirche, Württembergische Landesbibliothek Stuttgart, 15 May bis 22 Juli 1984.* Stuttgart: Calwer, 1984.

Falk, Franz, ed. *Die pfarramtlichen Aufzeichnungen (Liber consuetudinum) des Florentius Diel zu St. Christoph in Mainz (1491–1518).* Freiburg im Breisgau: Herder, 1904.

Fellmann, Walter, ed. *Hans Denck Schriften.* 3 vols. Gütersloh: Gütersloher, 1956–1960.

Fener, Georg. *Sturm wider ein layman thurn als Römischen predigers.* Augsburg: Grimm & Wirsung, 1521.

Finck, Salomon. *Gründliche und Nothwendige Antwort auff die ohn langsten ausgesprengte Berlinische newe Zeitungen oder Gesprechen/ Hansen Knorren/ und Benedict Haberechten/ etc. Wie auch Auff die zween Sacramentspiegel/ so unter dem Namen Salomo Fincken/ Lutherischen Spital Prediger zu Königsberg in Preussen.* Wittenberg: Helwig, 1614.

———. *Sacrament des Abendmals mit Aberglauben vnnd Menschentandt besudelt vnd solches ohne einigen grundt Göttliches Worts biß auff den heutigen Tag vortheidigen.* 2 vols. Frankfurt an der Oder: Hartman, 1615–16.

Firn, Anton. *Supplication eines Pfarrers und der Pfarrkinder zu St. Thoman.* Augsburg: Ulhart, 1524.

Flacius, Matthias. *Christlicher vnd bestendiger Grundt/ von der Waren/ Wesentlichen/ Eusserlichen gegenwart vnd muendlicher niessung deß Leibs vnd Bluts Christ/ im H. Abendmal.* N.p., 1575.

———. *Ein Buch, von waren und falschen Mitteldingen.* Magdeburg: Rödinger, 1550.

———. *Erklerung der schendlichen Suonde der jenigen die durch das Concilium Interim vnd Adiaphora von Christo zu Antichrist fallen.* Magdeburg: Rödinger, 1550.

Fridolin, Stefan. *Schatzbehalter der wahren Reichtümer des Heils*. Nuremberg: Koburger, 1491.

Fritzhans, Johann. *An ein ehrbarn, ehrsamen, weisen Rat und ganze christliche Gemein der Stadt Magdeburg, Gottes Wort belangende*. Wittenberg: Lufft, 1523.

———. *Wie man das klar hell Gotteswort predigen soll*. Zwickau: Gastel, 1524.

Gallus, Nikolaus. *Eine Disputation von Mitteldingen, vnd von itzigen verenderungen in kirchen, die Christlich vnd wol geordnent sind*. Magdeburg: Rödinger, 1550.

Gedicke, Simon. *Encaenia oder Einweihung . . . dreyer Kirchen im löblichen Ertzstift Magdeburg*. Magdeburg: Kirchner, 1597.

Gemigger, Laux. *Zu Lob dem Luther und Ehren der ganzen Christenheit*. Augsburg: Oeglin, 1521.

Gengenbach, Pamphilus. *Der evangelisch Bürger*. Basel: Gengenbach, 1524.

———. *Der Laienspiegel Sancti Pauli des alten Glaubens wider den neuen*. Basel: Gengenbach, 1522.

———. *Dies ist ein jämmerliche Klag über die Totenfresser*. Basel: Gengenbach, 1520.

———. *Von drien Christen, dem Römischen Christen, dem Böhemischen Christen, dem Thürckischen Christen*. Basel: Gengenbach, 1523.

Glentzer, Hans. *Ein hübsche Klag zu unserm Herren über alle Mißbräch geistlich und weltlich Stands*. Augsburg: Ramminger, 1523.

Greiffenberger, Hans. *Disz biechlin sagt von den falschen Kamisierern die sich auß thund vil guts mit fasten peten meße lesen füre andere*. Augsburg: Ulhart, 1523.

———. *Ein kurzer Begriff von guten Werken*. Augsburg: Ramminger, 1524.

———. *Ein Warnung vor dem Teufel der sich wider übt mit seinem Tändelmarkt unter einem gleißenden Schein*. Nuremberg: Gutknecht, 1524.

Greving, Joseph, ed. *Johann Ecks Pfarrbuch für U. L. Frau in Ingolstadt: Ein Beitrag zur Kenntnis der pfarrkirchlichen Verhältnisse im sechzehnten Jahrhundert*. Münster: Aschendorff, 1908.

Grumbach, Argula von. *Eine christenliche Schrifft ainer Erbarn Frawen*. Munich: Schobser, 1523.

———. *Wie ein christliche Frau des Adels in Bayern die Hoheschul zu Ingolstadt strafet*. Augsburg: Ulhart, 1523.

Grünpeck, Joseph. *Dialogus von dem Glauben der Christen und von dem Glauben des Machumeten*. Landshut: Weißenburger, 1522.

Grütsch, Konrad. *Quadragesimale Gritsch de tempore et de Sanctis*. Strasbourg, 1486.

Gümbel, Albrecht, ed. *Das Mesnerpflichtbuch von St. Lorenz in Nürnberg vom Jahre 1493*. Munich: Kaiser, 1928.

———, ed., *Das Mesnerpflichtbuch von St. Sebald in Nürnberg vom Jahre 1482*. Munich: Kaiser, 1929.

Günzburg, Johann Eberlin von. *Klag und Antwort von lutherischen und päpistischen Pfaffen über die Reformation, zu Regensburg ausgangen*. Nuremberg: Höltzel, 1524.

———. *Schöner Spiegel eines christlichen Lebens*. Strasbourg: Schwan, 1524.

———. *Wider die schender der Creaturen Gottes, durch weyhen oder segnen des Saltz, Wasser, Palmen, kraut, wachs, fewr, ayer, fladen etc*. Augsburg: Steiner, 1525.

———. *Wie sich eyn diener Gottes wortts ynn all seynem thun halten sol*. Wittenberg: Rhau-Grunenberg, 1525.

Güttel, Kaspar. *Dialogus oder Gesprächbüchlein von einem rechtgeschaffen Christenmenschen*. Augsburg: Otmar, 1523.

Hätzer, Ludwig. *Disputation gehalten zu Zürich zwischen Ulr. Zwinglin und Löwen Jud*. Zürich: Froschauer, 1523.

———. *Urteil Gottes, unsers Ehegemahls, wie man sich mit allen Götzen und Bildnissen halten soll*. Augsburg: Steiner, 1523.

Hedio, Caspar. *Von den zehenden Zwo trefflicher predig bescheen im Münster zu Straszburg*. Strasbourg: Köpfel, 1524.

Herbst, Hans. *Eyn Brüderliche und Christenliche Heyliger geschrifft gegrundte ermanung*. Nuremberg: Höltzel, 1524.

———. *Eyn gesprech von dem gemaynen Schwabacher Kasten*. Nuremberg: Höltzel, 1524.

Herold, Victor, ed. *Die brandenburgischen Kirchenvisitations-Abschiede und Register des XVI. und XVII Jahrhunderts*. Vol. 1: *Die Prignitz*. Berlin: Kommisionsverlag von Gsellius, 1928.

Herpff, Heinrich. *Sermones fratris Henrici herp . . . de tempore hyemales et festiuales*. Augsburg: Rynman, 1509.

Herrenberg, Gerhard von. *Expositiones textuales dubiorum*. Cologne: Quentell, 1497.

Heshusius, Tilemann. *Das Jesu Christi warer Leib vnd Blut im heiligen Abendmal gegenwertig sey/ wider den Rottengeist zu Bremen/ Doct. Albert Hardenberg*. Magdeburg: Kirchener, 1560.

———. *Treue Warnung für den Heidelbergischen Calvinischen Catechismum*. Eisleben: Gaubisch, 1564.

———. *Trostbüchlein, in hohen geistlichen Anfechtungen vnd schwermütiger Trawrigkeit*. Jena: Ernst von Gera, 1572.

Heyden, Helmut, ed. *Protokolle der Pommerschen Kirchenvisitationen*. 3 vols. Cologne: Böhlau, 1961–1964.

Hitzschold, Matthäus. *Ein sermon vom recht christlichen Leben*. Erfurt: Knappe, 1522.

———. *Von zweyerley menschen*. Wittenberg: n.p., 1523.

Hoffman, Simon. *Sermon, geschehn am Ostertag zu der Frühmesse zu Stolberg*. Erfurt: Buchfürer, 1523.

Hohenlohe, Sigismund von. *Creutz-Biechlinn*. Augsburg: Steiner, 1525.

Hubmaier, Balthasar. *Achtzehn Schlußreden*. Augsburg: Ramminger, 1524.

———. *Etlich Beschlußreden allen Christen von Unterricht der Meß*. Ulm: Hoffischer, 1525.

———. *Summ eines gantzen christenlichen Lebens*. Augsburg: Ramminger, 1525.

Hundt, Magnus. *Anthropologium de hominis dignitate et natura*. Leipzig: Stöckel, 1501.

———. *Introductionum in universalem Aristotelis physicen*. Leipzig: Stöckel, 1500.

Hürten, Heinz ed. *Cusanus-Texte V: Brixener Dokumente: Akten zur Reform des Bistums Brixen*. Heidelberg: Universitätsverlag, 1960.

Hutten, Ulrich von. *Clag vnd vormanung gegen dem übermässigen vnchristenlichen gewalt des Bapsts zu Rom*. Strasbourg: Schott, 1520.

Hüttner, Franz, ed. "Selbstbiographie des Stadtpfarrers Wolfgang Ammon (d. 1634)." *Archiv für Kulturgeschichte* 1 (1903): 50–98.

Janov, Matthias von. *Joan Husz von schedlickeit der menschen satzungen oder Tradition verdeutsch*. Altenburg: Kantz, 1525.

Jud, Leo. *Ein christenlich Widerfechtung wider Matthis Kretzen falsche Meß*. Zurich: Hager, 1524

Kannel, Eustasius. *Evangelisch Gesetz, wie es von Christo predigt*. Strasbourg: Prüss, 1524.

Kantz, Kaspar. *Von der evangelischen Mesß*. Strasbourg: Prüss, 1524.

Karlstadt, Andreas Bodenstein von. *Abtuung der Bilder*. Wittenberg: Schirlentz, 1522.

———. *Antwort, geweiht Wasser belangend*. Wittenberg: Lotter, 1521.

———. *Dialogus oder Gesprächbüchlein von dem Mißbrauch des hochwürdigen Sakraments*. Basel: Bebel, 1524.

———. *Ein nützliche Unterweisung wider der papistischen Messen Mißbrauch*. Augsburg: Ramminger, 1525.

———. *Ein Sermon vom Stand der christgläubigen Seelen*. Augsburg: Ulhart, 1523.

———. *Predigt von Empfahung des Heiligen Sakraments*. Augsburg: Otmar, 1522.

———. *Von Anbetung und Ehrerbietung der Zeichen des Neuen Testaments*. Augsburg: Ramminger, 1521.

———. *Von dem Neuen und Alten Testament*. Augsburg: Ulhart, 1525.

———. *Von dem Priestertum und Opfer Christi*. Jena: Buchfürer, 1523.

———. *Von dem Sabbat und geboten Feiertagen*. Augsburg: Ulhart, 1524.

———. *Von dem widerchristlichen Mißbrauch des Herren Brot und Kelch*. Augsburg: Steiner, 1524.

———. *Von geweihtem Wasser und Salz*. Leipzig: Schumann, 1520.

———. *Von päpstlicher Heiligkeit*. Wittenberg: Lotter, 1520.

———. *Wider die alte und neue papistische Messen*. Basel: Wolff, 1524.

———. *Wie sich der Glaube und Unglaub gegen dem Licht und Finsternis halten*. Basel: Wolff, 1524.

Kastl, Pseudo-Johannes von. *Ein nücz und schone ler von der aygen erkantnuß*. Edited by Renata Wagner. Munich: Beck, 1972.

Katechismus oder christlicher Underricht, wie der in Kirchen und Schulen der Churfürstl: Pfaltz getrieben wirdt. Heidelberg: Mayer, 1563.

Kayser, Karl, ed. *Die reformatorischen Visitationen in den welfischen Landen 1542–1544: Instruktionen, Protokolle, Abschiede und Berichte der Reformatoren*. Göttingen: Vandenhoeck & Ruprecht, 1897.

Kegler, Caspar. *Ein nützliches vnd tröstlichs Regiment wider dy Pestilenz*. Leipzig: Schumann, 1529.

Keller, Michael. *Etlicher Sermones von dem Nachtmahl Christi*. Augsburg: Ulhart, 1525.

Kettenbach, Heinrich. *Ain sermon oder predig von der christlichen kirchen*. Augsburg: Otmar, 1522.

———. *Ein new apologia*. Erfurt: n.p., 1523.

———. *Ein Sermon Bruoder Heinrichs zu der loblichen statt Vlm*. Bamberg: Erlinger, 1523.

———. *Ein sermon vom fasten vnd feyern*. Wittenberg: Rhau-Grunenberg, 1522.

———. *Eyn gesprech Bruder Hainrich von Kettenbach mit aim frommen alte mutterlin von Vlm*. Augsburg: Ramminger, 1523

———. *Eyn Sermon widder des Bapst Kuechen Predyger zu Vlm*. Erfurt: Loersfeld, 1523.

———. *Eyne Predigt auff den achten Sonntag nach dem Pfingstag*. Erfurt: Stürmer, 1525.

———. *Schutzrede, jedem Christen wohl zu wissen, wider das falsch Anklagen der Papisten*. Strasbourg: Köpfel, 1523.

———. *Vergleychung der Bäpst satzung, gegen der leer Christi Jhesu*. Strasbourg: Beck, 1523.

Kisswetter, Wolfgang. *Daß man das lauter, rein Euangelion ohn menschliche Zusatzunge predigen soll*. Altenburg: Kantz, 1525.

Klapper, Josef, ed. *Johannes von Neumarkt: Bischof und Hofkanzler: Religiöse Frührenaissance in Böhmen zur Zeit Kaiser Karls IV*. Leipzig: St. Benno, 1964.

Kolde, Theodor, ed. *Analecta Lutherana: Briefe und Aktenstücke zur Geschichte Luthers*. Gotha: Friedrich Perthes, 1883.

Korn, Gallus. *Ein Handlung, wie es einem Predigermönch zu Nürnberg von wegen der evangelischen Wahrheit gangen ist*. Augsburg: Nadler, 1522.

———. *Warum die kirch vier evangelisten hat*. Zwickau: Schönsperger, 1524

Kraffthеim, Johannes Crato von. *Ordnung der preservation/ wie man sich wider die erschreckliche seuche der pestilenz verwahren/ auch rath wie die erkant vnd curiert werden sol/ Mit einer lehr von dem vorsorg der geschwir/etc*. Breslau: Scharffenberg, 1555.

Krumpach, Nikolaus. *Eyn auserwöllt Byechlin*. Zwickau: Schönsperger, 1524.

Küchenmeisterei. Augsburg: Johann Schaur, 1494.

Landersdorfer, Anton, ed. *Das Bistum Freising in der Bayerischen Visitation des Jahres 1560*. Ottilien: St. Ottilien Verlag, 1991.

Landsperger, Johannes. *Ain nützlicher berücht von nyessung es hochwurdigen Sacraments*. Augsburg: Ramminger, 1524.

———. *Ein christenliche Betrachtung in der Meß*. Augsburg: Ulhart, 1524.

Lauterbach, Erhart. *Zwo Einweihungs Predigten*. Leipzig: Lamberg, 1608.

Leonhart, Sebastian. *Kurtze vnd einfeltige Beschreibung totivs cvrricvli vitae*. Dresden: n.p., 1592.

Leyser, Polycarp. *Christianismus, Papismus, et Calvinismus: das ist drei unterschiedliche Auslegungen des catechism Luthers*. Dresden: Stöckel, 1602.

Liber missarum specialis. Strasbourg: Prüss, 1503.

Linck, Wenceslaus. *Ain Epistel meinen lieben bruedern inn Christo*. Augsburg: Ramminger, 1523.

———. *Artickel vnd posiciones*. Grimma: Widemar, 1523.

———. *Die letzsten drey Psalmen von Orgelen, Paucken, Glocken, und der gleychen eüsserlichen Gotßdienst, ob und wie Got darynnen gelobt wyrdt*. Zwickau: Gastel, 1523.

———. *Dyalogus der auszgelauffen Münch*. Altenburg: Kantz, 1524.

———. *Ein heilsame Lere, wie das Herz . . . durch die sieben Seligkeit . . . auff das Wort Gottes gebauet wird*. Nuremberg: n.p., 1519.

———. *Eyn Sermon von anrueffunge der heyligen*. Wartburg: Gutknecht, 1523.

———. *Hie auff gottes wort allain als auff ainen bestendigen felsen*. Augsburg: Steiner, 1523.

———. *Sermon von dem Außgang der Kinder gottes auß des Entichrists gefengknuß*. Nuremberg: Hergot, 1524.

———. *Wie der grobe Mensch vnsers herren Esel sein sol*. Nuremberg: Gutknecht, 1519.

Locher, Johannes. *Artickel 15 durch grundt götlicher geschrifft*. Zwickau: Schönsperger, 1524.

———. *Gnadenreiches Privilegium christlicher freyheait allerley speyß*. Zwickau: Gastel, 1524.

Lonicer, Johann. *Von ererbyteung und anrüffung der Heiligen, so ferr die göttlich schrifft zeügknüsß gibt.* Strasbourg: Schott, 1523.

Lotzer, Sebastian. *Ain christlicher Sendbrief darin angetzaigt wirt, dz die layen macht vnd recht haben von dem hailigen wort gots reden, leren, vnd schreiben.* Augsburg: Ramminger, 1523.

———. *Ain vast haylsam trostlich christelich unüberwynndtliche beschyrmbüchlein.* Augsburg: Ramminger, 1524.

Luther, Martin. *D. Martin Luthers Werke: Kritische Gesamtausgabe.* 120 vols. Weimar: Böhlau, 1883–2009.

Magnus, Albertus. *Summa theologiae.* Volume 31. Edited by E. Borgnet. Paris: Vives, 1894.

Manuel, Niklaus. *Eyn Faß Nacht spyl vom Bapst vnd siner priesterschafft.* Zurich: Froschauer, 1522.

Marschalk, Haug. *Das heilig, ewig Wort Gottes.* Augsburg: Ramminger, 1523.

———. *Durch Betrachtung und Bekehrung der bösen Gebräuch in schweren Sünden ist gemacht dieser Spiegel der Blinden.* Augsburg: Ramminger, 1522.

———. *Ein edles, schönes Traktätlein von dem reinen himmlischen Wort.* Augsburg: Schönsperger, 1524.

Melanchthon, Philipp. *Vnderscheyd zwyschen weltlicher vnd christlicher fromkeyt.* Strasbourg: Schürer, 1522.

———. *Unterricht der Visitatoren an die Pfarrherrn im Kurfürstenthum zu Sachsen.* Nuremberg: Peypus, 1528.

———. *Von der Messe propositiones.* Altenburg: Kantz, 1525.

Melanchthon, Philipp, and Martin Luther. *Figur des antichristlichen Papsts und seiner Synagog.* Wittenberg: Rhau-Grunenberg, 1523.

Melhofer, Philipp. *Offenbarung der allerheimlichsten Heimlichkeit der jetzigen Baalpriester.* Augsburg: Ulhart, 1525.

———. *Von dem geistlichen Priestertum Christi und aller Gottgläubigen zehn Schlußreden.* Augsburg: Ulhart, 1525.

Meyer, Sebastian. *Von dem Pfründmarkt der Curtisanen vnd Tempelknechten.* Basel: Petri, 1521.

Mirus, Martin. *Encaenia oder Renovalia der Stifft-Kirchen zu Halberstadt.* Jena: Richtzenhan, 1591.

Missale ad notulam dominorum Teutonicorum. Nuremberg: Stuchs, 1499.

———. Hagenau: n.p., 1519.

Missale Argentiense. Basel: Wenssler, 1486.

Missale Augustense. Augsburg: Ratdolt, 1510.

———. Basel: Thum, 1510.

Missale Bambergense. Bamberg: Sensenschmidt, 1490.

———. Bamberg: Pfeyl, 1499.

Missale Basiliense. Basel: Koch, 1479.

Missale Brandenburgense. Nuremberg: Stuchs, 1494.

———. Leipzig: Lorr, 1516.

Missale Brixiense. Basel: n.p., 1511.

Missale Cisterciense. Strasbourg: Grüninger, 1487.

Missale Coloniense. Basel: Wenssler, 1487.
———. Cologne: Quentell, 1494.
———. Cologne: Bumgart, 1498.
Missale Constantiense. Augsburg: Ratdolt, 1505.
Missale Cracoviense. Nuremberg: n.p., 1493.
Missale diocesis Argentinensis. Hagenau: n.p., 1520.
Missale Eystettense. Eichstätt: Reyser, 1486.
———. Eichstätt: n.p., 1494.
Missale Halberstatense. Strasbourg: n.p, 1498.
———. Speyer: n.p., 1511.
Missale Havelbergense. Leipzig: Brandis, 1489.
Missale Herbipolense. Würzburg: Reyser, 1495, 1499.
Missale Hildensemense. Nuremberg: Stuchs, 1511.
Missale itinerantium. Cologne: n.p., 1503.
———. Cologne: Quentell, 1505.
———. Nuremberg: Höltzel, 1507.
———. Nuremberg: Huber, 1510.
Missale Magdeburg. Nuremberg: Stuchs, 1503.
Missale Merszburgn. Leipzig: Lotter, 1502.
Missale Misnense. Mainz: Schöffer, 1485.
———. Leipzig: Lotter, 1502.
Missale Moguntinum. Würzburg: Reyser, 1482.
———. Mainz: Schöffer, 1493.
———. Speyer: Drach, 1497.
———. Strasbourg: Prüss, 1510.
Missale Numburgense. Nuremberg: n.p., 1510.
Missale Ordinis Fratrum eremitarum sancti Augustini. Nuremberg: Order of the Observant Augustinian Hermits, 1491.
Missale Ordinis Praedicatorum. Venice: Frankfurt, 1484.
Missale Ordinis Sancti Benedicti. Hagenau: Anßhelmus, 1518.
Missale Pataviense. Passau: Petri, 1491.
———. Augsburg: Ratdolt, 1493, 1498.
———. Vienna: n.p., 1503, 1507, 1512.
———. Augsburg: n.p., 1505.
———. Winterburger: n.p., 1509.
———. Nuremberg: Heller & Hermann, 1514.
Missale Pragense. Leipzig: n.p., 1498.
Missale Ratisbonense. Regensburg: Sensenschmidt & Beckenhaub, 1485.
———. Bamberg: Petzensteiner, Sensenschmidt, 1492.
———. Bamberg: Pfeyl, 1500.
Missale Romanum. Nuremberg: Stuchs, 1484.
———. Basel: Wenssler, 1487.
Missale Salisburgense. Nuremberg: Stuchs, 1505.
———. Vienna: n.p., 1506, 1510.

———. Basel: n.p., 1510.

Missale secundum ordinem Carthusiensium. Giunta: n.p., 1509.

Missale speciale. Strasbourg: Beck, 1514.

Missale Wormatiense. Basel: Wenssler, 1490.

Monte Rocherii, Guido de. *Manipulus curatorum*. Augsburg: Christmann Heyny, 1481.

Motschiedler, Georg. *Ein newer Dialog oder gespräch zwischen einem verprentem/ vertirbnem Edelman und ainen Münch*. Nuremberg: Hergot, 1525.

Müncheberg, Lintholz von. *Textus trium librorum de anima*. Frankfurt an der Oder: Baumgarten, 1507.

Münster, Johann von. *Christliche und wohlgegründte Antwort des edlen und Ernvehsten Junckhern Johan von Münster zu Vortlage: Auff den Schmeichel und recht nach Scorpions Art an ihn gestelten brief Petri Michaelis Brillenmachers Jesuiten Mönchs zu Münster*. Bremen: Peters, 1591.

Müntzer, Thomas. *Ordnung und Berechnung des deutschen Amts zu Allstedt*. Eilenburg: Widemar, 1520.

Mykonius, Friedrich. *Eyn freüntlich ermanung vnd tröstung aller freündt vnd liebhaber gottis*. Zwickau: Schönsperger, 1524.

Nagel, Hans. *Von dem Glauben Gottes, der allein selig machet*. Augsburg: Steiner, 1525.

Oberndorf, Cuntz von. *Dialogus oder ein Gespräche wider Doktor Ecken Büchlein*. Leipzig: Stöckel, 1520.

Oberweimar, Florentina von. *Ein Geschicht wie Gott einer ehrbarn Klosterjungfrauen ausgeholfen hat*. Wittenberg: Cranach & Döring, 1524.

Obsequiale augustanum. Augsburg: Ratdolt, 1487.

Oechsner, Wolfgang. *Eyn kurtzer vnterricht von dem geplerre vnd mißbrauch der Seelmessen*. Nuremberg: Hergot, 1524.

Oecolampadius, Johannes. *Ain predig und ermanung . . . von wirdigen Ereenbietung dem Sacrament des fronleichnam Christi*. Augsburg: Grimm & Wirsung, 1521.

———. *Ein schöne Epistel an Kaspar Hedion*. Augsburg: Steiner, 1522.

Olearius, Johann. *Vorzeichnis mehr denn Zwey hundert Caluinischer Jrrthumb*. Halle: Gräber, 1597.

———. *Wider den Caluinischen Grewel der Verwüstung jn des Fürstenthumb Anhalt*. Halle: Gräber, 1597.

Olevianus, Kaspar. *Summ vnd jnnhalt vier predigten vom H. Abendmahl vnsers Heilands Jesu Christi: Darinn allein auß Gottes wort vnd nicht auß der vernunfft noch menschlichen Lehr, der rechte einfältige verstandt . . . wirdt fürgetragen*. Heidelberg: Mayer, 1564.

Opitius, Balthasar. *Eine Christliche Predigt/ zur einweihung des neuen Tempels auff S. Georgenthal*. Leipzig: Am Ende, 1613.

Ordinarius magdeburgensis. Leipzig: Brandis, 1485.

Ordo missalis Frisingensis. Augsburg: Ratdolt, 1502.

Osiander, Andreas. *Grund und Ursach aus der Heiligen Schrifft, wie und warum die Pröpst zu Nürnberg die Mißbrauch bei der heiligen Meß geändert haben*. Nuremberg: Höltzel, 1524.

Osiander, Andreas, and Dominikus Schleupner, Thomas Venatorius. *Ein gutt unterricht unnd getreuer rathschlag*. Bamberg: Erlinger, 1524.

Pallas, Karl, ed. *Die Registraturen der Kirchenvisitationen im ehemals sächsische Kurkreise.* 6 vols. Halle: Hendel, 1906–1918.

Paltz, Johannes von. *Coelifoedina.* Erfurt: Schenck, 1502.

Pankratius, Andreas. *Fünfzehn Predigten von der schrecklichen Plage der Pestilenz.* Hof: Pfeilschmidt, 1577.

Pareus, David. *Christlich vnd gründlich Bedencken vom Brot vnnd Brotbrechen im H. Abendmal des Herren.* Amberg: Forster, 1598.

———. *Summarische Erklärung, der wahren Catholischen Lehr, so in der Chur Pfaltz bey Rhein, vnd andern vom Bäpstlichen Sawerteyg geseuberten Kirchen bestendig vnd einmütiglich aus Gottes wort geübet wirdt.* Heidelberg: Harnisch, 1593.

Passau, Otto von. *Die vierundzwanzig Alten oder der goldene Thron.* Augsburg: Anton Sorg, 1480.

Peilicke, Johannes. *Philosophie naturalis Compendium.* Leipzig: Lotter, 1499.

Peringer, Diepold. *Des Christlichen Pawren getrewen radt/ wie die christglaubig seel ein gesprech mit dem menschlichen fleysch teglich halten vnd betrachten soll.* Zwickau: Schönsperger, 1524.

———. *Ein Sermon gepredigt von der Abgötterey: Gepredigt zu Kitzing im Franckenland auff vnsers Herren Fronleychnams tag.* Nuremberg: Hergot, 1524.

Pezel, Christoph. *Auffrichtige Rechenschafft von Lehr vnd Ceremonien, so jnn euangelischen Reformierten Kirchen/ anch der Richtschnur Goettliches Worts angestellet.* Bremen: Peters, 1592.

———. *Christliche vnd einfeltige Erklerung der notwendigen Lere vom heiligen Abendmal vnsers Herrn Jesu Christi.* Ursel: Heinrich, 1578.

Pfanner, Josef, ed. *Caritas Pirckheimer—Quellensammlung.* Landshut: Solanus-Druck, 1961.

Pfeffinger, Johannes. *Grüntlicher und warhafftiger Bericht der vorigen und jetzigen für und nach dem Kriege ergangen Handlungen von den Adiaphoris oder Mitteldingen.* Leipzig: Bapst, 1550.

Pfeiffer, Gerhard, ed. *Quellen zur Nürnberger Reformationsgeschichte: Von der Duldung liturgischer Änderungen bis zur Ausübung des Kirchenregiments durch Rat (Juni 1524-Juni 1525).* Nuremberg: Verein für bayerische Kirchengeschichte, 1968.

Rauscher, Hieronymus. *Hundert außerwelte, grosse, unverschempte, feiste, wolgemeste, erstunkene Papistische Lugen.* Regensburg: Geißler, 1562.

Reckenhofer, Martin. *Ein Urteil über ein Sermon, gepredigt wide die evangelische Lehr durch Johannem Freiburger.* Nuremberg: Hergot, 1524.

Reichert, Franz Rudolf, ed. *Die älteste deutsche Gesamtauslegung der Messe (Erstausgabe ca. 1480).* Münster: Aschendorff, 1967.

Reinhart, Martin. *Ein christlicher, brüderlicher Unterricht an die christliche Gemeine in Jena.* Zwickau: Gastel, 1523.

———. *Vnderrichte wie sich ein frumer Christ bey den Papistischen Messen/so yetz noch vil gehalten werden . . . halten soll.* Augsburg: Ulhart, 1524.

Reisch, Gregor. *Margarita philosophica, totius philosophiae rationalis, naturalis, et moralis principia.* Freiburg im Breisgau: Schott, 1503.

Reuter, Simon. *Antwort wider die Baalspfaffen.* Bamberg: Erlinger, 1523.

———. *Ein Christliche frage Simonis Reuters vonn Schlaytz, an alle Bischoffe vnnd anndere geystliche auch zum teyl weltliche regenten*. Bamber: Erlinger, 1523.

Reychart, Peter. *Ein christenlich Gesprächsbüchlein von zweien Weibern*. Augsburg: Steiner, 1523.

Rhegius, Urbanus. *Ain Sermon von dem hochwirdigen Sacrament des Altars*. Augsburg: Otmar, 1521.

———. *Das Blatten, Kutten, Kappen, Schern, Schmern/ Saltz/ Schmaltz vnd aller dergleichen Gott abschewlich seindt*. Worms: Schöffer, 1524.

———. *Underricht wie sich ain Christen mensch halten sol das er frucht der Meß erlang*. Augsburg: Grimm & Wirsung, 1522.

———. *Vom hochwürdigen Sakrament des Altars: Unterricht*. Augsburg: Ulhart, 1523.

———. *Von Kirchenweyhe*. Augsburg: Ramminger, 1522.

———. *Wie man christlich feyern sol*. Augsburg: Ramminger, 1522.

Richter, Aemilius Ludwig. *Die evangelischen Kirchenordnungen des sechzehnten Jahrhunderts: Urkunden und Regesten zur Geschichte des Rechts und der Verfassung der evangelischen Kirche in Deutschland*. Weimar: Landes-Industriecomptoirs, 1846. [reprint: Nieuwkoop: De Graf, 1967].

Rupe, Alanus de. *Unser lieben Frawen Psalter, vonn den dreien rosenkrenntzen, wie man die ordnen vnnd peten sol mitt vil bewerten exempeln eyn vast nutzlichs büchlin*. Augsburg: Zeissenmair, 1502.

Russ, Wolfgang. *Ein gütte nutzliche predig/ von dem rechtten guetten glauben*. Augsburg: Nadler, 1523.

———. *Ein Sermon, in welcher Mensch gereizt und ermahnt wird zu Lieb der evangelischen Lehre*. Zwickau: Schönsperger, 1523.

———. *Ein Sermon vom Unterschied der Werk der Menschen*. Strasbourg: Schürer, 1524.

Rychssner, Utz. *Ein hübsch Geprächsbüchlein von einem Pfaffen und einem Weber*. Augsburg: Steiner, 1524.

———. *Eine schöne Unterweyssung daß wir in Christo alle Brueder und Schwestern sind*. Augsburg: Steiner, 1524.

Sachs, Hans. *Dialogus des Inhalt ein Argument der Römischen wider das christlich Häuflein*. Nuremberg: Höltzel, 1524.

———. *Disputation zwischen einem Chorherren und Schuhmacher*. Augsburg: Ramminger, 1524.

———. *Ein Gespräch von den Scheinwerken der Geistlichen*. Augsburg: Ulhart, 1524.

Sack, Siegfried. *Von Christlicher Einweihung der Kirchen aus dem Exempel Salomonis . . . in der newen Kirchen in der Newenstadt Magdeburg*. Magdeburg: Roß, 1585.

Schenck, Jakob. *Sendtbrieff an seyne Geschwyhen*. Strasbourg: Schürer, 1524.

Schiller, Karl Martin, ed. *Hans Sachs: Werke in zwei Bänden*. Volume 1. Berlin: Aufbau, 1966.

Schilling, Anton, ed. "Die religiösen und kirchlichen Zustände der ehemaligen Reichsstadt Biberach unmittelbar vor Einführung der Reformation." *Freiburger Diözesan Archiv* 19 (1887): 1–191

Schwalb, Hans. *Beklagung eines Laien über viel Mißbrauch christlichen Lebens*. Augsburg: Ramminger, 1521.

Schwarzenberg, Johann von. *Beschwörung der alten teufelischen Schlangen mit dem göttlichen Wort.* Nuremberg: Hergot, 1525.

Schwenckfeld, Caspar von. *Ein christliche ermanung zu furdern das wortt Gottis an den herrn bischoff zu Breslaw.* Breslau: Lybisch, 1524.

Scultetus, Abraham. *De sensu et sensibilibus assertiones physicae, cum discussione problematum quorundam opticorum et astronomicorum.* Heidelberg: Smesmannus, 1591.

———. *Ethicorum libri duo, eiusdem studio laelli peregrine philosophi romani de noscendis et emendandis animi affectionibus.* Oberursel: Sutor, 1603.

———. *Kurtzer, aber schrifftmäßiger Bericht von den Götzen Bilder.* Heidelberg: Vögelin, 1620.

———. *Neue Zeitung aus Berlin in zweyen christlichen Gesprächen zweyer wandersleut/ Hans Knorren/ vnd Benedict Haberecht/ von dem jetzigen Zustand zu Berlin.* Pfirt: Knobloch, 1614.

Seebaß, Gottfried, ed. *Andreas Osiander Gesamtausgabe.* 10 vols. Gütersloh: Gütersloher Verlagshaus, 1975.

Sehling, Emil, et al., eds. *Die evangelische Kirchenordnungen des XVI. Jahrhunderts.* 22 vols. Tübingen: Mohr Siebeck, 1902–2017.

Selnecker, Nikolaus. *Bericht von der waren gegenwertigkeit des leibs vnd bluts vnsers Herrn.* Heidelberg: Mayer, 1565.

———. *Libellvs brevis et vtilis, de Coena Domini editus.* Strasbourg: Mylius, 1561.

———. *Paedagogia christiana: continens capita et locos doctrinas christianae.* Frankfurt: Brubach, 1565.

Sickingen, Franz von. *Ein Sendbrieff so der Edel.* Augsburg: Nadler, 1522.

Siegfried, Adam. *Einweihung der . . . newerbawten Asseburgischen Schloßkirchen zu Walhausen.* Eisleben: Gaubisch, 1616.

Sonnentaller, Johann. *Ursach, Warumb der vermeint geystlich huff mit yren patronen das Evangelion nit annimpt sunder schend det lester und verfolget mit kurtzer Contrafactur der pfafferey Müncherey Nonnerey.* Strasbourg: Prüß, 1524.

Spalatin, Georg. *Ceremonien vnd vngegründete mißbreuche y Gottisdienst abzuostellen.* Wittenberg: Weiss, 1525.

———. *Eyn Freundtliche Verwarnung vnd Bitt an eyn gantz Capitel die Vnchristliche Cerimonien zu fallen lassen.* Wittenberg: Weiss, 1525.

Spangenberg, Cyriacus. *Wider die Verleugner der Gegenwäartigkeit des Leibes Christi im Sacrament.* Ursel: Heinrich, 1583.

Spengler, Lazarus. *Hauptartikel durch welche gemaine Christenhait bißher verfürt worden ist.* Augsburg: Steiner, 1523.

———. *Schützred und christenliche antwurt ains erbarn liebhabers götlicher warhait der hailigen geschrifft, auf etlicher widersprechen.* Augsburg: Otmar, 1519.

———. *Verantwortung unnd auflösung etlicher vermainter Argument.* Augsburg: Steiner, 1524.

Stanberger, Balthasar. *Ein dialogus oder gesprech zwischen einem Prior, Leyenbruder und Bettler das wort gottes belanget.* Erfurt: Buchfürer, 1522.

Staupitz, Johann. *Ein nutzbarliches büchlein von der entlichen volziehung ewiger fürsehung.* Nuremberg: Peypus, 1517.

Staygmeyer, Hans. *Ein schöner dialogus oder Gespräch von einem Mönch und Becken.* Augsburg: Ulhart, 1524.

Steck, Max, ed. *Albrecht Dürer Schriften, Tagebücher, Briefe.* Stuttgart: Kohlhammer, 1961.

Steinhöwel, Heinrich. *Büchlein der Ordnung der Pestilenz.* Ulm: Johann Zainer, 1473.

Stifel, Michael. *Wider Doktor Murners falsch, erdicht Lied von dem Untergang christlichs Glaubens.* Strasbourg: Beck, 1522.

Stör, Thomas. *Von dem christlichen Weingarten.* Zwickau: Gastel, 1524.

Strauß, Jakob. *Ain trostliche verstendige leer über das wort sancti Pauli, der mensch soll sich selbs probieren, und also von dem brot essen, vnd von dem kelch trincken.* Augsburg: Otmar, 1522.

———. *Aufruhr, Zwietracht und Uneinigkeit zwischen wahren evangelischen Christen fürzukommen, unüberwindlich Lehr.* Nuremberg: Peypus, 1525.

———. *Ein kurz christenlich Unterricht des großen Irrtums, so im Heiligtum zu Ehren gehalten.* Erfurt: Buchfürer, 1523.

———. *Ein neüw wunderbarlich Beychtbuchlin.* Strasbourg: Schürer, 1523.

———. *Ein schöner, lieblicher Unterricht, zu bedenken und empfangen den Leib Christi, und sein roßenfarbes plut zu nyessen.* Augsburg: Schönsperger, 1524.

———. *Kurtz und verstendig leer, uber das wort. S. Pauli, zu den Römern.* Erfurt: Stürmer, 1523.

———. *Vnderricht D. Jacobo Straussen, wartzu die Bruderschaften nütz seyen.* Augsburg: Otmar, 1522.

———. *Von dem innerlichen und äusserlichen Tauf ein christliche Lehr.* Erfurt: Loersfeld, 1523.

———. *Wider den simoneischen Tauf und erkauften, erdichten Chrisam und Öl ein Sermon.* Augsburg: Ramminger, 1523.

Strigel, Victorinus. *Jn Philippi Melanchthonis Libellum de anima notae breves et ervditae.* Leipzig: Wipprecht, 1590.

Strigenitz, Gregor. *Esrae Predigtstül.* Leipzig: Schnellboltz, 1597.

St. Victor, Hugh of. *Didascalion: A Medieval Guide to the Arts.* Translated by Jerome Taylor. New York: Columbia University Press, 1991.

———. *On the Sacraments of the Christian Faith.* Translated by Roy Deferrari. Cambridge, Mass.: Medieval Academy of America, 1951.

Taurer, Abraham. *Hochnothwendigster Bericht wider den newen bildstürmischen carlstadtischen Geist im Fürstenthum Anhald.* Eisleben: Gaubisch, 1597.

Textus trium librorum de anima Aristotelis cum commentario secundum doctrinam venerabilis domini Alberti Magni. Cologne: Koelhoff, 1491.

Thorbecke, August, ed. *Statuten und Reformationen der Universität Heidelberg vom 16. bis 18. Jahrhundert.* Leipzig: Duncker & Humblot, 1891.

Ungerer, Edmund, ed. *Elsässische Altertümer in Burg und Haus, in Kloster und Kirche: Inventare vom Ausgang des Mittelalters bis zum dreissigjährigen Kriege aus Stadt und Bistum Strassburg.* 2 vols. Strasbourg: Trübner, 1913–1917.

Unzer, Matthias. *Kurtzer und einfältiger doch nützlicher und nothwendiger Bericht von der Pestilenz.* Halle: Hynitzsch, 1607.

Ursinus, Zacharias. *Gründtlicher bericht vom heiligen Abendmal unsers Herren Jesu Christi.* Heidelberg: Mayer, 1564.

Usingen, Bartholomäus Arnoldi von. *Exercitium de anima*. Erfurt, 1507.

Veesenmeyer, Karl Gustav, ed. *Sebastian Fischers Chronik, besonders von Ulmischen Sachen*. Ulm: Nübling, 1896.

Velde, Heymerich van den. *Problemata inter Albertum et Sanctum Thomam*. Cologne: Johann Landen, 1496.

Versehung eines Menschen Leib, Seel, Her und Gut. Nuremberg: Wagner, 1489.

Voegeli, Joerg. *Dry missiuen ains layeschen Burgers zu Constanz*. Konstanz: Schäffler, 1524.

Wagner, Philipp. *Einweihung des nawen chürfürstlichen Hauses die Augustusburgk genant*. Dresden: Stöckel, 1572.

Wann, Paul. *Sermones de tempore*. Passau: Petri, 1491

Watt, Joachim von. *Das Büchlein ist genant vom alten und neüwen Got, Glauben vnd Leer*. Strasbourg: Beck, 1521.

———. *Das Wolffgesang*. Augsburg: Ulhart, 1522.

Weida, Markus von. *Der Spiegel der hochloblichen Bruderschafft des Rosenkrantz Marie*. Leipzig: n.p., 1515.

Westphal, Joachim von. *Kurtzer begriff der Argument und Beweisungen, durch welche die Dienstbarkeit in Caeremonien von den Papisten und ihren Dienern zu leiden aufgelegt, verworffen, und verlegt wird*. Magdeburg: n.p., 1549.

———. *Verlegung des gründlichen Berichts der Adiaphoristen*. Magdeburg, 1551.

———. *Vier Predigten, das man den tewren schatz Göttlichs worts, unnd des rechten Gottesdiensts bewaren sol, widder die Papisten, Interimisten und Adiaphoristen*. Magdeburg: Lotter, 1550.

———. *Zwo Schrifften M. Joachimi Westphali, Pfarherrn zu Hamburg*. Magdeburg: Rödinger, 1550

Weyda, Ursula. *Wyder das vnchristlich schreyben vnd Lesterbuech des Apts Simon zuo Pegaw vnn seiner Brueder*. Zwickau: Schönsperger, 1524.

Williams, Ulla, and Werner Williams-Krapp, eds. *Die "Offenbarungen" der Katharina Tucher*. Tübingen: Max Niemeyer, 1998.

Willing, Johannes. *Ettliche Christliche predigten/ so in werendem Reichsztag zu Augspurg/ anno domini 1566*. Heidelberg: Agricola, 1567.

Witzel, Georg. *De Ceremoniis antiquae Ecclesiae*. Mainz: Behem, 1542.

———. *De traditione apostolica et ecclesiastica, daß die katholische Kirche Christi nicht allein was in der h. Schrift steht, sondern auch was sie bei den heiligen Vätern und ältesten Concilien göttlichs und löblichs funden, zu Gottes Dienst und Ehre ordentlich brauchen und beständiglich behalten möge*. Cologne: Quentel, 1549.

———. *Der heiligen Messen Brauch, wie er in der alten Kirchen vor tausend Jahren gewesen*. Mainz, Behem, 1541.

———. *Typus Ecclesiae Catholicae*. 5 vols. Cologne: Quentel and Calenius, 1559.

———. *Von den Eucharisty oder Meß, nach Answeisung der Schrift und der ältesten schrifterständigen h. Lehrer*. Leipzig: Schumann, 1534.

Wurm, Matthias. *Christlich Kurtz vermanung von fasten, feyrtage, beichten*. Strasbourg: Schwan, 1524.

———. *Christlicher bericht vnd vermannung Mathis Wurmen von Geydertheim*. Strasbourg: Schwan, 1524.

Zell, Katharina. *Den leidenen christglaubigen weybern der gemain zu Rentzingen*. Strasbourg: Knöpfel, 1524.

Ziegler, Clemens. *Ein fast schön büchlin in welchem yederman findet ein hellen und claren verstandt von dem leib und blut Christi*. Strasbourg: Schwan, 1525.

———. *Kurz Auszug Abgötterei*. Strasbourg: Schwan, 1524.

Zimmermann, Gerhard, and Gerd Heinrich, eds. *Die brandenburgischen Kirchenvisitations-Abschiede und -Register des XVI. und XVII. Jahrhunderts*. Vol. 2: *Das Land Ruppin*. Berlin: de Gruyter, 1963.

Zwingli, Huldrych. *Action oder Brauch des Nachtmals Gedechtnus oder Dancksagung Christi*. Zurich: Frochauer, 1525.

———. *Der Hirt*. Zurich: Froschauer, 1524.

———. *Ein klare underrichtung vom nachtmal Christi*. Zurich: Hager, 1526.

———. *Göttliche Ermahnung ehrsamen Eidgenossen Schweiz*. Augsburg: Grimm, 1522.

———. *Von clarheyt und gewüsse oder unbetrogliche des worts gottes*. Augsburg: Grimm & Wirsung, 1522.

———. *Von erkiesen und freyheit der speisen*. Basel: Petri, 1522.

Index

JACOB M. BAUM is an assistant professor of history at Texas Tech University.

Studies in Sensory History

Sonic Persuasion: Reading Sound in the Recorded Age *Greg Goodale*
The Deepest Sense: A Cultural History of Touch *Constance Classen*
Past Scents: Historical Perspectives on Smell *Jonathan Reinarz*
City of Noise: Sound and Nineteenth-Century Paris *Aimée Boutin*
Sensing Chicago: Noisemakers, Strikebreakers, and Muckrakers *Adam Mack*
Taste of the Nation: The New Deal Search for America's Food *Camille Bégin*
The Age of Noise in Britain: Hearing Modernity *James G. Mansell*
From Gluttony to Enlightenment: The World of Taste in Early Modern Europe *Viktoria von Hoffmann*
Reformation of the Senses: The Paradox of Religious Belief and Practice in Germany *Jacob M. Baum*

The University of Illinois Press
is a founding member of the
Association of American University Presses.

University of Illinois Press
1325 South Oak Street
Champaign, IL 61820-6903
www.press.uillinois.edu